Luther Holden

Holden's Manual of the Dissection of the Human Body

Luther Holden

Holden's Manual of the Dissection of the Human Body

ISBN/EAN: 9783742822123

Manufactured in Europe, USA, Canada, Australia, Japa

Cover: Foto ©Lupo / pixelio.de

Manufactured and distributed by brebook publishing software
(www.brebook.com)

Luther Holden

Holden's Manual of the Dissection of the Human Body

PREFACE

TO

THE THIRD EDITION.

—⧫—

WITHOUT DEPARTING from the original object of the Manual, new matter has been added here and there to this edition, more especially concerning the Anatomy of the Brain, the Organs of the Senses, and the Abdominal Viscera.

A few additional woodcuts have been introduced; and the order of dissection altered where it was considered advisable.

The author takes this opportunity of acknowledging that the real work of preparing this edition has been done by his colleague Mr. LANGTON, one of the Demonstrators of Anatomy at Saint Bartholomew's Hospital.

05 OUWER STREET
October 1868.

PREFACE

TO

THE SECOND EDITION.

—· ·◆—

IN THIS EDITION the author has most carefully revised the entire work. Considerable additional matter has been introduced. Many parts, which some students found obscure, have been entirely re-written.

The object of the author throughout has been to be as concise as possible, and to put the subject in as clear and practical a light as is compatible with the faithful handling of its natural difficulties.

It is hoped that the work, in its present form, is adapted, not only for students, but for members of the profession who wish to refresh their anatomical knowledge.

Most of the illustrations are the author's drawings from nature on wood; many he has taken from his own diagrams which he has found useful in teaching; others from photographs; and for some

he is indebted to the able pencil of Mr. GODART, the Librarian of
the Hospital. The engraving has been accurately executed by
Mr. JOYCE, of Bolt Court.

P.S.—The author suggests that students will find a great
advantage in colouring the woodcuts in light tints: the arteries
red, the veins blue, and the nerves yellow.

54 GOWER STREET:
   October 1861.

PREFACE

TO

THE FIRST EDITION.

+ ---

IF any apology be needed for the appearance of the present Manual, it may be stated, without any wish to disparage the labours of others, that the works of this kind hitherto published seem to the author open to one or the other of two objections;—either as being too systematic, and therefore not adapted for the dissecting-room, or as obscuring the more important features of anatomy by a multiplicity of minute and variable details.

In endeavouring to supply a presumed deficiency, the author has made it his special aim to direct the attention of the student to the prominent facts of anatomy, and to teach him the ground-work of the science; to trace the connection, and to point out the relative situation of parts, without perplexing him with minute descriptions.

A concise and accurate account is given of all the parts of the human body, the bones excepted, of which a competent knowledge is presupposed ; and directions are laid down for the best method of dissecting it.

The several regions of the body are treated of in the order considered most suitable for their examination; and the muscles, vessels, nerves, &c. are described, as they are successively exposed to view in the process of dissection.

The author has written the work entirely from actual observation : at the same time no available sources of information have been neglected, the highest authorities both English and Foreign having been carefully consulted. His acknowledgments are especially due to F. C. SKEY, Esq. F.R.S., Lecturer on Anatomy at St. Bartholomew's Hospital, for many valuable suggestions. He is also much indebted to his young friend, Mr. W. CLUBBE, for able assistance in dissections.

September 1851.

A MANUAL

DISSECTION OF THE HUMAN BODY.

— • —

DISSECTION OF THE SCALP.

An incision should be made from the nose along the mesial line to the occiput; another at right angles to the first from one side of the head to the other. These incisions must not divide more than the skin, that the subcutaneous vessels and nerves may not be injured.

Strata composing the scalp. The several strata of tissues covering the skull-cap are—1, the skin; 2, a thin layer of adipose tissue which contains the cutaneous vessels and nerves and the bulbs of the hair; and by which the skin is very closely connected to, 3, the broad thin tendon of the occipito-frontalis muscle (aponeurosis of the scalp); 4, an abundance of loose areolar tissue, which permits the free motion of the scalp upon, 5, the pericranium, or periosteum of the skull-cap.

Immediately beneath the skin, then, we expose the thin stratum of adipose tissue which connects it to the aponeurosis of the scalp. It forms a bed for the bulbs of the hair and for the ramifications of the cutaneous arteries. The toughness of this tissue, in which the arteries ramify, does not permit them to retract when divided; hence the hæmorrhage which follows incised wounds of the scalp; hence, also, the difficulty of drawing them out with the forceps. The blood-vessels of the scalp are derived, in front, from the

B

supra-orbital and *frontal* arteries, branches of the internal carotid;
on the sides, from the *temporal*; behind, from the *occipital* and
posterior auricular, branches of the external carotid. Trace the
leading trunks, and observe that they subdivide into branches,
which inosculate freely, and finally form a vascular network among
the bulbs of the hair. A few small branches here and there dip
down through the aponeurosis of the scalp to the pericranium.
The veins accompany the arteries.

Occipito-
frontalis
muscle.
     This cutaneous muscle is closely connected to the
scalp. It consists of two fleshy portions, one on the
occiput, the other on the forehead, connected by a broad
aponeurosis. The *origin* of the muscle takes place from the outer
two-thirds of the upper curve on the occipital bone, and the adjoining part of the mastoid process. The fibres ascend over the
back of the head, and terminate in the common aponeurosis. The
frontal portion, commencing in an arched form from the common
aponeurosis near the frontal suture, descends over the forehead,
and terminates partly in the skin of the brow, partly in the orbicularis and corrugator supercilii. Some fibres run down the nose
under the name of the *pyramidalis nasi*. The aponeurosis of the
scalp is continued over the temples and side of the head, gradually
changing from tendinous into fibro-cellular tissue. This muscle
enables us to move the scalp backwards and forwards. But its
chief action is as a muscle of expression. It elevates the brows,
and occasions those transverse wrinkles in the expression of surprise. Like the other muscles of expression, it is supplied by the
facial nerve.

Muscles of
the ear.
     There are several small muscles to move the cartilage
of the ear. In man they are thin and pale; but in
animals who possess a more delicate sense of hearing,
they are much more developed, for the purpose of quickly direct-
ing the cartilage of the ear towards the pulse of the air.

M. attollens
aurem.
     To indicate the position of this muscle the student
should draw down the upper part of the pinna of the
ear, when it will be found immediately under the ridge
of skin so produced. It arises from the aponeurosis of the scalp,

and is inserted into the cranial aspect of the upper part of the concha.

M. attrahens aurem.

The situation of this muscle, which is smaller than the preceding, is indicated by the prominence of skin, produced by drawing backwards the front part of the helix. It arises from the aponeurosis of the occipito-frontalis, and is inserted into the front of the helix.

M. retrahens aurem.

This muscle is exposed by reflecting the skin from the ridge produced by drawing the pinna forwards. It proceeds from the base of the mastoid process to the lower part of the concha. The retrahens and the attollens aurem are supplied by the auricular branch of the facial nerve; the attrahens by an offset from the temporal branch of the same nerve.

Nerves of the scalp.

The *supra-orbital nerve* is a branch of the ophthalmic division of the fifth. It emerges from the orbit through the notch of the frontal bone, and subdivides into branches, which are covered at first by the fibres of the orbicularis and occipito-frontalis; but they presently become subcutaneous: some of them may be traced over the top of the head as far as the occipital bone.

The *supra-trochlear nerve* is an offset from the frontal branch of the ophthalmic division of the fifth. It appears at the inner angle of the eyelids, and supplies the skin of the forehead.

The *superficial temporal nerves* ramify in company with the arteries of the same name. Some of them are derived from the superior, and some from the inferior maxillary division of the fifth pair; others from the facial.

The *posterior auricular nerve* is a branch of the facial, and runs with its corresponding artery behind the pinna of the ear, to supply the attollens and retrahens aurem, and the posterior belly of the occipito-frontalis.

The *great occipital nerve* is the posterior branch of the second cervical nerve. After passing through the complexus, it appears on the occiput with the occipital artery, and divides into wide-spreading branches, which supply the skin over the occiput.

The *small occipital nerve*, a branch of the anterior division of the second cervical (p. 15), runs along the posterior border of the insertion of the sterno-mastoid, and supplies the scalp.

Points of surgical interest. — Raise the aponeurosis of the scalp, and observe the quantity of loose areolar tissue which intervenes between it and the pericranium. This tissue never contains fat. There are some points of surgical interest concerning it :—1. Its looseness accounts for the extensive effusions of blood which one often sees after injuries on the head. 2. It admits of large flaps of the scalp being detached from the skull-cap; but these flaps do not mortify because they carry their blood-vessels with them. 3. In phlegmonous erysipelas of the scalp, it becomes infiltrated with pus and sloughs; hence the necessity of making incisions ; for the scalp will not lose its vitality, and liberate the sloughs like the skin of other parts under similar conditions, because its vessels run above the diseased tissue, and therefore its supply of blood is not cut off.

The *absorbent* vessels of the scalp run most of them backwards towards the occiput ; a few run towards the root of the zygoma, where they enter the absorbent glands in those situations respectively. Here, therefore, one finds glandular enlargements when the scalp is diseased.

To examine the brain and its membranes, the skull-cap must be removed about half an inch above the supra-orbital ridges in front, and on a level with the occipital protuberance behind. It is better to saw only through the outer table of the skull, and to break through the inner with a chisel. In this way the dura mater and the brain are less likely to be injured. On removing the skull we expose a tough fibrous membrane, *the dura mater,* which forms the most external of the membranes of the brain.

Meningeal arteries. — These arteries ramify between the skull and the dura mater. Their course may be traced by the grooves which they make in the bones. The most important is the ' *arteria meningea media,*' a branch of the internal maxillary artery. It enters the skull through the foramen spinosum, and divides into two principal branches; one runs in a groove along the anterior inferior angle of the parietal; the other curves backwards over the temporal bone, and subsequently ramifies on the parietal bone. The artery is accompanied by two veins, which empty themselves into the internal maxillary vein. The *arteria meningea parva* and a *meningeal branch* from the ascending pharyngeal artery also supply the dura mater and bones of the middle fossa. The other meningeal arteries are of insignificant size. The *anterior* come from the ethmoidal branches of the ophthalmic. The *posterior* come from the occipital and vertebral: these enter the skull through the foramen jugulare and the foramen magnum respectively.

The position of the meningeal arteries renders them liable to injury in fractures of the skull; hence extravasation of blood between the skull and dura mater is one of the common causes of compression of the brain.

Dura mater. This is so called from the notion that it gave rise to all the other membranes in the body. It is rough on its outer aspect, where it is more or less adherent to the inner surface of the skull. Internally it is smooth and shining, being lined by the parietal layer of the arachnoid membrane. Its remarkably tough and fibrous structure adapts it exceedingly well to the four purposes which it serves: 1. It forms the internal periosteum of the skull; 2. It forms, for the support of the lobes of the brain, three partitions—namely, the falx cerebri, the falx cerebelli, the tentorium cerebelli; 3. It forms the sinuses or venous canals which return the blood from the brain; 4. It forms sheaths for the nerves as they leave the skull.

Three partitions formed by dura mater. Of the partitions formed by the dura mater for the support of the lobes of the brain, two are vertical, and separate the two hemispheres of the cerebrum and those of the cerebellum; the third is nearly horizontal, and supports the posterior cerebral lobes.

Falx cerebri. The great partition is named, from its resemblance to the blade of a sickle, '*falx cerebri.*' It divides the cerebrum into two hemispheres—a right and a left. It begins in a point attached to the '*crista galli*,' and gradually penetrates deeper as it extends backwards. Its upper edge is convex and attached to the median groove on the inner aspect of the vertex of the skull; its inferior margin is concave and free, and runs along the upper aspect of the corpus callosum. From its base or broadest part proceeds the horizontal partition named '*tentorium cerebelli.*' This forms an arch for the support of the posterior cerebral lobes, so that they may not press upon the cerebellum beneath them. Observe that the tentorium is attached to the transverse ridge of the occipital bone, to the superior margin of the petrous part of the temporal bone, and to the posterior and anterior clinoid processes of the sphenoid.

Tentorium cerebelli.

The little partition which separates the lobes of the cerebellum is called '*falx cerebelli.*' It is placed vertically in the same line with the falx cerebri, and its point is attached to the edge of the foramen magnum.

Falx cerebelli.

It is one of the peculiarities of the cerebral circulation that the blood is returned through canals or 'sinuses' formed by the dura mater. These canals are produced by a splitting of the dura mater into two layers as shown in fig. 1, where 1 represents a vertical section through the superior longitudinal sinus. They are lined by the same smooth membrane as the rest of the venous system. Since their walls consist of unyielding structure, and are always on the stretch, it is obvious that they are admirably adapted to resist the pressure of the brain.

Sinuses of the dura mater.

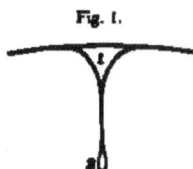

Fig. 1.

There are fifteen of these sinuses; five are pairs, and five are single, as follow :—

The five pairs of sinuses are,—	The five single sinuses are,—
The lateral.	The superior longitudinal.
The superior petrosal.	The inferior longitudinal.
The inferior petrosal.	The circular.
The cavernous.	The transverse.
The occipital.	The straight.

All of these eventually discharge their blood into the internal jugular veins.

Superior longitudinal sinus.   This runs along the upper edge of the falx cerebri (fig. 2). It begins very small at the crista galli, gradually increases in size in its course backwards, and opposite the tubercle of the occipital bone divides into the right

and left lateral sinuses, the right being in general the larger. Besides numerous veins from the cancellous texture of the skull-cap, the superior longitudinal sinus receives large veins from each hemisphere of the cerebrum. It is interesting to observe that these veins run from behind forwards, contrary to the current of blood in the sinus, and that they pass through the wall of the sinus very obliquely, like the ureter into the bladder.

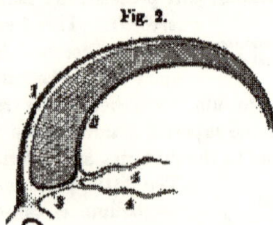

Fig. 2.

1. Superior longitudinal sinus.
2. Inferior longitudinal sinus.
3. Straight sinus.
4, 4. Venæ Galeni.

The probable object of this oblique entrance is to prevent regurgitation of blood from the sinus into the veins of the brain.

Cut open the superior longitudinal sinus: observe that it is triangular with its base upwards, and that its cavity is intersected in many places by slender fibrous cords, termed '*chordæ Willisii.*'[*] Their precise use is not understood.

Glandulæ Pacchioni.   In the neighbourhood of the superior longitudinal sinus we meet with small granulations, sometimes lying singly, sometimes in clusters. They are termed '*glandulæ Pacchioni,*'[†] and are found in three distinct situations:— 1, on the outside of the dura mater, often so large as to occasion depressions in the bones; 2, on the surface of the pia mater; 3, in the interior of the longitudinal sinus, covered by its lining membrane. Their size, number, and appearance differ in different

[*] So called after Willis, who first described them in his work De Cerebri Anatome, 1664.

[†] After the Italian anatomist, who first described them in 1705. These bodies would appear to originate in the subarachnoid cellular tissue, whence they, in their growth, either perforate the dura mater and hollow out the bones, or make their way into the longitudinal sinus.

subjects. Nothing is determined concerning their precise nature; but it is presumed that they are morbid products, since they are never observed in very young subjects.

The brain should now be removed, and preserved in spirit for future examination. Its anatomy with that of its remaining membranes will be described in a subsequent part of this work.

The other sinuses should now be examined.

Lateral sinuses. These are the two great sinuses through which all the blood from the brain is returned into the internal jugular veins. Their course is well marked in the dry skull. The right is commonly the larger. Each commences at the internal occipital protuberance, and proceeds at first horizontally outwards, enclosed between the layers of the tentorium, along a groove in the occipital bone and the posterior inferior angle of the parietal; it then descends along the mastoid portion of the temporal bone and again indenting the occipital, turns forwards to the foramen lacerum posterius, and terminates in the internal jugular vein.[*]

Inferior longitudinal sinus. This is of small size. It runs along the inferior free border of the falx cerebri, and terminates in the straight sinus at the anterior margin of the tentorium (fig. 2).

Straight sinus. This may be considered as the continuation of the preceding. It runs along the line of junction of the falx cerebri with the tentorium cerebelli, and terminates at the divergence of the two lateral sinuses. It receives the two 'venæ Galeni' (fig. 2), which return the blood from the lateral ventricles of the brain.

Cavernous sinus. This is so called because its interior is intersected by numerous threads. It extends along the side of the body of the sphenoid bone, outside the internal carotid artery. It receives the ophthalmic vein which leaves the orbit through the foramen lacerum orbitale; and it communicates with the circular sinus which surrounds the pituitary gland (fig. 3).

---

[*] It has in some subjects another outlet, through the foramen mastoideum, or else the posterior condyloid foramen.

Circular
sinus.

This surrounds the pituitary gland (P in the diagram), and communicates on each side with the cavernous.

Petrosal
sinuses.

These lead from the cavernous to the lateral. There are two on each side. The *superior* runs along the upper edge of the petrous bone; the *inferior* along the suture between the petrous and the occipital bones.

Fig. 3.

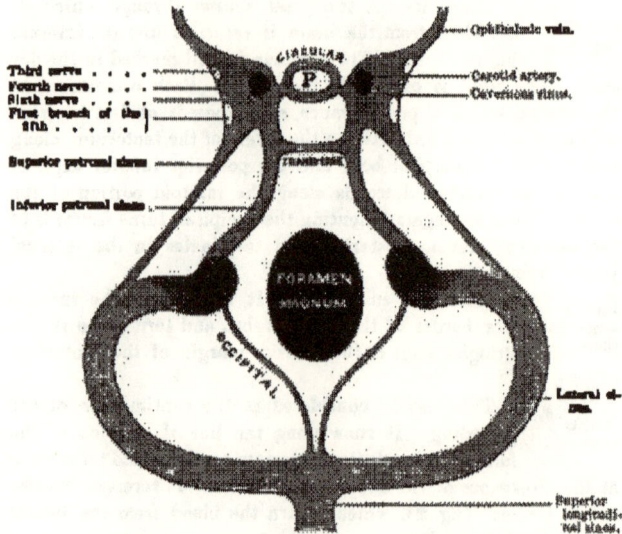

Ophthalmic vein.

Third nerve . . . .
Fourth nerve . . . .
Sixth nerve . . . .
First branch of the }
5th . . . . . .

Carotid artery.
Cavernous sinus.

Superior petrosal sinus

Inferior petrosal sinus

Lateral si-
nus.

Superior
longitudi-
nal sinus.

DIAGRAM OF THE VENOUS SINUSES AT THE BASE OF THE SKULL.

Transverse
sinus.

This extends from one inferior petrosal to the other, across the basilar process of the occipital bone.

Occipital
sinuses.

These are very small. They commence around the margin of the foramen magnum, run in the falx cerebelli, and open into the divergence of the lateral sinuses.*

* The meeting of the several sinuses opposite the spine of the occipital bone is

The student should now proceed to examine the nerves as they pass out of the base of the skull, and then to dissect the cavernous sinus.

Exit of the cranial nerves.   The cranial nerves proceed in pairs through the foramina at the base of the skull; they are named— first, second, third, fourth pair, &c., according to their order of succession from before backwards.

The *first pair* are the *olfactory nerves.* These cannot be seen, because the olfactory bulbs are removed with the brain, and torn from the delicate filaments which pass through the cribriform plate of the ethmoid bone.

The *second (optic nerve)* passes through the foramen opticum into the orbit accompanied by the ophthalmic artery.

The *third (motor oculi)* passes through the dura mater, close behind the anterior clinoid process, and enters the orbit through the sphenoidal fissure.

The *fourth (patheticus),* a small nerve, passes through the dura mater a little behind the posterior clinoid process. It then runs forwards through the sphenoidal fissure, when it lies above the third nerve, and is distributed to the superior oblique muscle.

The *fifth (trigeminal nerve)* passes through an aperture in the dura mater beneath the tentorium cerebelli, just above the point of the petrous portion of the temporal bone. Upon its larger or sensitive root, is developed a great ganglion called the ' *Gasserian ganglion.*' From this ganglion proceed the primary divisions of the nerve—namely, the *ophthalmic,* which passes through the sphenoidal fissure; the *superior maxillary,* through the foramen rotundum ; and the *inferior maxillary,* through the foramen ovale. The small motor root of the fifth lies beneath the ganglion, with which it has no communication, and accompanies the inferior maxillary division to supply the muscles of mastication.

The *sixth (abducens)* passes through the dura mater behind the

termed the ' *torcular Herophili,*' after the celebrated anatomist who first described it. It is a kind of triangular reservoir, with the base below, and presents six openings— namely, that of the superior longitudinal sinus, those of the two lateral and of the two occipital, and that of the straight sinus. The term ' *torcular*' is an incorrect version of the original word *ἑλκὶς* (a canal or gutter), employed by Herophilus.

body of the sphenoid, which it grooves. It enters the orbit through the sphenoidal fissure, and supplies the external rectus.

Fig. 4.

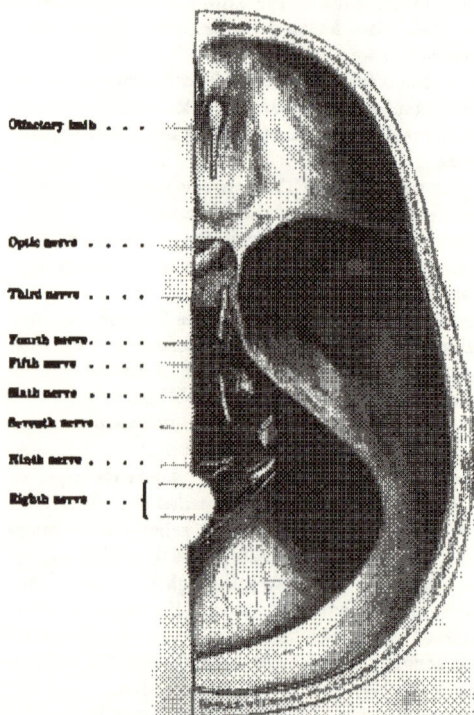

Olfactory bulb . . .
Optic nerve . . . .
Third nerve . . . .
Fourth nerve . . .
Fifth nerve . . . .
Sixth nerve . . . .
Seventh nerve . . .
Ninth nerve . . . .
Eighth nerve . .

EXIT OF THE CRANIAL NERVES.

The *seventh*, consisting of the *facial* and *auditory nerves*, passes through the meatus auditorius internus, in which they are connected by small offsets. The facial nerve lies internal to and above the auditory, before it enters the meatus auditorius.

The *eighth*, consisting of the *glosso-pharyngeal, pneumogastric,* and *spinal accessory*, passes through the anterior part of the foramen Jugulare. These three divisions do not all pass through the same tube of dura mater. The glosso-pharyngeal has a separate tube anterior to the other two, which have a common one.

The *ninth*, or *hypoglossal nerve*, passes through the anterior condyloid foramen in two fasciculi, which unite external to the skull.

We must now examine the cavernous sinus, and the nerves which course through its walls to the orbit—namely, the third, the fourth, the first division of the fifth, and the sixth.

Cavernous sinus. This sinus (fig. 3) lies by the side of the body of the sphenoid bone. In front it receives the ophthalmic vein, which comes through the sphenoidal fissure; behind, the superior and inferior petrosal sinuses run out of it; on the inner side it communicates with the circular sinus which surrounds the pituitary gland (P in the diagram).

In the outer wall of the cavernous sinus we trace from above downwards the third nerve, the fourth, the first division of the fifth, on their course to the orbit.[*] On its inner wall are situated the sixth nerve, and the internal carotid artery. These objects are said to be contained in the cavernous sinus; but they are not bathed by the blood of the sinus, because they are separated from it by the lining membrane.

Curves of the carotid artery. After the removal of the cavernous sinus, a good view is obtained of the remarkable curves, like the letter S, made by the carotid artery by the side of the sella turcica. The vessel enters the cranium at the apex of the petrous portion of the temporal bone, makes its sigmoid curves, and then passes through the dura mater, between the anterior clinoid process and the optic nerve; here it gives off the ophthalmic

[*] Such is the order in which the nerves are placed in the wall of the sinus. As they enter the orbit, the fourth nerve crosses over the third.

artery. While in the cavernous sinus, small branches (arteriæ receptaculi) arise from the carotid and supply the pituitary body, and the walls of the cavernous sinus.

Cavernous plexus. 　　The superior cervical ganglion of the sympathetic sends up with the carotid artery filaments, which form a plexus round it in its tortuous course through the carotid canal, and by the side of the sphenoid. After a careful dissection you may discover with the naked eye in this plexus, very small ganglia called *carotid* or *cavernous*; but they vary in number, size, and situation. Through these nerves a communication is established between the sympathetic and the nerves which enter the orbit.

THE DISSECTION OF THE NECK.

Make an incision through the skin, down the middle of the neck from the jaw to the sternum; a second along the clavicle to the acromion; a third along the base of the jaw as far as the mastoid process. Reflect the skin, and expose the cutaneous muscle called the '*platysma myoides*.' Between the platysma and the skin is a layer of adipose tissue, called the 'superficial fascia.' It varies in thickness in different subjects, but is generally more abundant at the upper part of the neck, especially in corpulent individuals, in whom it occasions a double chin.

Platysma myoides. 　　The *platysma myoides* is the cutaneous muscle of the neck. It arises from the subcutaneous tissue over the pectoralis major and deltoid muscles; thence proceeding over the clavicle and the side of the neck, its fibres become more closely aggregated, and terminate thus:—The anterior cross those of the opposite platysma, immediately below the symphysis of the jaw, and are lost in the skin of the chin; the middle are attached along the base of the jaw; the posterior cross the masseter muscle, and terminate partly in the subcutaneous tissue of the cheek, partly in the muscles at the corner of the mouth.

The platysma forms a strong muscular defence for the neck. It is also a muscle of expression.[*] It is supplied with nerves by the cervical plexus, and by the cervical branch of the facial nerve.

Cut through the platysma near the clavicle and turn it upwards. Beneath it lies the general investment of the neck, called the '*deep cervical fascia.*' Upon this fascia, we trace the superficial branches of the cervical plexus of nerves, the external jugular vein, and a smaller vein in front, called the anterior jugular. These superficial veins are so variable in size and course, that a general description only is applicable.

External jugular vein.   The external jugular vein is formed within the substance of the parotid gland by the junction of the temporal and internal maxillary veins. After receiving the transverse facial and posterior auricular veins, it appears at the lower border of the gland, crosses obliquely over the sterno-mastoid muscle (Fig. 5), to its posterior border, nearly as low down as the clavicle, where it pierces the deep cervical fascia and terminates in the subclavian vein. It is usually provided with two pairs of valves. A line drawn from the angle of the jaw to the middle of the clavicle would indicate its course. To trace the vein, during life, press upon it just above the clavicle; but do not be surprised if you fail to find it; it is sometimes wanting.

Near the angle of the jaw the external jugular vein communicates by a large branch with the internal jugular.

* If the entire muscle be permanently contracted it may occasion wry-neck, though distortion from such a cause is an exceedingly rare occurrence. A case in point is related by Mr. Gooch (*Chirurg. Works*), in which a complete cure was effected, after the failure of all ordinary means of relief, by the division of the platysma a little below the jaw.

The platysma myoides belongs to a class of muscles called '*cutaneous,*' from their office of moving the skin. There are not many in man, except upon the neck and face, and there is a little one (*palmaris brevis*) in the palm of the hand. To understand their use thoroughly we must refer to the lower orders of animals, in whom they fulfil very important functions, by moving not only the skin, but also its appendages. For instance, by muscles of this kind the hedgehog, porcupine, and animals of that family can roll themselves up and erect their quills: we are all familiar with the broad '*panniculus carnosus*' on the sides of herbivorous quadrupeds, which enables them to twitch their skins, and thus rid themselves from insects. In birds, too, these cutaneous muscles are extremely numerous, each feather having appropriate muscles to move it.

Before its termination the external jugular vein generally receives the supra-scapular, posterior scapular, and other unnamed veins: a disposition very unfavourable for the surgeon, because there is a *confluence of veins immediately over the subclavian artery* in the place where it is usually tied.

Fig. 5.

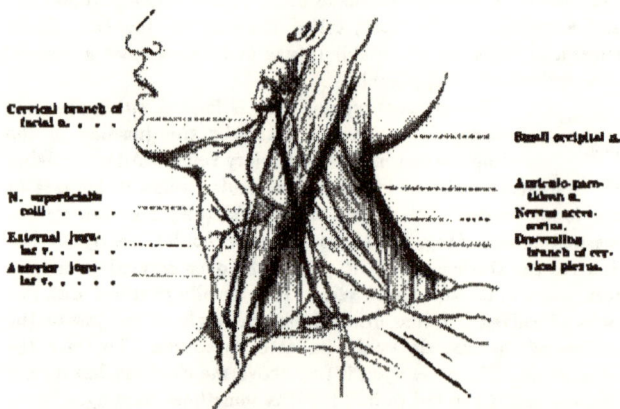

DIAGRAM OF THE SUPERFICIAL NERVES AND VEINS OF THE NECK.

Anterior jugular vein. The anterior jugular vein is situated more in the middle of the neck, and is much smaller than the external jugular. It commences by small branches below the chin, and runs down the front of the neck, nearly to the sternum: it then curves outwards, beneath the sterno-mastoid muscle, and opens either into the external jugular or the subclavian vein. We commonly meet with two anterior jugular veins, one on either side; immediately above the sternum they communicate by a transverse branch.

The size of the anterior jugular vein is inversely proportionate to that of the external jugular. When the external jugular is small, or terminates in the internal jugular, then the anterior jugular becomes an important supplemental vein, and attains considerable size. It is not uncommon to find it a quarter of an inch in diameter, and we have seen it nearly half an inch. These varieties should be remembered in tracheotomy.

Superficial absorbent glands are sometimes found near the cutaneous veins of the neck. They are small, and escape observation unless enlarged by disease. One or two are situated over the sterno-mastoid muscle; others near the mesial line.

Cutaneous nerves of the neck.   The cutaneous nerves of the neck are the superficial branches of the cervical plexus: the plexus itself cannot at present be seen. It lies under the sterno-mastoid muscle, close to the transverse processes of the four upper cervical vertebræ, and is formed by the communications of the anterior divisions of the four upper cervical nerves. The cutaneous branches of the plexus emerge beneath the posterior border of the sterno-mastoid, and take different directions. We divide and name them thus (fig. 5):

Cutaneous branches of the cervical plexus.	Ascending branches	Auriculo-parotidean.
		Small occipital.
	Transverse branch	Superficialis colli.
	Descending branches	Sternal.
		Clavicular.
		Acromial.

The *auriculo-parotidean n.* comes from the second and third cervical nerves, and ascends obliquely over the sterno-mastoid muscle, near the external jugular vein, towards the parotid gland. Near the gland it divides into two principal branches, of which the anterior is distributed to the skin over the gland and the side of the cheek; the posterior ascends to the cartilage of the ear, and ramifies chiefly upon its occipital surface. Other filaments communicate in the substance of the parotid gland with branches of the portio dura, or facial nerve.

The *small occipital nerve* comes from the second cervical nerve. It runs near the posterior border of the sterno-mastoid muscle to the occiput, where it supplies the back of the scalp. It also sends off a branch which is distributed to the skin of the side of the head. Beneath the sterno-mastoid this nerve commonly forms a loop which embraces the nervus accessorius, and sends a branch to it.

The *transverse* branch, called the *n. superficialis colli*, comes from the second and third cervical nerves. It passes forwards over the sterno-mastoid muscle, and supplies the front of the neck. Some of its filaments ascend towards the jaw, and join the cervical branch of the facial nerve; other filaments descend and supply the skin in front of the neck as low as the sternum.

The *descending* branches are derived from the third and fourth cervical nerves, and divide into three branches, which cross over the clavicle, and supply the skin of the front of the chest and shoulder. Of these, one, called the *sternal*, supplies the skin over the upper part of the sternum; another, the *clavicular*, passes over the middle of the clavicle, and is distributed to the skin over the pectoral muscle, the mammary gland, and the nipple; the third, named *acromial*, crosses over the acromion to supply the skin of the shoulder. Reviewing these cutaneous branches of the cervical plexus, we find that they have a very wide distribution, for they supply the skin covering the following parts—viz., the ear, the back of the scalp, the side of the cheek, the parotid gland, the front and side of the neck, the upper and front part of the chest and shoulder.

Cervical branch of the facial nerve.
Look for this branch beneath the fascia near the angle of the jaw (p. 15). It leaves the parotid gland, and divides into filaments which curve forwards below the jaw; some of these join the transverse branch of the cervical plexus; others supply the platysma.

Cervical fascia.
Now turn your attention to the membranous investment called the '*cervical fascia*,' which encloses the several structures of the neck. In some subjects the fascia is very thin; in others, with strong muscles, it is proportionably dense and resisting. It is always relatively stronger in particular situations, for the more effective protection of the parts beneath; for instance, in front of the trachea, in the form above the clavicle, and below the angle of the jaw. It not only covers the soft parts of the neck collectively, but, by its inflections, forms separate

c

sheaths for the muscles, vessels, and glands. It isolates them, and
keeps them in their proper relative position. A lengthened
description of its numerous layers would be not only extremely
tedious, but unintelligible, without considerable knowledge of the
anatomy of the neck. We propose, therefore, to give only a
general outline of the fascia, and of its principal layers, commencing from behind.

Tracing it from behind, we find that the cervical fascia (sometimes called deep cervical or muscular fascia of the neck) is
attached to the ligamentum nuchæ and to the spinous and transverse processes of the cervical vertebræ. From these attachments
it passes forwards to the posterior border of the sterno-mastoid,
where it splits into two layers, which invest that muscle and reunite at its anterior border. It then passes towards the mesial
line, where it becomes continuous with the corresponding fascia of
the opposite side. The layer which lies in front of the sterno-
mastoid is attached above to the base of the inferior maxilla, to
the zygoma, to the mastoid process, and the superior curved line of
the occipital bone. Traced downwards, we find it attached to the
clavicle and to the upper border of the sternum. In the middle
line it is closely connected to the hyoid bone, and below the thyroid
body divides into two layers, one being attached to the front of the
upper border of the sternum, the other to the back of the upper
border of the same bone. Between these layers there is a well-
marked interval, in which are contained more or less fat, and one
or two small absorbent glands. This layer forms investing sheaths
for the depressor muscles of the os hyoides and larynx. The other
layer—viz., that which passes beneath the sterno-mastoid—forms
the common sheath for the carotid artery, internal jugular vein,
and the pneumo-gastric nerve, which lie behind this muscle; it
proceeds inwards as a thin layer, and is continued behind the
pharynx (constituting the *pra vertebral fascia*) to join the fascia of
the opposite side. Below, it is attached to the first rib, to which it
binds down the intermediate tendon of the omo-hyoid; and still
further down it is continuous with the external coat of the aorta
and the pericardium. It may, also, be traced under the clavicle

along the axillary vessels and nerves into the axilla. Above it is attached to the angle of the lower jaw, from which it extends backwards to the styloid process, and forms the 'stylo-maxillary' ligament. Thence it is attached to the base of the skull, the petrous portion of the temporal bone, and the basilar process of the occipital bone.

A correct knowledge of the attachments of the principal layers of the cervical fascia is essential to a right understanding of the course which pus takes when it forms in the neck. For instance, suppose the pus to be formed at the lower part of the neck. If it be seated immediately under the superficial layer (which is attached to the clavicle), it may burrow beneath the clavicle into the axilla. But if it be seated beneath the deep layer (which is attached to the first rib), then it becomes a more serious affair, since the pus may readily travel through the loose tissue by the side of the pharynx, and make its way into the chest, where it will probably burrow down the anterior or the posterior mediastinum, and burst into the trachea or the œsophagus.

Besides forming sheaths for the several structures of the neck, there are other purposes to which the cervical fascia is subservient. The firm attachment of its layers to the sternum, the first rib, and the clavicle, forms a fibrous barrier at the upper opening of the chest, which supports the soft parts, and prevents their yielding to the pressure of the atmosphere during inspiration. Dr. Allan Burns[*] first pointed out this important function of the cervical fascia, and has recorded a case exemplifying the results of its destruction by disease.

Moreover, the great veins at the root of the neck, namely, the internal jugular, subclavian, and innominate, are so closely united by the cervical fascia to the adjacent bones and muscles, that when divided they gape. They are, as the French express it, 'canalisées,' and are therefore better able to resist the pressure of the atmosphere, which tends to render them flaccid and impervious during inspiration. But this anatomical disposition of the

[*] Surgical Anatomy of the Head and Neck.

great veins makes them more liable to the entrance of air when wounded. Many deaths are recorded, resulting from the sudden entrance of air into the veins during operations about the neck, or even the axilla.

Sterno-cleido-mastoideus. The sterno-cleido-mastoideus *arises* by a round tendon from the upper part of the sternum, and by fleshy fibres, from the sternal third of the clavicle. It is *inserted* by a thin aponeurosis into the mastoid process, and about the outer half of the superior curved ridge of the occipital bone.

The sternal origin of the muscle is at first separated from the clavicular by a slight interval: subsequently the sternal fibres gradually overlap the clavicular. The muscle is confined by its strong sheath of fascia, in such a manner that it forms a slight curve, with the convexity forwards. Observe especially that its front border overlaps the common carotid artery; along this border we make the incision in the operation of tying the vessel.

Action of sterno-mastoid. When both sterno-mastoidei act simultaneously, they draw the head and neck forwards, and are therefore especially concerned in raising the head from the recumbent position. When one sterno-mastoid acts singly, it turns the head obliquely towards the opposite shoulder; in this action it co-operates with the splenius of the other side.* On emergency, the sterno-mastoid acts as a muscle of inspiration, by raising the sternum, its fixed point being, in this case, at the head. The sterno-mastoid is supplied with nerves by the n. accessorius, and by deep branches of the cervical plexus. It has three nutrient arteries, an upper mastoid, a middle, and a lower.

The upper mastoid artery, a branch of the occipital, enters the muscle with the n. accessorius; the middle mastoid is a branch

* The single action of the muscle is well seen when it becomes rigid and causes a wry neck. Other means of relief failing, the division of the muscle near its origin is sometimes beneficial in curing the distortion. In deciding as to the propriety of this operation, we should be careful to examine the condition of the other muscles, lest, after having divided the sterno-mastoid, we should be disappointed in removing the deformity.

of the superior thyroid; the lower mastoid is a branch of the supra-scapular.

Anatomists avail themselves of the sterno-mastoid muscle, to divide the neck on each side into two great triangles, an anterior and a posterior (fig. 6). The base of the anterior triangle is formed by the jaw, its sides by the mesial line and the front border of the sterno-mastoid. The posterior has the clavicle for the base, while the sides are defined by the hind border of the sterno-mastoid, and the free border of the trapezius.

Triangles of the neck.

The omo-hyoid muscle, which crosses the neck under the sterno-mastoid, subdivides these great primary triangles into four smaller ones (fig. 6), of unequal size: an anterior superior, an anterior inferior, a posterior superior, and a posterior inferior. The direction of the omo-hyoid muscle renders their boundaries at once obvious.

The fat and cellular tissue must now be carefully removed from the posterior triangle. The following muscles will be seen forming its floor, viz., beginning from above, the splenius capitis, the levator anguli scapulæ, the scalenus medius and posticus. This triangle is subdivided into two unequal parts by the posterior belly of the omo-hyoid—an upper or occipital and a lower or clavicular. In the upper triangle are found the superficial branches of the cervical plexus, and passing obliquely downwards from beneath the sterno-mastoid is the spinal accessory nerve, which enters the under part of the trapezius. The transversalis colli (posterior scapular) artery and vein, and its branch the superficialis colli (which chiefly supplies the trapezius), cross transversely outwards the lower part of the space. A chain of lymphatic glands is also found along the posterior border of the sterno-mastoid.

Contents of posterior triangle.

The upper part of the sterno-mastoid is traversed obliquely by a large nerve called the spinal accessory or n. accessorius. This nerve, one of the three divisions of the eighth pair of cerebral nerves, arises from the cervical portion of the spinal cord by a series of filaments from the lateral tract as

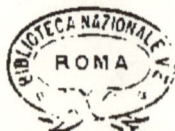

Nervus accessorius.

low down as the sixth cervical vertebra. It ascends between the
ligamentum denticulatum and the posterior roots of the spinal
nerves, through the foramen magnum into the skull. It leaves
the skull through the foramen lacerum posterius, runs behind the
internal jugular vein, then passes obliquely through the upper
third of the sterno-mastoid, and crosses the posterior triangle of

Fig. 8.

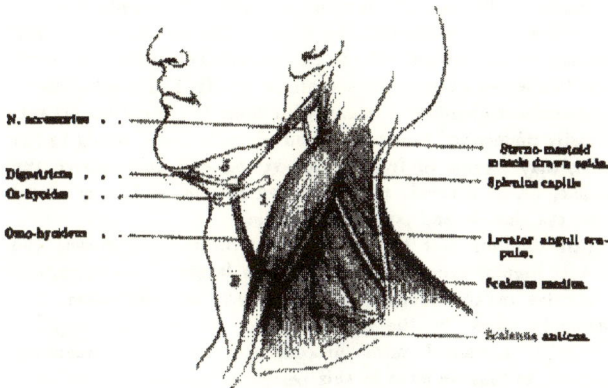

TRIANGLES OF THE NECK.

the neck to the under surface of the trapezius, to which it is distributed. The nervus accessorius supplies also the sterno-mastoid,
and, after leaving the muscle, is joined by branches from the
second and third cervical nerves. The upper mastoid artery, a
branch of the occipital, runs into the sterno-mastoid with the
nerve.

Supra-
clavicular
triangle.   The supra-clavicular triangle is bounded below by the
clavicle, in front by the outer border of the sterno-mastoid, and above by the posterior portion of the omo-
hyoid muscle. The area of the triangle thus formed will vary in
proportion to the obliquity of the omo-hyoid muscle, and the extent
to which the sterno-mastoid is attached to the clavicle; the trapezius must also be taken into the account, for in some instances it

comes so far forwards as almost to meet the sterno-mastoid. The depth of the vessels and nerves contained in this space depends not only upon the degree to which the clavicle arches forwards, but varies with the elevation and depression of the shoulder.

Immediately beneath the skin covering this region we find the platysma myoides, the descending branches of the cervical plexus, and a layer of fascia which binds down the omo-hyoid muscle to the clavicle. Beneath this is a deeper layer of fascia, which covers the subclavian vessels and the brachial plexus of nerves, and descends with them beneath the clavicle into the axilla. Between these two layers we meet with more or less fat and areolar tissue, and absorbent glands continuous with those in the axilla. It will be easily understood how a collection of matter, originating in the axilla, may ascend in front of the vessels and point above the clavicle, or, *vice versâ*, matter formed in the neck may travel under the clavicle and point in the axilla.

Near the posterior border of the sterno-mastoid muscle the external jugular vein passes through both layers of the fascia, and terminates in the subclavian: but before its termination it is commonly joined by the supra-scapular, the posterior scapular, and other unnamed veins proceeding from the surrounding muscles; so that we have in this particular situation a *confluence of veins*, which, when large or distended, are exceedingly embarrassing.

The fascia and the glands should be removed, and the following objects carefully dissected. Behind and nearly parallel with the clavicle is the supra-scapular (transversalis humeri) artery, a branch of the thyroid axis. A little higher is the transversalis colli, or posterior scapular (commonly a branch of the thyroid axis), which crosses the lower part of the neck towards the posterior superior angle of the scapula. Both these arteries, *the last particularly*, are very irregular in respect to their origin. Search for the outer border of the scalenus anticus, which descends from the transverse processes of the cerebral vertebræ to the first rib: running down perpendicularly upon it is seen the phrenic nerve. The subclavian vein lies upon the first rib in front

of the insertion of the muscle. The subclavian artery, which
appears behind the outer border of the scalenus anticus, must be
fairly exposed, care being taken to preserve the small branch
which proceeds from the brachial plexus to the subclavius muscle.
The large nerves constituting the brachial plexus will be found
emerging between the scalenus anticus and medius, higher than
the subclavian artery.

Anterior
triangle.

The anterior triangle must now be dissected. And
first examine the flat muscles in front of the neck,
which pull down the larynx; namely, the sterno-hyoid,
sterno-thyroid, and omo-hyoid.[*] Remove the fascia which covers
them, disturbing them as little as possible, and take care of the
nerves (branches of the descendens noni), which enter their outer
borders.

Sterno-
hyoid.

The sterno-hyoid *arises* from the back part of the
sternum and sterno-clavicular ligament, and is inserted
into the lower border of the body of the os-hyoides.
This is the most superficial of the muscles in front of the neck.
We cut in the mesial line between these muscles in laryngotomy.

Sterno-
thyroid.

The sterno-thyroid *arises* from the back part of the
sternum, below the origin of the sterno-hyoid and the
cartilage of the first rib, and is *inserted* into the oblique
ridge on the ala of the thyroid cartilage. This muscle is situated
immediately under, and is much broader than, the sterno-hyoid.

Notice that the two sterno-hyoid muscles converge as they
ascend to their insertions, and that opposite the cricoid cartilage
and the two or three upper rings of the trachea they are in contact
with one another. The sterno-thyroid, however, diverge to their
insertions and are in contact below, the result of which is that the
trachea is completely covered in front by muscular fibres.

Omo-hyoid.

The omo-hyoid *arises* from the upper border of the
scapula, and from the ligament over the notch, and is

---

[*] The sterno-hyoid and sterno-thyroid muscles often present slight transverse
tendinous lines. These tendinous intersections are quite rudimentary in man; but in
some animals with long necks, e. g. the giraffe, they are so developed that each depressor muscle is composed of alternations of muscle and tendon.

inserted into the body of the os-hyoides near the great cornu. This muscle is digastric; that is, it consists of two fleshy portions connected by a tendon. From the scapula it comes nearly hori-

Fig. 7.

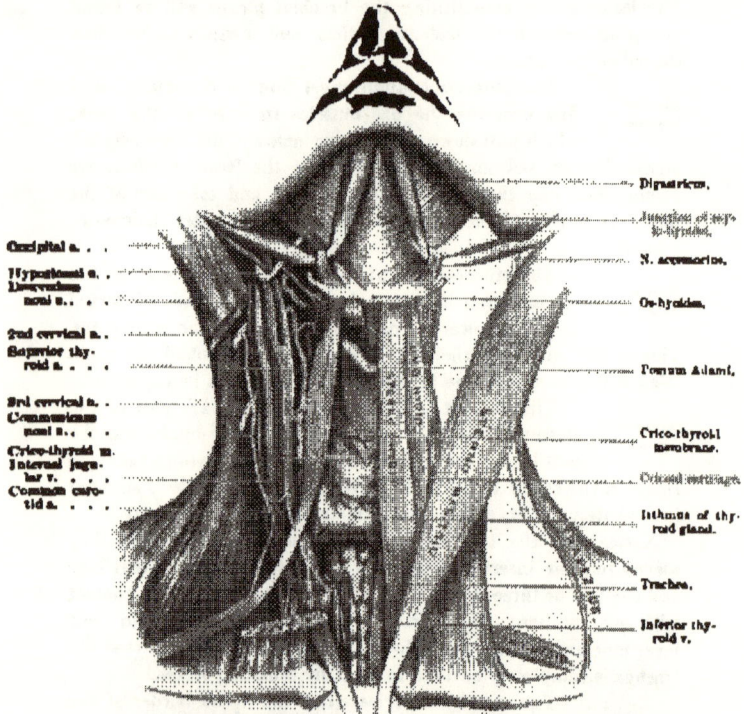

CENTRAL LINE OF THE NECK.—COURSE AND RELATIONS OF COMMON CAROTID A.

zontally forwards across the lower part of the neck, and passes beneath the sterno-mastoid, over the sheath of the great vessels of the neck; then, changing its direction, it ascends nearly vertically close to the outer border of the sterno-hyoid. Thus the muscle does not proceed straight from origin to insertion, but forms an obtuse angle beneath the sterno-mastoid muscle. The intermediate tendon is situated at the angle, and is bound down to the first rib by a process of the deep cervical fascia. The object of this peculiar direction of the omo-hyoid appears to be to keep tense that part of the cervical fascia which covers the apex of the lung, and thus to resist atmospheric pressure.

Action of the depressor muscles.

The sterno-hyoid, sterno-thyroid, and omo-hyoid muscles, co-operate in fixing the larynx and os-hyoides, e. g. in sucking, or they depress the larynx after it has been raised in deglutition. Again, they depress it in the utterance of grave notes. That the larynx is raised or depressed according to the height of the note may be ascertained by placing the finger upon it while we go through the gamut.

These depressor muscles are all supplied with nerves (fig. 7, p. 25) by the 'descendens noni' (a branch of the ninth, or hypoglossal), and by the 'communicantes noni' (branches of the cervical plexus). The descendens noni sends a separate branch to each belly of the omo-hyoid. They are supplied with blood by the superior thyroid artery.

Thyro-hyoid.

The thyro-hyoid arises from the oblique line on the ala of the thyroid cartilage, and runs up to be *inserted* into the body and half the great cornu of the os-hyoides. This muscle is a continuation of the sterno-thyroid. It is supplied by a special branch from the hypoglossal nerve. It covers the thyro-hyoid membrane, and the superior laryngeal nerve and artery as they enter the larynx.

The sterno-mastoid muscle must now be reflected from its origin to examine the course and relations of the common carotid artery. This done, notice the strong layer of fascia which lies under the sterno-mastoid, and forms the under part of its sheath. It is attached to the angle of the jaw, thence descends over and protects the great vessels of the neck, and is firmly connected to the clavicle and first rib. This fascia prevents matter from coming to the surface, when suppuration takes place by the side of the pharynx.

Remove this fascia, taking care not to cut away the descendens noni and communicantes noni nerves, which cross the sheath of the common carotid. Dissect out any absorbent glands which lie about the sheath of the great vessels.

Course and relations of the common carotid. The common carotid arises on the right side from the arteria innominata behind the right sterno-clavicular articulation; on the left, from the arch of the aorta.

It ascends in front of the bodies of the cervical vertebræ, by the side of the trachea, thyroid gland, and larynx, as high as the upper border of the thyroid cartilage, and then divides into the external and internal carotid. Thus a line drawn from the sternal end of the clavicle to a point midway between the mastoid process and the angle of the jaw, will nearly indicate its course. It is contained in a sheath of cervical fascia. In the same sheath are the internal jugular vein and the pneumogastric nerve. The vein lies on the outer side of, and parallel with, the artery: the nerve lies behind, and between the artery and the vein. Behind the sheath is the sympathetic nerve. Lastly, along the vertebral column the sheath lies successively upon the longus colli and the rectus capitis anticus major muscles.

At the lower part of the neck the carotid artery is deeply seated; it is covered by the superficial fascia, platysma myoides, deep fascia, the sternal portion of the sterno-mastoid, the sterno-hyoid, and thyroid muscles, and about two inches above the clavicle it is crossed by the omo-hyoid. Above this point the artery becomes more superficial, and is covered by the platysma, cervical fasciæ, and only slightly overlapped by the sterno-mastoid. Lying immediately upon the sheath of the artery, we find the descendens noni joined by the communicantes noni nerves. The sheath is crossed by three veins; namely, the facial, the superior, and middle thyroid-veins, which empty themselves into the internal jugular. This is the general rule, and especial attention should be directed to it, because the veins are liable to be overlooked and injured in the operation of tying the carotid.

It is plain that it is easier to tie the common carotid above the omo-hyoid than below it. We make an incision (three inches long)

down the inner border of the sterno-mastoid ; we cut through the
platysma and cervical fascia, draw aside the overlapping edge of
the sterno-mastoid, and expose the sheath of the vessel. We then
make a small opening in the sheath large enough to admit the
aneurismal needle, and tie the vessel, taking care not to include
the pneumogastric or descendens noni nerves in the ligature.

In what
respects the
left carotid
differs from
the right.
In the first part of its course the left carotid differs
from the right in the following particulars:—
1. It arises from the arch of the aorta, is therefore
longer and deeper seated than the right, and is covered
by the first bone of the sternum.

2. It is crossed by the left brachio-cephalic vein.

3. It is in close relation with the œsophagus.

4. It is in close relation with the left recurrent nerve.

5. It is in close relation with the thoracic duct.

Division
of the
common
carotid.
The common carotid at its division is often a little
bulbous. This dilatation is sometimes so marked, that
during life we have seen it mistaken for an incipient
aneurism. It is necessary to be aware that the carotid
sometimes divides much lower than usual. Several times we have
seen the division as low as the level of the cricoid cartilage.

Internal
jugular
vein.
The internal jugular vein returns the blood from the
brain. Leaving the skull at the foramen jugulare, the
vein descends on the outer side of the carotid, but in
the sheath with it, and joins the subclavian vein at nearly a right
angle to form the brachio-cephalic. In its course down the neck
it receives the pharyngeal, occipital, lingual, facial, superior and
middle thyroid veins.

Previous to its termination the internal jugular advances slightly
to meet the subclavian vein, so that it lies on a plane a little anterior to the carotid. Besides which, the direction of the vein being
perpendicular, and that of the artery oblique, there is necessarily a
small interval between them at the lower part of the neck, more
especially on the right side. In this interval we find the pneumogastric nerve, and, deeper, the vertebral artery. Here, too, on the
left side, we look for the thoracic duct.

The descendens noni (p. 25), a branch of the hypoglossal, runs down obliquely over the sheath of the carotid to supply the depressor muscles of the os-hyoides.

Descendens noni.

Trace the nerve upwards, and see that it leaves the
hypoglossal where this nerve curves round the occipital, or perhaps
the mastoid artery. For a short distance the descendens noni lies
within the carotid sheath; but about the level of the os-hyoides it
comes through the sheath, and crosses obliquely the carotid, from
the outer to the inner side. The descendens noni is reinforced by
one or more nerves termed communicantes noni (derived from the
second and third cervical nerves). These communicating branches
descend on the outer side of the internal jugular vein, and form
generally two loops in front of the carotid sheath. From these
loops the nerves proceed to the anterior and posterior bellies of
the omo-hyoid, the sterno-hyoid, and sterno-thyroid muscles. A
small branch may sometimes be traced proceeding from the descendens noni into the chest to join the cardiac and phrenic nerves.

In some subjects the descendens noni seems to be wanting; but
look carefully, and you will probably discover it concealed *within*
the carotid sheath: in such case the reinforcing loops from the
cervical nerves will be found behind the internal jugular vein.

Let us now examine the thyroid body, and, to expose it, let us
reflect the sterno-hyoid and thyroid muscles from their insertions
so that they can be replaced if necessary. Afterwards we will examine the absorbent glands of the neck, and then survey the
objects in the central line of the neck, from the jaw to the
sternum.

Thyroid body.

This very vascular gland-like substance lies over the
front and sides of the upper part of the trachea, and
extends upwards on each side of the larynx. It con-
sists of two lateral lobes, connected a little below the cricoid cartilage by a transverse portion called the 'isthmus.' Each lobe is
conical, about two inches in length, with the base opposite the
sixth or seventh ring of the trachea, and the apex by the side of
the thyroid cartilage. Its anterior surface is covered by the
sterno-hyoid, sterno-thyroid, and omo-hyoid muscles; its deep

surface clasps the sides of the trachea and larynx, and usually extends so far backwards as to be in contact with the pharynx. Its external border overlaps, in most cases partially, but sometimes completely, the common carotid artery, particularly on the right side; and there are instances in which the lobe is deeply grooved by the vessel.

The isthmus lies over the second and third rings of the trachea. This portion of the organ varies much in its dimensions. In some instances there is no transverse portion. This corresponds with the normal disposition in most of the lower orders of mammalia; but in man, it is a failure in the union of the two halves by which the organ is originally developed.[*] Generally, the vertical measurement is about half an inch. Between its upper border and the cricoid cartilage is a space about four or five lines in extent, where the trachea is free; this space, therefore, is the more preferable situation for tracheotomy. But the vertical measurement of this isthmus is sometimes of very considerable length. We have seen it covering the trachea almost down to the sternum.[†]

The thyroid body is closely connected, by fibrous tissue, to the sides of the trachea and cricoid cartilage. Hence it rises and falls with the larynx in deglutition.

Taken as a whole, the thyroid varies in size in different individuals and at different periods of life. It is relatively larger in the child than the adult, in the female than the male. In old

[*] Concerning the development of the lateral halves and central portion of the thyroid body, see a paper by Callender in the Proceedings of the Royal Society, 1867.

[†] From the upper part of the isthmus, or from the adjacent border of either lobe, most commonly the left, a conical prolongation of the thyroid body, called 'the pyramid,' frequently ascends in front of the crico-thyroid membrane, as high as the 'pomum Adami,' and is connected to the body of the os-hyoides by fibrous tissue. In some subjects we may observe a few muscular fibres passing from the os-hyoides to the pyramid. This constitutes the 'levator glandulæ thyroideæ' (see preparation in Museum of St. Barth. Hosp., Patholog. Series, No. 11) of some anatomists. There are instances in which the pyramid is double; and, lastly, I have seen a considerable portion of this thyroid substance lying over the crico-thyroid membrane, completely isolated from the rest of the organ. These varieties deserve notice, because any one portion of this structure may become enlarged independent of the rest, and occasion a bronchocele.

age it diminishes in size, becomes firmer, and occasionally contains earthy matter.

But by far the most notable considerations in respect to the thyroid body are the number, the large size, and the free inosculations of its blood-vessels. In fact, it appears to be composed of a tissue of arteries and veins. The superior thyroid arteries come from the external carotid and enter the front surface of the apex of each lobe; the inferior thyroid come from the subclavian, and enter the under surface of the base. An artery, called the middle thyroid, is observed in some subjects; it comes from the arteria innominata, or the arch of the aorta, and ascends directly in front of the trachea to the isthmus.

Its veins are equally large, and form a plexus upon it. The superior and middle thyroid veins cross the common carotid, and open into the internal jugular. The inferior thyroid veins, two in number, descend over the front of the trachea, communicate freely with each other, and terminate in the left brachio-cephalic vein. When you perform tracheotomy, bear in mind the size of these inferior thyroid veins, and the possible existence of a middle thyroid artery.

Its nerves are furnished by the laryngeal branch of the pneumogastric and the middle and inferior cervical ganglia of the sympathetic. They accompany the arteries.

The thyroid body weighs from one to two ounces, and belongs to the class of ductless glands, since no excretory duct has been discovered. It is invested by a thin covering of condensed cellular tissue which penetrates into it, imperfectly dividing it into lobes and supporting the vessels as they enter it. It consists of a multitude of cells, which vary in size, and do not communicate with each other. Some of them may be recognised with the naked eye; but the greater number require the aid of the microscope. In hypertrophy of the gland we sometimes see them as large as a horsebean, or even larger. These cells are lined by a limitary membrane and contain a glairy transparent fluid, in which are found a large number of nuclei and nucleated cells. The arteries ramify most minutely

upon their walls. Of its functions nothing is with certainty
known. The presumption is, that it is concerned in the elabora-
tion of the blood.

An enlargement of the thyroid body is termed a ' Bronchocele.'
If the relation of its lobes to the trachea and œsophagus be properly understood, it is easy to predicate the consequences which
may result from their enlargement. The nature and severity of
the symptoms will to a certain extent be determined by the part
of the organ affected. If the isthmus be enlarged, difficulty in
breathing will probably be the prominent symptom; and an enlargement of the left lobe is more likely to produce a difficulty in
swallowing, on account of the inclination of the œsophagus towards
the left side.

An instance is related by Allen Burns in which the isthmus was
placed between the trachea and the œsophagus. It must be
obvious that enlargement of a part so situated would occasion great
difficulty in swallowing. I have seen two cases in which the lateral
lobes projected so far inwards that they completely embraced the
back of the œsophagus.

Small absorbent glands are observed about the thyroid body,
especially in front of the trachea; one is often situated over the
crico-thyroid membrane. These glands, if enlarged by disease,
might be mistaken for a small bronchocele.

Deep
cervical
absorbent
glands.
     In the areolar tissue which surrounds the great
vessels of the neck, we meet with a series of absorbent
glands, called the deep cervical. They form an uninterrupted chain (whence their name *glandulæ con-
catenatæ*), from the base of the skull, along the side of the neck,
to the clavicle, beneath which they are continuous with the
thoracic and the axillary glands. Some of these glands lie anterior
to the common carotid artery, others, between it and the spine.
This disposition explains the well-known fact, that, when these
glands are enlarged, the great vessels and nerves of the neck are
liable to become imbedded in their substance.

The glands are particularly numerous near the division of the
common carotid, by the side of the pharynx, and the posterior

belly of the digastricus. The absorbents connected with them come from all parts of the head and neck. These vessels unite, to form, on both sides of the neck, one or more absorbent trunks, called the jugular. On the left side this jugular trunk joins the thoracic duct, or opens by a separate orifice into the left subclavian vein: on the right it always opens into the subclavian vein.

The contiguity of the glands to the great vessels and nerves of the neck explains the symptoms produced by their enlargement. The tumour may be so situated as to be raised and depressed by the pulsation of the carotid, and thus simulate an aneurism. A careful examination, however, will distinguish between a real and an apparent pulsation. By grasping the tumour we become sensible that the rising and falling do not depend upon any variation of its magnitude, but upon the impulse derived from the artery; consequently, if the tumour be lifted from the vessel, all feeling of pulsation ceases.

Survey of the central line of the neck. Study well the parts in the central line of the neck (fig. 7, p. 25). Beginning at the chin, we observe the insertions of the digastric muscles. Below these is the junction, or 'raphé,' of the mylo-hyoid muscles. Then comes the os-hyoides. Below the os-hyoides comes the thyro-hyoid membrane, attached above to the upper border of the hyoid bone and below to the thyroid cartilage. Below this is the pomum Adami, or notch of the thyroid cartilage. Below the thyroid cartilage is the cricoid. These two cartilages are connected by the crico-thyroid membrane. Below the cricoid c. is the trachea. This is crossed by the isthmus of the thyroid body, and lower down it is covered by the inferior thyroid veins.

Now the chief surgical interest lies just above and below the cricoid cartilage. We can feel this cartilage very plainly in the living subject at any age, no matter how fat. In laryngotomy, the crico-thyroid membrane is divided transversely. The membrane should be divided *close* to the edge of the cricoid c., for two reasons:—1. In order to be farther from the vocal cords. 2. To avoid the crico-thyroid artery which crosses the middle of the membrane. If more room be required, the cricoid cartilage should be divided longitudinally.

In tracheotomy, the trachea is opened by a perpendicular incision, either above the isthmus of the thyroid body, or below it. The operation above the isthmus, if there be space enough for the introduction of the canula, is the easier and safer of the two; for here the trachea is nearer to the surface, and no large blood-vessels are, generally speaking, in the way. The space available measures from a quarter to half an inch; and the isthmus is not so firmly adherent to the trachea as to prevent its being drawn downwards for a short distance. However, it is right to state, that in one case out of every eight or ten, there is *no* available space.

Tracheotomy below the isthmus is neither an easy nor a safe operation, for many reasons: 1. The trachea recedes from the surface as it descends, so that just above the sternum it is nearly an inch and a half from the skin. 2. The large inferior thyroid veins are in the way. 3. A middle thyroid artery may run up in front of the trachea, direct from the arteria innominata. 4. The arteria innominata itself lies sometimes upon the trachea higher than usual, and may, therefore, be in danger. 5. The left brachio-cephalic vein in some cases crosses the trachea above the edge of the sternum instead of below it. The celebrated French surgeon Béclard used to relate in his lectures the following occurrence :— A student had fallen into the Seine, and was nearly drowned. As he was recovering very gradually, some kind friends attempted to accelerate the process by making an opening into the trachea. In so doing they wounded the brachio-cephalic vein. Blood poured into the trachea, and the result was instantly fatal.

Some surgeons advocate the practice of dividing the isthmus vertically, in order to get at the trachea beneath it. Let such surgeons remember that an artery, which would bleed freely if divided, generally runs along the upper edge of the isthmus. The artery is a branch of the superior thyroid, and inosculates with a corresponding branch on the opposite side.

Whoever pays attention to this subject in the dissecting-room

will soon be convinced of the fact, that not only largo veins but
largo arteries occasionally cross the crico-thyroid membrane as well
as the trachea. Every winter session convinces me more and
more of the necessity of cutting *cautiously* down to, and fairly ex-
posing the air tube, before we venture to open it.

Dissection
of the
submaxil-
lary re-
gion, or
the digas-
tric tri-
angle.
When the platysma and the cervical fascia have been
removed from their attachment to the jaw, the most
conspicuous object is the submaxillary gland. Observe
that the fascia forms for it a complete case. Beneath
the jaw we find several absorbent glands, of which some
lie superficial to the salivary gland, others beneath it.
These glands receive the absorbents of the face, the
tonsils, and the tongue.

A little dissection will expose a muscle called the 'digastricus,'
consisting of two distinct portions connected by a tendon. They
form, with the body of the jaw, a triangle, called the 'digastric,'
of which we propose to examine the contents. And first of the
digastric muscle itself.

Digastricus.
The digastricus consists of two muscular bellies
united by an intermediate tendon. It *arises* from the
digastric fossa of the temporal bone, and is *inserted* close to the
symphysis of the lower jaw. Raise the submaxillary gland to
see the intermediate tendon of the digastricus, the angle which it
forms, and how it is fastened by aponeurosis to the body and
greater cornu of the os-hyoides. Observe also that this aponeurosis
is connected in the mesial line with its fellow of the opposite side,
so that a fibrous expansion occupies the interval between the
anterior portions of the digastrici.

The chief action of the digastricus is to depress the lower jaw.
But if the lower jaw be fixed, then the muscle raises the os-hyoides,
as in deglutition.

The posterior belly of the digastricus is supplied by a nerve
from the facial; the anterior belly by a branch from the mylo-
hyoidean nerve (which comes from the third division of the fifth
pair).

D 3

Stylo-hyoideus. The stylo-hyoideus *arises* from the styloid process of the temporal bone, and is *inserted* into the body of the os-hyoides. This muscle runs close along the posterior belly of the digastricus. Most frequently the digastric tendon runs through the substance of it. Its nerve comes from the facial

Fig. 8.

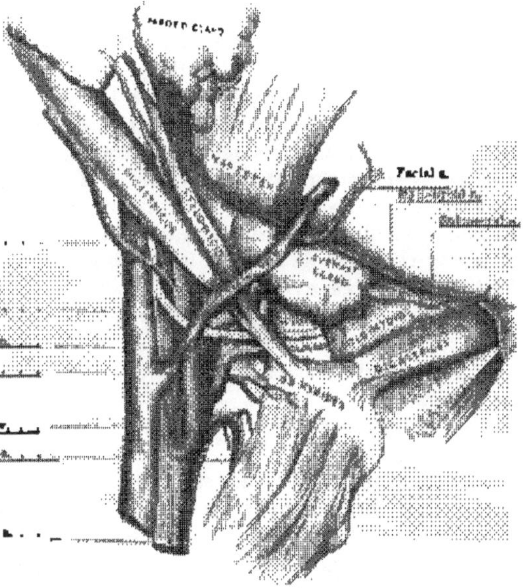

DIGASTRIC TRIANGLE AND CONTENTS.

close to its exit from the stylo-mastoid foramen. Its action is to raise and draw back the os-hyoides.

The digastric triangle is bounded above by the body of the lower jaw, parotid gland, and mastoid process of the temporal bone; behind by the posterior belly of the digastricus; and in front by the anterior belly. The objects we have to examine in this triangle are twelve in number, as follow:—

1. Submaxillary gland.
2. Facial vein.
3. Facial artery.
4. Submental artery.
5. Mylo-hyoideus nerve.
6. Submaxillary absorbent glands.

7. Stylo-maxillary ligament.
8. Part of the parotid gland.
9. Part of the external carotid artery.
10. Mylo-hyoideus muscle.
11. Hypoglossal nerve.
12. Part of the hyo-glossus muscle.

Submaxillary salivary gland.

In the ordinary position of the head, the sub-maxillary gland is partially concealed by the jaw, but when the head falls back the gland is more exposed. It is about the size of a chestnut, and is divided into several lobes. Its upper margin is covered by the body of the jaw; its lower margin overlaps the side of the os-hyoides. Its cutaneous surface is flat, but the lobes on its deep surface are irregular, and often continuous with those of the sublingual gland. By raising the gland we find that it lies upon the mylo-hyoideus, the hyo-glossus, the stylo-glossus, the tendon of the digastricus, and a portion of the hypoglossal nerve, seen above the tendon. The facial artery lies in a groove on its upper border; and it is separated from the parotid gland, which is situated behind it, by the stylo-maxillary ligament. Mark these relations well, because they are of importance, as we shall presently explain, in tying the lingual artery.

The duct of the gland (Wharton's duct *) passes from its under surface, runs forwards under the mylo-hyoideus and upon the hyo-glossus muscle; it then passes beneath the gustatory nerve, and subsequently runs between the sublingual gland and the genio-hyo-glossus, to open into the floor of the mouth, by the side of the frænum linguæ. Its length is about two inches; its dimensions are not equal throughout, for it is dilated about the middle, and contracted at the orifice. Saliva, collected in the dilated portion, is sometimes spirted to a considerable distance out of the

* Thom. Wharton, Adenographia, seu glandularum totius corporis descriptio. 12mo. Amstel., 1669.

narrow orifice, in consequence of the sudden contraction of the neighbouring muscles.

An abnormal dilatation of the submaxillary duct is called a 'ranula.' It makes a tumour with semi-transparent walls, perceptible beneath the tongue. In some cases, however, what appears to be a 'ranula' is in reality a cyst formed in the loose areolar tissue under the tongue, or an enlargement of one of the small bursæ which are normally placed here.*

Facial vein. The facial vein does not accompany the facial artery. It leaves the face at the anterior edge of the masseter m., then runs over the submaxillary gland, the digastricus and stylo-hyoideus and the carotid artery, to join the internal jugular. This is the rule—but there are frequent exceptions. The principal point to remember is, that the vein runs superficial to the gland, and that we must be cautious in opening abscesses under the jaw.

Facial artery. The facial artery is the third branch of the external carotid. It runs tortuously under the hypoglossal nerve, the posterior belly of the digastricus and stylo-hyoideus, and underneath or through the substance of the submaxillary gland to the face, where it appears at the anterior border of the masseter. Below the jaw the facial gives off the four following branches:—

1. *The ascending or inferior palatine artery* runs up between the stylo-glossus and the stylo-pharyngeus m. to the soft palate and tonsils, and inosculates with the *descending* palatine, a branch of the internal maxillary.

2. The *tonsillar* runs up between the internal pterygoid and the stylo-glossus m., then, perforating the superior constrictor, supplies the tonsil and root of the tongue.

3. *Glandular* branches to the submaxillary gland.

4. The *submental* runs forwards upon the mylo-hyoideus muscle, under the inferior maxilla, turns over the chin, and inosculates with the terminal branches of the inferior dental and inferior

* These sublingual bursæ were first described by Fleischmann, De noris sublingua burnis, Nuremberg, 1811.

labial. It supplies the mylo-hyoideus, the anterior belly of the digastricus, and the sublingual absorbent glands.

Mylo-hyoidean nerve. Look for the mylo-hyoidean nerve near the submental artery. The nerve comes from the inferior dental (before its entrance into the dental foramen), and running along a groove on the inner side of the jaw, advances between the bone and the internal pterygoid m., to supply the mylo-hyoideus and the anterior belly of the digastricus.

The submaxillary absorbent glands receive the absorbent vessels of the face and the tongue. We often see them enlarged in cancer of the tongue and cancer of the lower lip. It is worth remembering that there are absorbent glands in the mesial line below the chin.

Mylo-hyoideus. The mylo-hyoideus *arises* from the mylo-hyoid ridge of the lower jaw, as far back as the last molar tooth, and is *inserted* into the body of the os-hyoides. Its fibres pass obliquely downwards and forwards, the posterior only are inserted into the body of the os-hyoides, the anterior being attached to a median tendinous line, termed a '*raphé.*' Thus the muscles of opposite sides form a muscular floor for the mouth. It is supplied with nerves by the mylo-hyoid branch of the dental, with blood by the submental a. The muscles of opposite sides conjointly elevate the os-hyoides and the floor of the mouth—as in deglutition.

Stylo-maxillary ligament. This is simply a deep layer of the cervical fascia, extending from the angle of the jaw to the styloid process. It is a broad sheet of fascia, and separates the submaxillary gland from the parotid. It is continuous with the fascia covering the pharynx; this gives it a surgical interest, because it prevents accumulations of matter formed near the tonsils and upper part of the pharynx from coming to the surface.

The remaining objects seen in the submaxillary triangle, namely, the parotid gland, the external carotid, the hypoglossal nerve, and the hyo-glossus muscle, will be described presently when they can be better seen. Your attention should now be directed

to a piece of surgical anatomy, which will enable you readily to
find and tie the lingual artery. It is this :—

A horizontal incision being made along the body and greater
cornu of the os-hyoides through the skin, the platysma, and
the cervical fascia, you will come at once upon the lower edge
of the submaxillary gland. Lift up the gland, which can be easily
done, and underneath it you will observe that the tendon of the
digastricus makes two sides of a triangle, of which the base is
formed by the hypoglossal nerve crossing the hyo-glossus m.
Within this little triangle, cut transversely through the fibres of
the hyoglossus, and under them is the lingual artery. The first
time you perform this operation on the dead subject, you will
probably miss the artery and cut (through the middle constrictor)
into the pharynx.

The facial vessels must now be divided immediately below the
jaw. Reflect the anterior belly of the digastricus from its insertion; detach the mylo-hyoideus from the middle line and the
os-hyoides, and turn it over the body of the jaw, taking care not
to injure the muscle and structures beneath. The lower jaw must
now be sawn through, a little to the dissector's side of the symphysis, and the bone drawn upwards by hooks. The tongue should
be drawn out of the mouth, and fastened by hooks. The os-
hyoides should be drawn down by means of hooks, so as to put the
parts on the stretch. All this done, we have to make out the
following objects, represented in fig. 9, p. 41.

1. Genio-hyoideus.	6. Sublingual gland.
2. Hyo-glossus.	7. Hypoglossal nerve.
3. Stylo-glossus.	8. Gustatory nerve.
4. Genio-hyo-glossus.	9. Submaxillary ganglion.
5. Submaxillary duct.	10. Lingual artery.

Genio-
hyoideus.   The genio-hyoideus *arises* from the inferior tubercle
behind the symphysis of the jaw, and is *inserted* into
the front of the body of the os-hyoides. This round
muscle is situated in the mesial line, parallel to its fellow. Its
nerve comes from the hypoglossal, and its blood from the
lingual artery. Its action is to draw the os-hyoides forwards and

upwards; and if the hyoid bone be fixed, it depresses the lower jaw.

Hyo-glossus. The hyo-glossus *arises* from the body, the greater and lesser cornua of the os-hyoides, and is *inserted* into the posterior two-thirds of the side of the tongue. It is a square and flat muscle, and its fibres ascend nearly perpendicularly from origin to insertion. Its nerve comes from the hypoglossal, and its blood from the lingual artery. Its action (with that of its fellow)

Fig. 9.

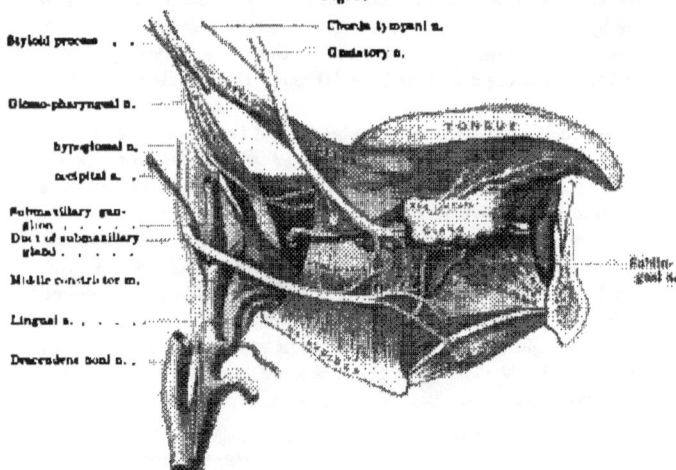

MUSCLES, VESSELS, AND NERVES OF THE TONGUE.

is to depress the tongue. Observe the several objects which lie *upon* the hyo-glossus; namely, the hypoglossal and gustatory nerves, the submaxillary ganglion, the duct of the submaxillary gland, and the sublingual gland. *Beneath* the hyo-glossus muscle lie the lingual artery, part of the middle constrictor of the pharynx, part of the genio-hyo-glossus, the lingualis muscle, and the glosso-pharyngeal nerve.

The genio-hyo-glossus *arises* by a tendon from the
upper tubercle behind the symphysis of the lower jaw,
Genio-hyo-glossus. and is *inserted* into the os-hyoides and the tongue from
the base to the apex. It is the largest and most important
of the muscles of the tongue. It is fan-shaped, with the apex
attached to the symphysis: thence its fibres radiate into the entire
length of the tongue. It derives its nerves from the hypoglossal,
and its blood from the lingual artery. Its action is various. The
posterior fibres, by raising the os-hyoides and drawing forwards
the base of the tongue, protrude the tongue out of the mouth;
the anterior draw the tongue back again. When every part of the
muscle acts, it draws down the whole tongue, and is therefore one
of the chief muscles concerned in suction.

The stylo-glossus, a long and slender muscle, *arises*
Stylo-glossus. from the apex of the styloid process and the stylo-
maxillary ligament, and is *inserted* along the side of
the tongue. It runs outside the hyo-glossus nearly to the tip of
the tongue. Its nerve comes from the hypoglossal. Its action is
to retract the tongue.

The hypoglossal, or ninth cerebral nerve, is the *motor*
Hypo-glossal nerve. nerve of the muscles of the tongue. It arises (by
several roots) from the front of the medulla oblongata
between the pyramid and the olive. After leaving the skull
through the anterior condyloid foramen, it lies beneath the internal
jugular vein and internal carotid artery, where it is intimately
connected with the pneumogastric nerve; it then comes up
between the artery and vein, and, immediately below the posterior
belly of the digastricus, curves forwards round the occipital, over
both carotid and facial arteries. It then crosses the hyo-glossus
muscle, and passing beneath the mylo-hyoid, divides into branches
which supply all the muscles of the tongue; namely, the stylo-
glossus, hyo-glossus, genio-hyo-glossus, lingualis, and the genio-
hyoideus. As it curves round the occipital artery, the hypoglossal
nerve sends the 'descendens noni' to the depressors of the
os-hyoides (p. 25). It also sends a nerve to the thyro-hyoideus,
which proceeds from it where it crosses over the external carotid.

Near the anterior border of the hyo-glossus, it communicates with the gustatory nerve. (Fig. 9.)

The hypoglossal at its origin is purely a *motor* nerve. But after leaving the skull, it receives communications from the first two cervical nerves. These communications are important physiologically for two reasons :—1. They account for the hypoglossal nerve containing sensitive fibres. 2. They contribute the greater part of the filaments of the 'descendens noni.' It is also connected with the pneumogastric and sympathetic nerves at the base of the skull.

Sublingual salivary gland. — The sublingual gland lies immediately beneath the mucous membrane of the floor of the mouth. Its shape is oblong, with the long axis (about an inch and a half) directed from before backwards. It rests upon the upper surface of the mylo-hyoid muscle, and towards the mesial line it is in contact with the hyo-glossus and the genio-hyo-glossus.

The ducts of the sublingual gland (ducts of Rivinus[a]) vary in number from eight to twenty. They terminate by minute openings behind the orifice of the submaxillary duct, along a ridge upon the floor of the mouth. The ducts of some of the lobes terminate in the submaxillary duct.

The duct of the submaxillary gland may now be traced across the hyo-glossus, and under the gustatory nerve to the floor of the mouth.

Gustatory nerve. — This nerve is a branch of the inferior maxillary or third division of the fifth pair of cerebral nerves. It descends between the ramus of the jaw and the internal pterygoid muscle, comes forwards over the superior constrictor of the pharynx and along the upper part of the hyo-glossus, crossing at an acute angle over the duct of the submaxillary gland. Having reached the under part of the tongue, the nerve divides into filaments which supply the papillæ on its anterior three-fourths.

Submaxillary ganglion. — Look at the lower border of the gustatory nerve before it crosses the submaxillary duct: you will find a small ganglion, about the size of a pin's head. Like the other ganglia in connection with the branches of the fifth pair,

[a] Aug. Quirin. Rivinus, de Dyspepsia. Lips. 1678.

it receives nerve-filaments of three different kinds—viz. motor, sensitive, and sympathetic. Its motor root is the chorda tympani, which, apparently a branch of the gustatory, is derived from the facial nerve (a nerve of motion). Its sensitive roots proceed from the gustatory; and its connection with the sympathetic system of nerves is established by a branch which comes from the 'nervi molles' round the facial artery. Thus provided with nerves, the ganglion supplies the submaxillary and sublingual glands and their ducts.

The lingual artery is generally the second branch of the external carotid. Curving slightly upwards from its origin, the artery soon runs forwards beneath the hyo-glossus muscle, parallel to the os-hyoides. At the anterior edge of the hyo-glossus it ascends to the under surface of the tongue, and is continued forwards to the apex of the tongue under the name of 'ranine.' The curves made by the artery are for the purpose of allowing the elongation of the tongue. Under the hyo-glossus, the artery lies upon the middle constrictor of the pharynx, and the genio-hyo-glossus muscles; in the substance of the tongue, it lies between the genio-hyo-glossus and the lingualis. Its branches are as follow:—

Lingual artery.

1. The *hyoid*, a small artery which runs along the upper border of the hyoid bone, supplying the muscles and anastomosing with its fellow.

2. The *dorsales linguæ*, two or more, which run under the hyo glossus to the back of the tongue.

3. The *sublingual*, arising near the anterior border of the hyo-glossus, supplies the sublingual gland, the mylo-hyoideus, and the mucous membrane of the mouth and gums. This artery generally gives off the little artery of the 'frænum linguæ,' which is sometimes wounded in cutting the frænum in children who are tongue-tied; especially when we neglect the rule of pointing the scissors downwards and backwards.

4. The *ranine* is the termination of the lingual artery. As it runs forwards to the tip of the tongue along the outer side of the genio-hyo-glossus, it distributes branches to the tongue, and at the tip inosculates slightly with its fellow.

The *lingual vein* runs over the hyo-glossus, and terminates in the internal jugular.

The best place for finding and tying the lingual artery has already been mentioned. The rule laid down is trustworthy only when the artery runs its normal course. I have known an instance in which a good anatomist failed in an attempt to tie the lingual artery, because the vessel arose from the facial behind the sub-maxillary gland, and then passed through the mylo-hyoideus to reach the tongue.

Study next the course and relations of the external carotid artery, and its branches in the neck. In preparing a view of them, observe that nearly all the veins lie in front of their corresponding arteries.

Course and relations of the external carotid artery.
The external carotid arises from the common carotid about the level of the upper border of the thyroid cartilage. It ascends beneath the hypoglossal nerve, the facial and lingual veins, the posterior belly of the digastricus and stylo-hyoideus, enters the parotid gland, where it lies beneath the facial nerve and external jugular vein, and terminates near the neck of the jaw, by dividing into the temporal and internal maxillary arteries.

Notice the relative position which the external and internal carotids bear to each other. The external lies at first on the same plane with, but nearer to the side of the pharynx than the internal. The external, however, soon changes its position, and crosses obliquely in front of the internal to reach the space between the angle of the jaw and the mastoid process. The internal carotid ascends perpendicularly by the *side of the pharynx* to the base of the skull.

The external is separated from the internal carotid by the stylo-glossus and stylo-pharyngeus muscles, the glosso-pharyngeal nerve, and the stylo-hyoid ligament.

The external carotid gives off the following branches:—

1. The superior thyroid.	5. The posterior auricular.
2. The lingual.	6. The internal maxillary.
3. The facial.	7. The temporal.
4. The occipital.	8. The ascending pharyngeal.

The superior thyroid, the first branch of the external
carotid, arises just below the great cornu of the os-
hyoides. It runs beneath the omo-hyoid, sterno-hyoid,
and sterno-thyroid muscles to the upper and front
surface of the thyroid body, in which it terminates. Its branches
are the four following:—

1. The *hyoid*, a small muscular branch, runs horizontally inwards below the greater cornu of the os-hyoides, and anastomoses
with its fellow.

2. The *superior laryngeal* branch, accompanied by the superior laryngeal nerve, runs beneath the thyro-hyoid muscle,
perforates the thyro-hyoid membrane (sometimes the thyroid
cartilage), and supplies the muscles and the mucous membrane
of the larynx.

3. The *sterno-mastoid*, a small branch variable as to origin,
descends over the sheath of the carotid artery to the mastoid
muscle.

4. The *crico-thyroid*, an artery of great interest in reference to
the operation of laryngotomy, crosses the crico-thyroid membrane,
and communicates with a corresponding branch on the opposite
side (fig. 7, p. 25). One or two small branches pass through the
membrane to the interior of the larynx. It is important to know
that the crico-thyroid artery often varies in direction and size. In
most cases it is small, and runs across the centre of the membrane;
we should therefore be least likely to wound it in laryngotomy, by
dividing the membrane close to the cricoid cartilage. But it is
by no means infrequent to find this artery of considerable size,
taking an oblique or a perpendicular direction in front of the
membrane, and finally distributed to one of the lobes of the
thyroid body. I have seen several instances in which the membrane was crossed by the main trunk of the superior thyroid.
These facts should establish the practical rule in laryngotomy, not
to make an opening into the larynx until we have fairly exposed
the parts, and ascertained whether any large artery lies in the
way.

Among the many arterial inosculations about the thyroid body are two which deserve notice ; the one is formed between the two superior thyroid arteries along the upper border of the isthmus, the other takes place along the back part of the lateral lobe between the superior and inferior thyroid.

The *superior thyroid vein* crosses the sheath of the common carotid, and joins the internal jugular.

The superior laryngeal nerve, mentioned as accompanying the superior laryngeal artery, comes from the inferior ganglion of the pneumogastric. It descends by the side of the pharynx, behind both carotid arteries, enters the larynx through the thyro-hyoid membrane, and supplies the mucous membrane of the larynx with its exquisite sensibility. Some of its branches may be traced upwards to supply the epiglottis and base of the tongue; others descend to the 'rima glottidis;' and a large branch passes down behind the ala of the thyroid cartilage to join the recurrent laryngeal nerve.

Before it enters the larynx, the nerve sends the 'external laryngeal' branch to supply the crico-thyroid muscle.

Lingual artery.   The lingual artery and its branches have been described (p. 44).

Facial artery.   The facial artery and its branches below the jaw have been described (p. 38).

Occipital artery.   The occipital artery, the fourth branch of the external carotid, runs backwards along the lower border of the digastricus towards the mastoid process. It then passes under all the muscles inserted into the mastoid process—namely, the sterno-mastoid, the splenius capitis, and the trachelo-mastoid. Arrived at the back of the head, the artery runs superficial to the complexus, and divides into wide-spreading branches for the supply of the scalp. Observe that in the first part of its course, the occipital artery crosses over the internal carotid artery, the internal jugular vein, the spinal accessory nerve, and is itself crossed by the hypoglossal nerve. It sends off the three following branches :—

1. The *sterno-mastoid*, which enters the muscle with the nervus accessorius.

2. The *posterior meningeal* ascends with the internal jugular vein, and enters the cranium through the foramen jugulare to supply the dura mater.

3. The *princeps cervicis*, which we shall see better hereafter, runs down the back of the neck under the complexus, supplies this muscle and the semi-spinalis colli.

The *occipital vein* usually terminates in the internal jugular, sometimes in the external.

Posterior auricular artery.   The posterior auricular artery, the fifth branch of the external carotid, arises above the digastric muscle, and runs, under cover of the parotid gland, to the furrow between the cartilage of the ear and the mastoid process. Above the mastoid process it divides into two branches, a posterior which inosculates with the occipital, and an anterior which communicates with the temporal. It supplies the back of the scalp and the cartilage of the ear. Its only named branch is the *stylomastoid*, a very constant little artery, which runs through the stylo-mastoid foramen to the tympanum of the ear.

Posterior auricular nerve.   The posterior auricular nerve lies close to the corresponding artery. It is the first branch of the facial after its exit from the stylo-mastoid foramen. It runs behind the ear and divides into an auricular branch which supplies the retrahens and attollens aurem, and an occipital branch distributed to the posterior belly of the occipito-frontalis.

Ascending pharyngeal artery.   This artery arises near the division of the common carotid. It ascends between the internal carotid and the side of the pharynx to the base of the skull, lying upon the rectus capitis anticus major. It gives off some pharyngeal branches which supply the constrictor muscles. It then enters the pharynx above the free border of the superior constrictor, and terminates on the soft palate, the Eustachian tube, and the tonsils. It gives off a *meningeal branch*, which passes through the foramen lacerum medium to the dura mater in the middle fossa.

The examination of the two remaining branches of the external carotid—namely, the internal maxillary and temporal, must be for the present postponed. Meantime, let us make out the deep cervical plexus and its branches.

Cervical plexus of nerves. This plexus is formed by the anterior branches of the four upper cervical nerves. It consists of a series of loop-like communications, which take place between these nerves, close to the transverse processes of the four upper cervical vertebræ. The plexus is situated behind the sterno-mastoid and internal jugular vein, and lies in front of the scalenus medius and the levator anguli scapulæ.

The plexus gives off *superficial* and *deep* branches. The superficial branches have been already described (p. 16).

The deep branches may be divided into an internal and an external series.

INTERNAL SERIES.—1. The *phrenic* arises from the third, fourth, and fifth cervical nerves, and passes through the thorax to be distributed to the diaphragm.

2. The *communicantes noni* come from the second and third cervical nerves, wind round the internal jugular vein, and join the descendens noni in front of the carotid sheath, supplying the depressor muscles of the os-hyoides and larynx.

3. *Muscular* branches to the recti antici and lateralis and longus colli muscles.

4. Branches which communicate with the pneumogastric, hypoglossal, and sympathetic nerves, and one to join the fifth cervical.

EXTERNAL SERIES.—1. One or more branches to the nervus accessorius.

2. Muscular branches to supply the trapezius, levator anguli scapulæ, scalenus medius, and sterno-mastoid.

The clavicle should now be sawn through the middle, and the sternal half raised with the sterno-mastoid attached, so that the bone can be replaced, to study its relation to the subjacent parts. The scalene muscles and the subclavian artery throughout its whole course must next be carefully dissected.

The scalene muscles, so called from their resemblance to a scalene triangle, extend from the transverse processes of the cervical vertebræ to the first and second ribs. They may be con-

sidered as intercostal muscles, since the transverse processes of the
cervical vertebræ are but rudimentary ribs. Anatomists describe
them as three separate muscles—an anterior, a middle, and a
posterior; the anterior and middle are attached to the first rib, the
posterior to the second. In plan and purpose these three muscles
are one.

Scalenus anticus. The scalenus anticus *arises* from the anterior tubercles
of the transverse processes of the third, fourth, fifth, and
sixth cervical vertebræ, and is *inserted* by a flat tendon into the
tubercle on the *inner* border of the first rib.

Scalenus medius. The scalenus medius *arises* from the posterior
tubercles of the transverse processes of the six lower
cervical vertebræ, and is *inserted* into the first rib behind the
scalenus anticus.

Scalenus posticus. The scalenus posticus *arises* from the posterior
tubercles of the transverse processes of the two or three
lower cervical vertebræ, and is *inserted* into the second rib between
its tubercle and angle.

The scalene muscles are important agents in raising the thorax,
in a deep inspiration. Take a deep breath, and you can easily feel
them contracting. They can bend the cervical portion of the
spine, if their lower attachment be the fixed point, as in rising
from the recumbent position.

The scalenus anticus is just one of those muscles about which
we ought to know well all that lies in front of it, and all that lies
behind it. In front of it are, the phrenic nerve, the subclavian
vein, the supra-scapular and posterior scapular arteries. Behind
it are the subclavian artery and the five nerves which form the
brachial plexus.

Make your finger familiar with the feel of the tubercle on the
first rib, to which the scalenus anticus is attached. This tubercle
is the best guide to the subclavian artery, for it guides you to the
outer edge of the scalenus anticus, where you must look for the
vessel. Is the scalenus anticus entirely concealed from view by the
sterno-mastoid or not? This will depend upon the breadth of the
clavicular attachment of the sterno-mastoid. As a general rule, it

may be said, that the scalene muscle *is* concealed by the sterno-mastoid, and that consequently, in tying the subclavian artery, it will greatly facilitate the operation, if the clavicular origin of the muscle be partially divided.

Phrenic nerve. The phrenic nerve runs down in front of the scalenus anticus, from the outer to the inner border. It arises from the third, fourth, and fifth cervical nerves, but chiefly from the fourth. It enters the chest between the subclavian artery and vein, crosses in front of the internal mammary artery, and continues its course between the pericardium and pleura, in front of the root of the lung, to the diaphragm, which it supplies.

When the spinal cord is injured above the fourth cervical vertebra, the origin of the phrenic is implicated; therefore the diaphragm, as well as the other muscles of inspiration, are paralysed. Death is the immediate result.[*]

COURSE AND RELATIONS OF THE SUBCLAVIAN ARTERIES.

The left subclavian artery differs from the right, not only in its origin, but in the relations of the first part of its course. The right should, therefore, be examined first, and then the differences between it and left.

Right subclavian artery. The right subclavian artery is one of the two great branches into which the arteria innominata divides behind the sterno-clavicular joint. It runs outwards behind the scalenus anticus, then inclines downwards over the

---

[*] The phrenic nerve is frequently joined by a filament from that branch of the brachial plexus which supplies the subclavius muscle. It is important to be aware that cases sometimes occur in which this seemingly insignificant filament is a branch of considerable size, and forms the greater portion of the phrenic itself. I have met with many instances in which this accessory branch was larger than the regular trunk; in all of them it crossed over the subclavian artery in the third part of its course, and would probably have been injured in the operation of tying this vessel. That such an accident has actually happened is recorded by Bransby Cooper in his surgical lectures. He speaks of having injured this accessory branch of the phrenic in tying the subclavian artery. The patient had incessant spasm of the diaphragm till he died.

first rib, at the lower border of which it takes the name of 'axillary.' The artery describes a curve, of which the greatest convexity is between the scalene muscles. The height to which the arch ascends varies. Generally, it rises higher in women than in men, on the right side than on the left.

To study its relations more precisely, the course of the subclavian is divided into three parts :—1. The part which intervenes between its origin and the inner border of the scalenus anticus. 2. That which lies behind the scalenus. 3. That which intervenes between the outer border of the scalenus and the lower border of the first rib.

The *first* portion of the artery lies deeply in the neck and passes upwards and outwards to the inner border of the scalenus anticus. It is covered by the skin, platysma, superficial and deep fasciæ, the sternal end of the clavicle, the sterno-mastoid, sterno-hyoid, and sterno-thyroid muscles, and a layer of deep fascia, continued from the inner border of the scalenus anticus. It is crossed by the internal jugular and vertebral veins, by the pneumogastric and phrenic nerves, and by some cardiac filaments of the sympathetic. Behind the artery are the recurrent branch of the pneumogastric, the sympathetic nerve, the apex of the lung and the pleura. Three branches arise from this portion of the subclavian—viz., the vertebral, internal mammary, and thyroid axis.

In the *second* part of its course, the artery lies between the scalene muscles. It is covered by skin, platysma, and superficial fascia, by the clavicular origin of the sterno-mastoid, the deep cervical fascia, and by the scalenus anticus and phrenic nerve which separate it from the subclavian vein. Behind the artery is the scalenus medius; above it, is the brachial plexus. Only one branch, the superior intercostal, is given off from this part of the artery.

In the *third* part of its course, the artery passes downwards and outwards, and lies upon the surface of the first rib. Here it is covered by the skin, platysma, and two layers of the cervical fascia; subsequently by the supra-scapular artery, the clavicle, the subclavius muscle, with its nerve; and, what is of much more consequence, it is here crossed by the external jugular and (often) the supra and posterior scapular veins; so that we have here a con-

Fig. 10.

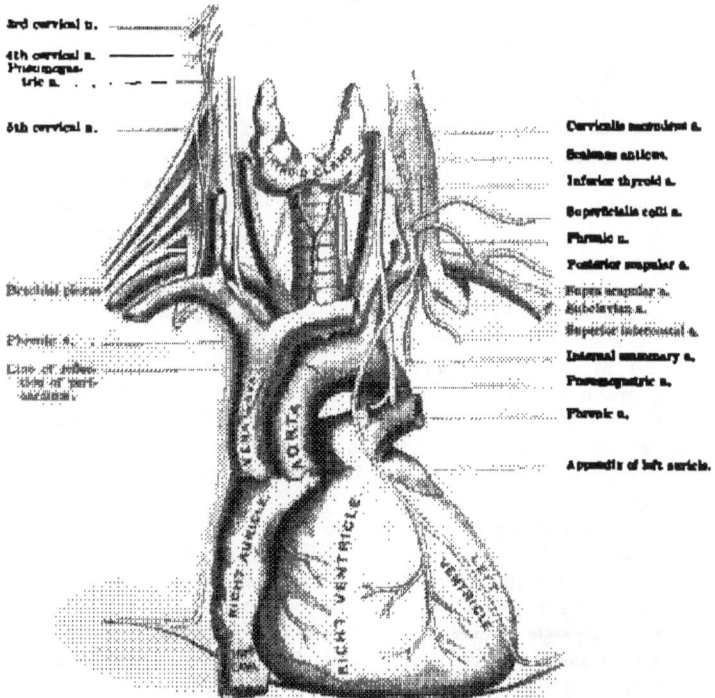

3rd cervical n.

4th cervical n.
Pneumogastric n.

5th cervical n.

Brachial plexus

Phrenic n.

Line of attachment of pericardium

Cervicalis ascendens a.

Scalenus anticus.

Inferior thyroid a.

Superficialis colli a.

Phrenic n.

Posterior scapular a.

Supra scapular a.
Subclavian a.

Superior intercostal a.

Internal mammary a.

Pneumogastric n.

Phrenic n.

Appendix of left auricle.

fluence of large veins in front of the artery. The subclavian vein is situated below the artery, but on a plane anterior to it. Above the artery and to its outer side, are the trunk nerves of the brachial plexus. One of these nerves (the conjoined fifth and

sixth cervical) runs so nearly parallel with the artery, and on
a plane anterior to it, that it is quite possible to mistake the
nerve for the artery, in the operation of tying it. I have heard
a hospital surgeon of great experience say, that he had seen this
mistake committed three times during life. Behind the artery
is the scalenus medius, and below it the first rib. In this part
of its course, the artery as a rule gives off no branches; the most
frequent exceptions are the posterior scapular, and supra-scen-
pular.

The left subclavian is the last of the three great branches which
arise from the arch of the aorta. It ascends nearly
Left subcla-   vertically out of the chest, and then arches in front of
vian artery.
the apex of the lung and pleura to reach the inner
border of the scalenus anticus, behind which it runs over the
first rib.

In the first part of its course, the left subclavian lies deeply in
the chest, near the spine. On its left side it is covered by the
pleura; on its right side are the thoracic duct, the œsophagus and
the trachea: the pneumogastric, phrenic, and sympathetic nerves,
and the left carotid artery run nearly parallel with it: the left
brachio-cephalic vein crosses in front of it. Behind it, is the
longus colli muscle and the inferior cervical ganglion.

Arrived at the level of the upper part of the chest, the left
subclavian arches, like the right, over the apex of the lung, and
has similar relations—namely, in front, it is covered by the sternal
end of the clavicle, the sterno-mastoid, sterno-hyoid, and sterno-
thyroid muscles, and by the internal jugular and vertebral veins:
behind it, are the apex of the lung and the pleura.

Behind the scalenus anticus, and on the surface of the first rib,
the relations of the left subclavian are similar to those of the right
(p. 52).

The left subclavian, then, differs from the right only in the first
part of its course. Now what are these differences?

1. The left subclavian comes direct from the arch of the aorta,
and is therefore longer, deeper in the chest, and more vertical
than the right, which comes from the arteria innominata.

2. The left subclavian is in close relation with the œsophagus and the thoracic duct: the right is not.

3. The left subclavian is crossed by the left brachio-cephalic vein.

4. The left subclavian has the phrenic, pneumogastric, and sympathetic nerves nearly parallel with it; on the right side, these nerves cross the artery at a nearly right angle.

5. The left subclavian is not embraced by the recurrent laryngeal nerve, like the right subclavian.

The thoracic duct bears an important relation to the left subclavian. It ascends from the chest to the left of the œsophagus and *behind* the artery; then arches behind the internal jugular vein, and terminates in the subclavian vein at its junction with the jugular. The duct is so thin and transparent that it easily escapes observation; it is most readily found by raising the subclavian vein close to its junction with the jugular, and searching with the handle of the scalpel on the inner side of the scalenus anticus, in front of the vertebral vein.

Before tracing the branches of the subclavian artery, consider some points relating to the operation of tying it.

To tie the artery in the first part of its course, namely, on the inner edge of the scalenus anticus, is an operation of great difficulty and danger, even with the parts in a normal position. The great depth at which the artery is placed, the size and close proximity of its numerous branches, the large veins by which it is covered, its connection with the pneumogastric, recurrent laryngeal, phrenic, and sympathetic nerves, and above all its close contiguity with the pleura, form a combination of circumstances so formidable that one cannot be surprised the operation has never been performed with a favourable result.

In the second part of its course, namely, between the scalene muscles, the artery is more accessible. It would be necessary to divide the clavicular origin of the sterno-mastoid, the cervical fascia, and the scalenus anticus, to reach the vessel; the phrenic nerve and the subclavian vein would be the chief objects exposed to injury. This operation was performed first and with success by

Dupuytren in the year 1819. More recently it has been performed
by Dr. Warren, of Boston. The patient recovered, though the
pleura was wounded.[*]

But in the last part of its course, that is, on the outer side of
the scalenus, the artery may be tied with comparative facility.
The incision should be made from three to four inches in length,
parallel with the upper border of the clavicle. We divide the
platysma, some of the supra-clavicular nerves, and the cervical
fascia. The external jugular vein must be drawn to the outer
side, or divided and tied at both ends. With the finger and the
handle of the scalpel we then make our way down to the outer
edge of the scalenus anticus, behind which the artery will be found
lying upon the first rib. Remember the tubercle on the inner edge
of the rib which indicates the insertion of the scalenus: this
tubercle is the best guide to the artery. It will be necessary to
divide a layer of fascia which immediately covers the vessel before
the needle can be introduced around it. Mr. Ramsden of St.
Bartholomew's Hospital was the first who tied the subclavian in
the third part of its course, in the year 1809; since that time the
operation has been repeatedly performed, with most favourable
results.

In the hands of a surgeon possessed of a practical knowledge of
anatomy the operation is easy, provided all circumstances be
favourable; but circumstances are often very unfavourable. It
often happens that the aneurismal or other tumour, on account of
which the operation is performed, raises the clavicle beyond its
natural level, and so disturbs the parts, that to expose the artery
and place a ligature around it becomes exceedingly difficult.
Under such circumstances one cannot be surprised that even distinguished anatomists have committed mistakes. Sir Astley
Cooper[†] failed in one instance. Dupuytren perforated the artery
with the point of the needle, and included one of the nerves in the
ligature: fatal hæmorrhage was the result.[‡] I was present at an

---

[*] Med. Chirurg. Trans., vol. xxix. p. 25.
[†] London Medical Review, vol. ii. p. 300.
[‡] Edinburgh Med. and Surg. Journal, vol. xvi. 1820.

operation in which the large nerve (a branch of the brachial plexus)
which runs parallel with and on a plain anterior to the artery was
mistaken for it and tied; the surgeon being deceived by the pulsation communicated to the nerve.

Branches of
the subcla-
vian artery.

The branches of the subclavian extend so far, that in
the present dissection we can trace them only for a short
distance. They are four in number:—

1. The vertebral.
2. The thyroid axis, which gives off the inferior thyroid, supra-
scapular, posterior-scapular, and cervicalis ascendens.
3. The internal mammary.
4. The superior intercostal, which gives off the deep cervical.

As a rule, three branches are given off from the subclavian in
the first part of its course—the vertebral, internal mammary, and
thyroid axis—and one from the second part, the superior intercostal. The most frequent deviation is, that the posterior scapular
(transversalis colli) arises from the subclavian in the third part of
its course.*

Vertebral
artery.

This, the first and largest branch, arises from the
upper part of the subclavian. For a short distance it
lies in the interval between the scalenus anticus and the
longus colli. Here it enters the foramen in the transverse process
of the sixth cervical vertebra, and ascends through the foramina
in the transverse processes of the succeeding vertebræ. In the
interval between the axis and the atlas, the artery makes a sigmoid
curve, that it may not be stretched in the rotation of the head.
Having traversed the foramen of the atlas, the artery curves
backwards along the groove in its arch, perforates the posterior
occipito-atlantoid ligament and the dura mater, then enters the
skull through the foramen magnum, and unites with its fellow

* With reference to the origin of the posterior scapular (transversalis colli) artery,
I made special observations during the winter session of 1858-59. I found that this
artery was given off most frequently, not by the thyroid axis, but by the subclavian
in the third part of its course. Under these circumstances the superficialis colli a.
generally came from the thyroid axis.

near the lower border of the 'pons Varolii,' to form the basilar
artery.

The vertebral artery is accompanied by slender nerves from the
inferior cervical ganglion of the sympathetic. These nerves communicate with the spinal nerves forming the brachial plexus.

Destined for the brain, the vertebral gives off no branches in
the neck, except a few small ones to the deeply-seated muscles;
it furnishes, however, to the spinal cord and its membranes small
arteries which pass through the intervertebral foramina.

The *vertebral vein* is formed by small branches from the muscles
near the foramen magnum. It descends in front of the artery
through the foramina in the transverse processes, and joins the
brachio-cephalic vein. It receives the veins from the cervical
portion of the spinal cord. In some subjects it communicates with
the lateral sinus by a branch through the posterior condyloid
foramen.

The cervical nerves pass through the intervertebral foramina
behind the vertebral artery, so that the artery runs behind its
vein, and in front of the nerves.

Thyroid
axis.

The *thyroid axis* arises from the subclavian near the
inner edge of the scalenus anticus, and after a course of
a quarter of an inch divides into four branches, which
take different directions; namely, the inferior thyroid, the posterior
scapular, the supra-scapular, and the ascending cervical.

The *inferior thyroid* artery ascends tortuously behind the
sheath of the common carotid and the sympathetic nerve, to the
deep surface of the thyroid body, in which it communicates freely
with the superior thyroid and with its fellow. It gives small
branches to the trachea, the œsophagus, and the larynx.

The *ascending cervical* artery usually arises from the inferior
thyroid. It ascends close to the spine, between the scalenus
anticus and the rectus capitis anticus major, and terminates in
small branches, some of which supply these muscles; others enter
the intervertebral foramina, and supply the spinal cord and its
membranes.

The *supra-scapular* artery (transversalis humeri) runs outwards over the scalenus anticus, then directly *beneath* and parallel with the clavicle; crossing over the third part of the subclavian artery to the superior border of the scapula, it passes *above* the transverse ligament which bridges over the notch, and divides into branches, some of which ramify above, others below, the spine of this bone. It inosculates freely in the infra-spinous fossa with the 'dorsalis scapulæ,' a branch of the subscapular, and with the posterior scapular artery. Near the notch, it is joined by the supra-scapular nerve, which runs *through* it.

The *posterior scapular* (transversalis colli) artery, of which the normal origin is said to be from the thyroid axis, very frequently arises from the subclavian in the last part of its course. It is larger than the preceding artery, and runs tortuously across the side of the neck (higher than the supra-scapular), over the scalene muscles and the great nerves of the brachial plexus (sometimes between them), and disappears beneath the trapezius and the levator anguli scapulæ to reach the posterior angle of the scapula. It then runs beneath the rhomboid muscles, in which it is lost. In the space between the sterno-mastoid and trapezius, the posterior scapular gives off the 'superficialis colli.' This vessel proceeds tortuously across the posterior triangle of the neck to the under surface of the trapezius, which, with the levator anguli scapulæ, it principally supplies.

The *superficialis colli* often comes direct from the thyroid axis, when the posterior scapular arises from the last part of the subclavian.

The veins corresponding to the supra-scapular and posterior scapular arteries terminate in the external jugular, sometimes in the subclavian. The middle thyroid vein crosses in front of the common carotid artery, and joins the internal jugular.

This artery arises from the subclavian opposite to the thyroid axis. It enters the chest behind the subclavian vein,

Internal mammary.

and descends behind the cartilages of the ribs, about half an inch from the sternum. Its further progress will be examined in the dissection of the chest. The corresponding vein most frequently terminates in the brachio-cephalic.

Superior intercostal.
This artery is given off by the subclavian behind the scalenus anticus, so that you must divide the muscle to see it. It descends into the chest behind the pleura, passing over the necks of the first and second ribs, and furnishes the arteries of the two upper intercostal spaces. It usually inoscu-

Fig. 11.

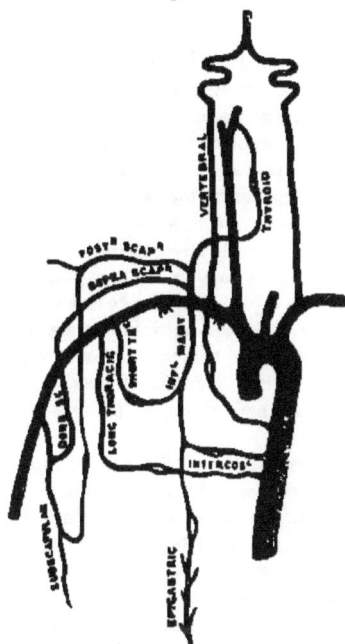

DIAGRAM TO SHOW THE INOSCULATIONS OF THE SUBCLAVIAN ARTERY.

lates with the first inter-costal branch of the aorta. The corresponding vein terminates on the right side in the vena azygos; on the left in the brachio-cephalic.

Deep cervical.
This artery arises from the superior inter-costal, seldom direct from the subclavian. It goes to the back of the neck between the first rib and the transverse process of the last cervical vertebra, and ascends between the complexus and the semi-spinalis colli, both of which it supplies. It sometimes inosculates with the 'prin-ceps cervicis,' a branch of the occipital a.

To test your knowledge of the branches of the sub-clavian artery, reflect upon the answer to the follow-ing question :—If the ar-tery were tied in the *first part* of its course before it gives off any branches, how would the arm be supplied with blood? The answer is, by five collateral channels, as follow :—1. By the com-

munications between the superior and inferior thyroid : 2. By the
communication between the two vertebral: 3. By the communications between the internal mammary and the intercostals and
the epigastric: 4. By the communications between the thoracic
branches of the axillary, and the intercostal branches of the aorta :
5. By the communications between the superior intercostal and
the aortic intercostal. These inosculations are shown in the
diagram, p. 60.

Again, if the subclavian were tied in the *third* part of its course,
the circulation would be carried on by the communications :—1.
Between the supra-scapular and dorsalis scapulæ (branch of subscapular): 2. Between the posterior scapular and the subscapular :
3. Between the long and short thoracic on the one hand, and the
internal mammary and aortic intercostals on the other.

Subclavian
vein.
The subclavian vein does not form an arch like the
artery, but proceeds in a nearly straight line over the
first rib to join the internal jugular. Throughout its
whole course the vein is situated on a plane anterior to and a little
lower than the artery, from which it is separated by the scalenus
anticus, the phrenic and pneumogastric nerves. It has a valve
just before its junction with the internal jugular. It receives the
anterior jugular, external jugular, and through it the supra-
scapular and posterior-scapular veins.

Brachial
plexus
of nerves.
The large nerves forming the plexus which supplies
the upper extremity are the anterior divisions of the
four lower cervical and the first dorsal. Emerging
from the intervertebral foramina they appear between the anterior
and middle scalene muscles, and pass with the subclavian artery
into the axilla. To this bundle of nerves the name 'plexus' is
given, on account of their mutual communications. The plexus
at its root is wide, and situated higher than the subclavian artery,
and nearly on the same plane ; but as the plexus descends beneath
the clavicle its component nerves converge, and in the axilla, completely surround the artery.

The plexus is crossed superficially by the omo-hyoid muscle,
and by the supra-scapular and posterior scapular arteries.

The arrangement of the nerves in the formation of the plexus is usually thus :—The fifth and sixth cervical unite to form a single cord ; the eighth cervical and the first dorsal form another cord ;

Fig. 12.

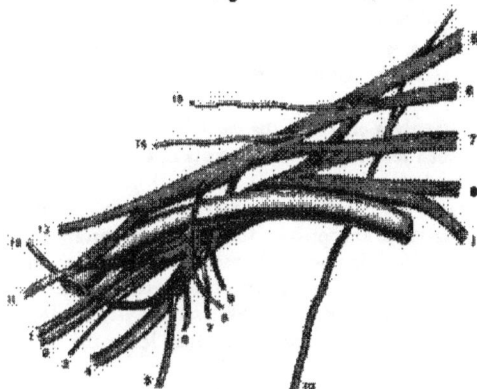

DIAGRAM OF THE BRACHIAL PLEXUS OF NERVES, AND THEIR RELATION TO THE AXILLARY ARTERY.

1, Ulnar.
2. Internal cutaneous.
3. Lesser int. cutaneous (n. of Wrisberg).
4. Musculo-spiral.
5. N. to latissimus dorsi.
6. N. to teres major.
7. N. to subscapularis.
8-9. Anterior thoracic n. to pectoral muscles.
10. N. to serratus magnus.
11. Median.
12. Circumflex.
13. External cutaneous.
14. Supra-scapular.
15. Posterior scapular.

the seventh cervical runs for a short distance alone, and then splits into two branches, one of which joins the cord formed by the fifth and sixth cervical, the other, that formed by the eighth cervical and first dorsal. The branch joining the trunk formed by the eighth cervical and first dorsal usually receives a large reinforcement from the conjoined fifth and sixth cervical. Thus two great trunks are formed, which lie for some distance above and to the outer side of the subclavian artery. Beneath the clavicle, a third cord is formed by the junction of a fasciculus from each of the two primary trunks, so that in the axilla there are three large cords, one external to the axillary artery, one internal to it, the third behind it.*

The plexus gives off above the clavicle the following nerves:—

a. A branch forming one of the roots of the phrenic arises from the fifth cervical.

b. *Nerve to the subclavius m.*—This proceeds from the fifth and sixth cervical, and crosses the subclavian artery in the third part of its course. It frequently sends a filament, which passes in front of the subclavian vein to join the phrenic nerve.

c. *Nerves* to the *scalene* and the *longus colli* muscles are given off from the lower cervical nerves as they leave the intervertebral foramina.

d. *Nerve* to the *rhomboid muscles.*—This arises from the fifth and sixth cervical nerves, and accompanies the posterior scapular artery, beneath the levator anguli scapulæ, which, as well as the rhomboid muscles, it supplies.

e. The *supra-scapular* nerve arises from the cord formed by the fifth, sixth, and seventh cervical n., runs to the upper border of the scapula, where it meets with the corresponding artery, and then passing through the notch in the scapula, terminates in the supra-spinatus and infra-spinatus m.

f. The *nerve* (called *external respiratory* by Sir C. Bell) to the *serratus magnus* arises from the fifth and sixth cervical, appears between the middle and posterior scalene muscles, then descends behind the plexus and the subclavian vessels to the outer surface of the serratus magnus, to which it is exclusively distributed.

* This seems, from a number of dissections, to be the most frequent arrangement of the nerves forming the brachial plexus. This arrangement is, however, very variable, often differing on the two sides in the same subject.

It only remains to be observed that the upper cord of the brachial plexus receives a branch from the lower cord of the cervical, and that each of its component nerves communicate by slender filaments with the sympathetic system.

Below the clavicle the plexus divides into branches for the supply of the arm; namely, the anterior thoracic nerves (two in number, to the pectoralis major and minor), the subscapular (three in number, to the subscapularis, the latissimus dorsi, and teres major), the circumflex (to the deltoid and teres minor), the median, the musculo-spiral, the ulnar, the external cutaneous, the internal cutaneous, and the lesser internal cutaneous (nerve of Wrisberg).

DISSECTION OF THE FACE.

Much practice is required to make a good dissection of the face. The muscles of expression are numerous and complicated; they are interwoven with the subcutaneous tissue and closely united to the skin: their fibres are often pale and indistinct. The face is amply supplied with motor and sensitive nerves, of which the ramifications extend far and wide. Therefore you must not be discouraged, if in a first attempt you fail to make a satisfactory display of the parts.

The cheeks and nostrils should be distended with horse-hair, and the lips sewn together.

Make an incision down the mesial line of the face; another from the chin along the base of the lower jaw to the angle, then prolong it in front of the ear to the zygoma. Reflect the skin from below upwards. Each muscle as it is cleaned must be put on the stretch by hooks.

The nerve which supplies all the muscles of the face is the ' portio dura,' or facial division of the seventh cerebral nerve. It emerges from the stylo-mastoid foramen, and divides into branches, which pass through the parotid gland, forming a plexus termed the ' pes anserinus.'

The sensitive nerves of the face are supplied by the three

divisions of the fifth cerebral nerve; namely, the supra-orbital, the infra-orbital, and the mental. No other nerve takes any share in conferring sensation upon the face except the auriculo-parotidean branch of the cervical plexus (p. 16), which supplies the skin covering the parotid gland and part of the cheek.

The skin covering the cartilages of the nose is supplied by a small nerve called the *naso-lobular*. It is the terminal branch of the nasal division of the ophthalmic nerve. It appears between the bone and the cartilage, lying under the compressor naris m.

Musculus risorius (Santorini). This muscle arises from the fascia over the masseter m., and passes forwards to be inserted into the angle of the mouth, where it intermingles with the orbicularis oris and other muscles in this situation. It produces the smile, not of good humour, but of derision.

It is convenient to arrange the muscles of the face under three heads; appertaining respectively to the mouth, the nose, the eye-brows and lids. Begin with those of the mouth.

The muscles of the mouth are arranged thus: there is an orbicular or sphincter muscle surrounding the lips; from this, as from a common centre, muscles diverge and are fixed into the surrounding bones. They are named elevators, depressors, &c., according to their respective action.

Orbicularis oris. This muscle, nearly an inch in breadth, surrounds the mouth. Its size and thickness in different individuals, produce the variety in the prominence of the lips. Observe that its fibres do not surround the mouth in one unbroken series (excepting a thin fasciculus which is said to pass around the free margin of the lips), but that those of the upper and lower lip decussate at the angles of the mouth, and intermingle with the fibres of the buccinator and other muscles which converge from different parts of the face. The cutaneous surface of the muscle is intimately connected with the lips and the surrounding skin; the deep surface is separated from the mucous membrane by the labial glands and the coronary vessels.

The 'orbicularis' is the antagonist of all the muscles which

F

move the lips. Upon a nice balance of their opposite actions depends the play of the mouth.*

Depressor anguli oris.   This muscle *arises* from the oblique line of the lower jaw below the foramen mentale, and is *inserted* into the angle of the mouth, intermingling with the zygomatic muscles. It is an important muscle in the expression of sorrowful emotions. We see its action when children cry.

Depressor labii inferioris, or quadratus menti.   This muscle *arises* from the oblique line of the lower jaw, and is *inserted* into the lower lip. It covers the vessels and nerves which come through the foramen mentale. It must therefore be divided in cutting through the nerve in cases of neuralgia.

Levator menti.   This muscle *arises* from the lower jaw below the incisor teeth, and is inserted into the skin of the chin. To see it properly, evert the lower lip and remove the mucous membrane on either side of the frænum. There are two of them, one for each side. Their action is well shown when we shave.

Zygomaticus major and minor.   The Z. major *arises* from the outer surface of the malar bone, passes obliquely downwards and is *inserted* into the angle of the mouth, joining the depressor anguli oris. The Z. minor *arises* from the outer surface of the malar bone, in front of the preceding, and is *inserted* into the angle of the mouth, joining the levator labii superioris. The action of the zygomatici is seen in laughing.

Before examining the orbicularis palpebrarum, notice the tendo oculi. To make the tendon more apparent the tarsal cartilages should be drawn outwards.

Tendo oculi.   This tendon is about two lines† in length, and is readily felt at the inner angle of the eye by drawing

---

* In strong muscular lips the upper part of the orbicularis sends a small subcutaneous slip of muscle from each side along the septum nasi nearly to the apex. The interval between the two slips corresponds to the furrow which leads from the nose to the lip. This is the 'naso-labialis' or 'depressor septi narium' of Haller and Albinus.

† A line is the twelfth part of an inch.

the eyelids outwards. It is fixed to the nasal process of the superior maxillary bone, in front of the lachrymal groove, passes outwards, and divides into two portions, one of which is attached to the upper, the other to the lower tarsal cartilage. The tendon crosses the lachrymal sac a little above the centre, and furnishes a tendinous expansion which covers the sac and is attached to the margin of the bony groove. To see this expansion we must reflect that portion of the orbicularis palpebrarum which covers the sac.

In puncturing the lachrymal sac the knife is introduced below the tendon, in a direction downwards, outwards, and a little backwards. We have to divide the skin, a few fibres of the orbicularis, and the fibrous expansion from the tendo oculi. The angular artery and vein are situated on the inner side of the incision.

Orbicularis oculi. This muscle *arises* from the tendo oculi, from the nasal process of the superior maxillary bone, and from the internal angular process of the frontal; it is inserted into the skin of the brow, temple, and cheek.

This broad sphincter muscle surrounds the margin of the orbit and eyelids, and its fibres are divided into two portions, an external or orbital and an inner or palpebral. Its orbital fibres take a wide sweep, passing uninterruptedly around the orbit, and mingle on the forehead with the occipito-frontalis; on the cheek with the zygomaticus minor, and the levator labii superioris.

The fibres which belong to the eyelids (orbicularis palpebrarum) are thin and pale. They arise from the tendo oculi, and form, over each eyelid, a series of elliptical curves which meet at the external canthus of the lids, and are attached to the external tarsal ligament and malar bone. The degree of their curvature becomes less as they approach the margin of the lids, so that some fibres proceed close to the lashes. This was first pointed out by Riolanus,[*] and described as the ' musculus ciliaris.'[†]

---

[*] Anthropologia, lib. v. cap. 10.

[†] Strictly speaking the ciliary muscle arises from the two little divisions of the tendo oculi, and is inserted, at the external canthus, into the fibrous tissue which unites the two tarsal cartilages.

No fat is ever found on the eyelids; nothing intervenes between the skin and the muscle but loose areolar tissue, that there may be no impediment to the free play of the lids.

The orbicular muscle not only shuts the eye but protects it. When the eye is threatened by a blow, the muscle suddenly contracts, presses the eye back into the orbit, and contracts the skin of the brow and cheek so as to form a soft cushion in front of the orbit. The cushion itself may be severely bruised, as is seen in a 'black eye'; but the globe itself is rarely injured. When the eye is closed, as in winking, the palpebral portion of the muscle contracts. Observe this movement attentively, and see that the lids are drawn slightly inwards as well as closed. The object of this inward motion is to direct the tears towards the inner angle of the eyelids, where they are absorbed by the puncta lachrymalia.

Since the orbicular muscle is supplied by the facial nerve, it is affected in facial palsy, and the patient cannot shut the eye.

Corrugator supercilii. This arises from the superciliary ridge of the frontal bone, passes outwards, and is inserted into the under surface of the orbicularis oculi. It lies concealed beneath the orbicularis, and is the proper muscle of frowning.

Pyramidalis nasi. This is situated on the bridge of the nose, on each side of the mesial line, and is regarded as a prolongation of the occipito-frontalis. It mingles with the fibres of the compressor nasi, and its action is to elevate the skin of the nose, as in the expression of surprise.

The present being a good opportunity to examine the structure of the eyelids, postpone for the present the dissection of the remaining muscles of the face.

STRUCTURE OF THE EYELIDS.—The eyelids are composed of different tissues arranged in successive strata one beneath the other. There are—1, the skin; 2, the orbicularis palpebrarum; 3, the expanded tendon of the levator palpebræ (in the upper lid only); 4, the tarsal cartilage and the palpebral ligament which extends from the margin of the orbit to the inner free margins of these cartilages; 5, Meibomian glands; 6, mucous membrane. These structures are separated by areolar tissue, which for good reasons never contains fat.

The *skin* of the eyelids is remarkably smooth and delicate. It is abundantly supplied with sensitive nerves by branches of the fifth pair—namely, by the supra-orbital, supra-trochlear, infra-trochlear, lachrymal, and infra-orbital nerves.

The *orbicularis palpebrarum* has been already described (p. 67). It is supplied with nerves by the facial.

The *levator palpebræ* arises from the back of the orbit, gradually becomes broader, and terminates in a thin aponeurosis, which unites with the broad tarsal ligament, and is lost on the upper surface of the superior tarsal cartilage.

Tarsal cartilages and ligaments. These are plates of fibro-cartilage which support and give figure to the eyelids. There is one for each lid, and they are connected at the angles (commissures or canthi) of the lids through the medium of fibrous tissue. One can best examine them by everting the lids. Each cartilage resembles its lid in form. The upper is the larger, is broad in the middle, and gradually becomes narrower at either end. The lower is nearly of uniform breadth throughout. Both are thicker on the nasal than the temporal side. They are connected to the margin of the orbit, and maintained in position by the tendo oculi, and by what are called the *broad tarsal* or *palpebral ligaments*: these ligaments are continuations from the periosteum of the orbit to the tarsal cartilages. There are two of them, termed upper and lower, and proceeding to each cartilage respectively. When an abscess forms in the areolar tissue of the lids, these ligaments prevent the matter from making its way into the orbit.

Each tarsal cartilage is moreover attached to the malar bone, by means of a ligament, called the *external tarsal ligament*.

The ciliary margin is the thickest part of the tarsal cartilages. It is generally stated that the inner edge of each is sloped or beveled off; and that, when the lids are closed, there is formed, with the globe of the eye, a triangular channel. This channel is said to conduct the tears to the puncta lacrymalia. According to our observation, this channel does not exist: for when the lids are closed, their margins are in such accurate apposition, that not the slightest interstice can be discovered between them.

The *puncta lacrymalia* are two pin-holes apertures, easily discovered on the margin of the lids, close to the inner angle. They are the orifices of the canals, called *canaliculi*, which pass inwards, and convey the tears into the lachrymal sac. Observe that their orifices are directed backwards. In facial palsy, the tensor tarsi being affected, the puncta lose their proper direction, and the tears flow over the cheek.

In the introduction of probes for the purpose of opening the contracted puncta, or of slitting up the lachrymal duct, it is necessary to know the exact direction of these tubes. (*See* diagram.)

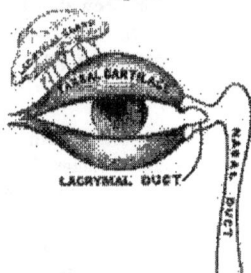

Fig. 13.

By passing a bristle into one of them, we find that it does not run straight from the punctum to the sac, but that it proceeds for a short distance perpendicularly, and then, dilating into a small pouch, makes a sharp bend inwards to the lachrymal sac. In the majority of cases, the tubes open into the sac by a common orifice. When, from any cause, the tears are secreted in greater quantity than usual, they overflow and trickle down the cheek.

The *eyelashes* (cilia) are planted in two or more rows along the edge of the tarsal cartilages. The eyelashes of the upper lid are longer and more numerous than in the lower; and their convexity is directed downwards, while those of the lower lid have an opposite curve. The bulbs of the lashes are situated between the tarsal cartilage and the fibres of the ciliary muscle. They are supplied with blood by the palpebral branches of the ophthalmic, which run parallel and close to the free borders of the lids under the ciliary muscle.

These sebaceous glands, so called after the anatomist * who first

* H. Meibom, De vasis palpebrarum novis. Helmstedt, 1666.

Meibomian glands. described them, are situated on the under surface of each of the tarsal cartilages. In the upper lid there are about thirty; not so many in the lower. On everting the lid, they are seen running in longitudinal rows in grooves of the cartilage. Under the microscope, one sees that they consist of a central tube, round the sides of which are a number of openings leading to short cæcal dilatations. The orifices of these glands are situated on the free margin of the lid behind the lashes. Their use is to secrete an unctuous substance, which prevents the lids from sticking together.

Caruncula lacrymalis. This name is given to a small reddish body situated at the inner corner of the eye. It is composed of an aggregation of sebaceous glands covered by mucous membrane. In some instances minute hairs grow upon it. Its use is, probably, to support the inner junction of the eyelids. When the caruncle is diminished in size by disease, the puncta lacrymalia become displaced, and the tears run down the cheek.

External to the caruncula lacrymalis is a slight vertical fold of conjunctiva, 'plica semilunaris,' which is by some considered to be a rudimentary membrana nictitans (third eyelid found in birds).

The conjunctival coat of the eyelid will be described with the anatomy of the eye. Observe at present, that it is more vascular than the conjunctival coat of the eye, and that it presents a number of minute papillæ, which, when enlarged and aggregated by inflammation, give rise to the disease called 'granular lids.'

Such, in outline, is the structure of the eyelids. Their use is best described by Socrates, who, in answer to the question whether animals were made by chance or design, replies:—'Think you not that it looks like the work of prescience, because the sight is delicate, to have guarded it with eyelids, which open when we want to see, but shut when we go to sleep; to have fenced these lids with eyelashes, which, like a sieve, strain the dusty wind, and hinder it from hurting the eyes; and over the eyes to have placed eyebrows, as eaves, to carry off the sweat of the brow from disturbing the sight?" *

The dissection of the muscles of the face must now be continued. In order to see the origin of the elevators of the upper lip and nose, the lower circumference of the orbicularis oculi must be raised.

Levator labii superioris alæque nasi.
This *arises* from the superior maxillary bone near its orbital margin, and passing downwards divides into two portions, an inner *inserted* into the side of the nose, an outer into the upper lip. It acts chiefly in expressing the smile of derision, and the scornful affections of the mind. Its habitual use occasions corresponding permanent folds in the skin, which are, to a certain extent, indicative of the feelings and passions.

Levator labii superioris.
This *arises* from the lower margin of the orbit above the infra-orbital foramen, and is *inserted* into the upper lip. It is nearly an inch in breadth at its origin, and it covers the infra-orbital vessels and nerves.

Levator anguli oris.
This muscle, which is covered by the levator labii superioris, *arises* from the canine fossa of the superior maxilla, below the infra-orbital foramen, and is *inserted* into the angle of the mouth, superficial to the buccinator, its fibres blending with those of the orbicularis oris, zygomatici, and depressor anguli oris.

Two muscles belonging to the nose must now be examined—the triangularis or compressor nasi, and the depressor labii superioris

Compressor nasi.
This muscle is triangular, and *arises* by its apex from the superior maxillary bone, internal to the canine fossa, and is attached by a broad thin aponeurosis which spreads over the dorsum of the nose and joins its fellow. The

* Xenophon's Memorabilia. b. 1. c. iv.: Οὗ δοκεῖ σοι καὶ τάδε προνοίας ἔργα δουλεῖναι, τ). ἐπεὶ ἀσθενὴς μέν ἐστιν ἡ ὄψις, βλεφάροις αὐτὴν θυρῶσαι, ἃ, ὅταν μὲν αὐτῇ χρῆσθαί τι δέῃ, ἀναπεράννυται, ἐν δ’ τῷ ὕπνῳ συγκλείεται; ὡς δ’ ἂν μηδὲ ἄνεμοι βλάπτωσιν, ἠθμὸν βλεφαρίδας ἐμφῦσαι· ὀφρύσι τε διαγεατῶσαι τὰ ὑπὲρ τῶν ὀμμάτων ὡς μηδ’ ὁ ἐκ τῆς κεφαλῆς ἱδρὼς κακουργῇ·

origin of this muscle is concealed by the levator labii superioris alæque nasi.

Depressor labii superioris or depressor alæ nasi. This *arises* from the superior maxilla, above the second incisor tooth, and is *inserted* into the septum and ala of the nose. It is situated between the mucous membrane and the muscular structure of the upper lip.

To expose it, the upper lip must be everted and the mucous membrane removed.

Besides the muscles above described, we find, in connection with the cartilages of the ala of the nose, pale muscular fibres, in which no definite arrangement can be traced. They constitute the '*dilatator narium anterior*' and the '*dilatator narium posterior*' of some anatomists. By acting upon the cartilages of the nose, these little muscles contribute in some degree to express the condition of the mind. Some of them dilate the nostrils; for instance, in dyspnœa: others contract them, as in smelling.

Buccinator. The buccinator *arises* from the alveolar borders of the upper and lower jaws, corresponding to the molar teeth, and from the pterygo-maxillary ligament. The fibres pass forwards and are inserted into the angle of the mouth and the muscular structure of the lips; the central fibres decussate, i.e. the lower fibres pass upwards along the upper lip, and the upper fibres pass downwards along the lower lip.

The buccinator is the great muscle of the cheek. It forms with the superior constrictor of the pharynx, a continuous muscular wall for the side of the mouth and pharynx. The bond of connection between the buccinator and the superior constrictor, is the 'so-called' pterygo-maxillary ligament. Now this ligament (see diagram) extends from the hamular process vertically to the posterior extremity of the mylo-hyoid ridge of the lower jaw near the last molar. To call it a ligament seems a misnomer: it is simply a fibrous intersection between the two muscles.

The duct of the parotid gland passes obliquely through the buccinator into the mouth, opposite the second molar of the upper jaw.

The chief use of the buccinator is to keep the food between the teeth during mastication. It can also widen the mouth. Its power of expelling air from the mouth, as in whistling or playing on a wind instrument, has given rise to its peculiar name. It is

Fig. 14.

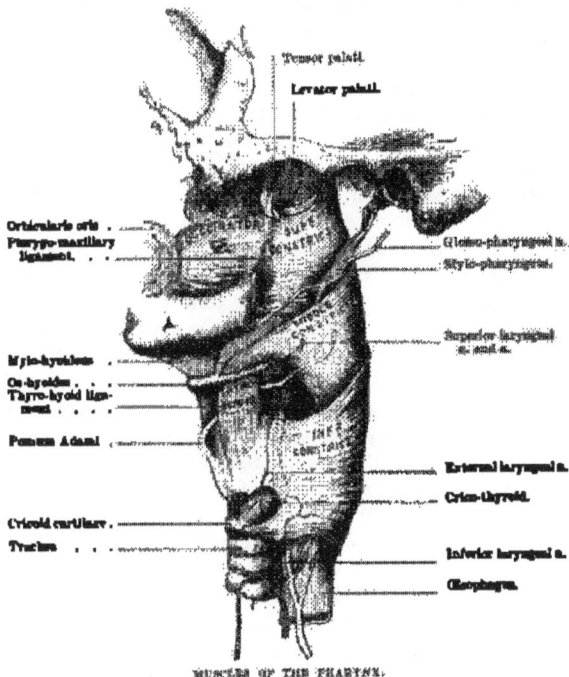

MUSCLES OF THE PHARYNX.

supplied by the facial nerve, and is, therefore, affected in facial paralysis.

Buccal fascia.   The buccinator muscle is covered by a layer of fibrous tissue, which adheres closely to its surface, and is attached to the alveolar border of the upper and lower jaw. This structure is thin over the anterior part of the muscle, but more dense behind, where it is continuous with the aponeurosis of the pharynx. It is called the 'bucco-pharyngeal' fascia, since it supports and strengthens the muscular walls of these cavities. In consequence of the resistance of this fascia, abscesses do not readily burst into the mouth or the pharynx.

Molar glands.
The molar glands, three or four in number, situated immediately outside the posterior part of the bucci- nator, are about the size of a split pea, and their secretion is conveyed to the mouth by separate ducts near the last molar teeth.

Between the buccinator and the masseter there is in almost all subjects an accumulation of fat. It is found, beneath the zygoma especially, in large round masses, and may be turned out with the handle of the scalpel. It fills up the zygomatic fossa, and being soft and elastic, does not present the least obstacle to the free movements of the jaw. Its absorption in emaciated individuals occasions the sinking of the cheek.

Facial artery.
The facial (external maxillary) artery is the third branch of the external carotid. It runs tortuously be- neath the hypoglossal nerve, the posterior belly of the digastricus, and the stylo-hyoideus, next *through* the substance of the submaxillary gland, and mounts over the base of the jaw at the *anterior edge of the masseter* muscle. Up to this point we traced it in the dissection of the neck (page 38). It now ascends tortuously near the corner of the mouth and the ala of the nose, towards the inner angle of the eye, where, much diminished in size, it inosculates with the terminal branch of the ophthalmic, a branch of the internal carotid. In the first part of its course, the facial artery is covered only by the platysma; above the corner of the mouth it is crossed by a few fibres of the orbicularis oris and the zygomatici; still higher it is covered by some of the fibres of the elevators of the upper lip and the nose. It lies successively upon the buccinator, levator anguli oris, and levator labii superioris muscles. In its course along the face it gives off the following branches :—

a. The *inferior labial* artery passes inwards under the depressor anguli oris and inosculates with the mental branch of the inferior dental and the inferior coronary artery.

b. The *inferior coronary* artery comes off near the angle of the mouth, runs tortuously along the lower lip, between the mucous membrane and the orbicularis muscle, and inosculates with its fellow.

c. The *superior coronary* proceeds along the upper lip close to the mucous membrane, and inosculates with its fellow; thus a complete arterial circle is formed round the mouth. These arteries can be felt pulsating on the inner side of the lip, near the free border. From this circle numerous branches pass off to the papillæ of the lips, and the labial glands. The superior coronary gives off a small branch (artery of the septum) which ascends along the septum to the apex of the nose.

d. The *lateral artery of the nose*, a branch of considerable size, arises opposite the ala nasi, ramifies upon the external surface of the nose, and inosculates with the nasal branch of the ophthalmic artery.

e. The *angular artery*, which may be regarded as the termination of the facial, inosculates on the inner side of the tendo oculi with the ophthalmic.

The facial artery supplies numerous branches to the muscles of the face, and inosculates with the transversalis faciei, infra-orbital, and mental arteries.

The facial artery and its branches are surrounded by a minute plexus of nerves (nervi molles), invisible to the naked eye. They are derived from the superior cervical ganglion of the sympathetic, and exert a powerful influence over the contraction and dilatation of the capillary vessels, and thus occasion those sudden changes in the countenance indicative of certain mental emotions, e. g. blushing or sudden paleness.*

* M. Bernard and Brown Séquard have proved by experiment that if the branches of the sympathetic, which accompany the facial artery, be divided, the capillary vessels of the face, being deprived of their contractile power, become immediately distended with blood, and the temperature of the face is raised.

The *facial vein* does not run with the artery, but takes a straight course from the inner angle of the eye to the anterior edge of the masseter. In this course it descends beneath the zygomatic muscles, over the termination of the parotid duct, and at the anterior border of the masseter passes over the jaw, behind the facial artery, and joins the internal jugular.

The facial vein is a continuation of the frontal, which descends over the forehead, and, after receiving the supra-orbital, takes the name of angular at the corner of the eye. It communicates with the ophthalmic vein, receives the veins of the eyelids, the external parts of the nose, the coronary veins, and others from the muscles of the face. Near the angle of the mouth it is often increased in size by a large vein which comes from a venous plexus deeply seated behind the superior maxillary bone.

Arteria transversalis faciei.
This artery arises from the temporal or the external carotid in the substance of the parotid gland. It runs forwards across the masseter above the parotid duct, and is distributed to the glandula socia parotidis, and the masseter. It anastomoses with the infra-orbital and facial. It is seldom of large size, except when it supplies those parts which usually receive blood from the facial. We have seen it as large as a goose-quill, furnishing the coronary and the nasal arteries; the facial itself not being larger than a sewing thread.

Your attention must now be directed to the parotid gland; its boundaries, its deep relations, the course of its duct, and the objects contained within the gland.

Parotid gland.
The parotid, the largest of the salivary glands, occupies the space between the ramus of the jaw and the mastoid process. It is bounded above by the zygoma; below by the sterno-mastoid, and digastric muscles; behind by the meatus auditorius and the mastoid process; in front, it lies over the ascending ramus of the jaw, and is prolonged for some distance over the masseter. It is separated from the submaxillary gland by the stylo-maxillary ligament; sometimes the two glands are directly continuous.

The superficial surface of the gland is flat, and covered by a

strong layer of fascia, a continuation of the cervical. It not only
envelopes the gland, but sends down numerous partitions which
form a framework for its lobes. The density of this sheath explains the pain caused by inflammation of the gland, the tardi-
ness with which abscesses within it make their way to the surface,
and the propriety of an early opening.

The deep surface of the gland is irregular, and moulded upon
the subjacent parts. Thus, it passes inwards between the neck of
the jaw and the internal lateral ligament; it extends upwards and
occupies the posterior part of the glenoid cavity; below, it reaches
the styloid process, and sometimes penetrates deep enough to
touch the internal jugular vein.

That portion of the gland which lies on the masseter muscle is
called ' glandula socia parotidis.' It varies in size in different
subjects; and is situated chiefly above the parotid duct, into which
it pours its secretion by one or two smaller ducts.

The *duct* of the parotid gland (ductus Stenonis [*]) is thick and
strong, and about two inches long. In this respect it differs from
the duct of the submaxillary gland, which is less exposed to injury. It runs transversely forwards over the masseter, about an
inch below the zygoma, perforates the buccinator obliquely, and
opens into the mouth opposite the second molar tooth of the upper
jaw. Near its termination it is crossed by the zygomaticus major
and the facial vein. After perforating the buccinator, the duct
passes for a short distance between the muscle and the mucous
membrane. Its orifice is small and contracted compared with the
diameter of the rest of the duct, which will admit a crow-quill; it
is not easily found in the mouth, being concealed by a fold of
mucous membrane.

Since it is desirable, in operations about the face, to avoid injuring the parotid duct, it is well to know that the precise direction of the duct corresponds with a line drawn from the middle of
the lobule of the ear to a point midway between the nose and the
upper lip.

---

[*] Nic. Steno, De glandulis oris, &c. Lugd. Bat. 1661.

On cutting into the substance of the parotid gland, the following objects are seen in its interior, proceeding in the order of
their depth from the surface :—

1. Two or more small absorbent glands.

2. The 'pes anserinus,' or primary branches of the facial
nerve.

3. Branches from the auriculo-parotidean and temporo-auricular
nerves which communicate here with the facial.

4. The external jugular vein formed by the junction of the
internal maxillary and temporal veins.

5. The external carotid, which, after giving many branches to
the gland, divides opposite the neck of the jaw, into the internal
maxillary and temporal arteries.*

The absorbent glands about the parotid deserve notice, because
they are liable to become enlarged, and simulate disease of the
parotid itself. An absorbent gland lies close to the root of the
zygoma, in front of the cartilage of the ear ; this gland is sometimes affected in disease of the external tunics of the eye ; e.g.
in purulent ophthalmia : also in affections of the scalp.

To display the plexus of nerves (pes anserinus), formed by the
branches of the facial in the parotid gland, find one of the larger
branches, say one of the malar, on the face, and trace this into
the substance of the gland, as a clue to the others.

Portio dura
or facial
nerve.
 This is the motor nerve of the face. It supplies all
the muscles of expression, except those which move the
eyes. It arises immediately below the ' pons Varolii,'
from the lateral tract of the medulla oblongata. The nerve enters
the meatus auditorius internus, lying upon the auditory nerve,
traverses a tortuous bony canal (aqueductus Fallopii) in the

* Reviewing the intricate and deep connections of the parotid gland, one cannot
but conclude that it is almost, if not quite, impracticable to remove it entirely during
life. If this conclusion be correct, even in the normal condition of the gland, what
must it be when the gland is enlarged by disease? John Bell, however, relates a
case in which he was induced to attempt the extirpation of a diseased parotid (Principles of Surgery, vol. iii. p. 262). Other surgeons, too, of more modern date, have
attempted the same thing. It is not unlikely that they have mistaken a tumour in
the substance of the parotid for disease of the parotid itself.

petrous portion of the temporal bone, and leaves the skull at the stylo-mastoid foramen. Its course and connections in the temporal bone will be investigated hereafter: at present we must trace the facial part of the nerve.

Having emerged from the stylo-mastoid foramen, the nerve enters the parotid gland, and soon divides into two primary branches, named, from their distribution, *temporo-facial* and *cervico-facial*. These primary branches cross over the external carotid, and the external jugular vein, and form, by their communications within the substance of the parotid, the plexus called '*pes anserinus*,' from its resemblance to the skeleton of a goose's foot. The plexus and the direction of its ramifications must be carefully made out, for you may have to remove tumours formed in the interior of the parotid; you may find the nerves spread over the tumour, and you must dissect between the nerves without injuring them.

Close to the stylo-mastoid foramen, the facial nerve sends off its *posterior auricular* branch (p. 3), which ascends behind the ear and supplies the retrahens and attollens aurem m. and the posterior belly of the occipito-frontalis; it also gives off a branch to the posterior belly of the digastricus and another to the stylo-hyoideus. In this situation it communicates by filaments with the glosso-pharyngeal, pneumogastric, and auriculo-parotidean nerves.

The *temporo-facial* division crosses the external carotid and the neck of the jaw, receives two or more communications from the temporo-auricular (branch of the fifth), and subdivides into temporal, malar, and infra-orbital branches.

The *temporal* branches ascend over the zygoma, supply the frontalis, the attrahens aurem, the orbicularis palpebrarum, the corrugator supercilii, and tensor tarsi, and communicate with filaments of the supra-orbital nerve.

The *malar* branches cross the malar bone, supply the orbicularis oculi, and communicate with filaments of the lacrymal and superior maxillary nerves.

The *infra-orbital* branches proceed transversely forwards beneath the zygomatici over the masseter, and supply the elevators of the upper lip and the muscles of the nose. Beneath the levator labii superioris we find a free communication with the infra-orbital branches of the superior maxillary nerve (second division of the fifth).

The *cervico-facial* division, joined by filaments from the auriculo-parotidean (branch of cervical plexus), descends towards the angle of the jaw, and subdivides into buccal, supra- and infra-maxillary branches.

The *buccal* branches pass forwards over the masseter parallel with the parotid duct, and supply the buccinator: they communicate with the buccal branch of the inferior maxillary nerve (second division of the fifth).

The *supra-maxillary* branches advance over the masseter and facial artery, and run under the depressor muscles of the lower lip, all of which they supply. Some of the filaments communicate with the mental branch of the dental nerve.

The *infra-maxillary* or cervical branches, one or more in number, were dissected with the neck (p. 17). They arch forwards below the jaw, covered by the platysma, and communicate with the superficialis colli (branch of the cervical plexus).

Respecting the function of the facial nerve, it is necessary to remember that though at its origin it is purely a motor nerve, yet after leaving the stylo-mastoid foramen it becomes a compound nerve, in consequence of the filaments which it receives from the temporo-auricular branch of the fifth, and from the auriculo-parotidean branch of the cervical plexus. These communications explain the pain which is often felt in facial paralysis along the track of the facial nerves.

Sensitive nerves of the face.   These are the supra-orbital, the infra-orbital, and the mental, all branches of the fifth pair.

The *supra-orbital* nerve is a branch of the first division of the fifth pair. It leaves the orbit through the supra-orbital notch, and is at first covered by the orbicularis and occipito-frontalis. But it presently divides into wide-spreading branches, which supply the skin of the forehead and scalp. The supra-orbital artery is a branch of the ophthalmic.

The *infra-orbital nerve* is the terminal branch of the superior maxillary or second division of the fifth nerve. It emerges with its artery from the infra-orbital foramen, covered by the levator labii superioris. The nerve immediately divides into several branches, *palpebral, nasal,* and *labial*; the palpebral, ascending beneath the orbicularis, supply the lower eyelid, and communicate with the facial: the nasal pass inwards to supply the nose and join the nasal branch of the first division of the fifth; the labial, by far the most numerous, descend into the upper lip, and eventually terminate in lashes of filaments, which endow the papillae of the lip with exquisite sensibility.

The *infra-orbital artery* is the terminal branch of the internal maxillary; it supplies the muscles and skin, and inosculates with branches of the facial.

The *mental nerve* is a branch of the inferior maxillary or third division of the fifth. It emerges from the mental foramen in the lower jaw, in a direction upwards and backwards, beneath the depressor labii inferioris. It soon divides into a number of branches, some of which supply the skin of the chin, but the greater number terminate in the papillae of the lower lip.

The *mental artery* is a branch of the inferior dental. It supplies the gums and the chin, and inosculates with the sub-mental and inferior coronary arteries.

MUSCLES OF MASTICATION.—TEMPORAL AND SPHENO-MAXILLARY REGIONS.

In this dissection, the parts should be examined in the following order:—

1. Superficial arteries and nerves of the temple.
2. Masseter muscle.
3. Temporal aponeurosis.
4. Temporal muscle.

5. Pterygoid muscles.
6. Internal maxillary artery and branches.
7. Inferior maxillary nerve and branches.

Reflect the skin of the temple from below upwards. Under the skin you come upon a layer of tough fibro-cellular tissue, continuous, above, with the aponeurosis of the scalp, below, with the fascia covering the masseter and the parotid gland. In this tissue are contained the superficial temporal vessels and nerves.

This is the smaller of the two terminal branches of the external carotid. Arising in the substance of the parotid gland near the neck of the jaw, it passes over the root of the zygoma close to the meatus auditorius, ascends for about an inch and a half upon the temporal fascia, and there divides into an anterior and a posterior branch. Above the zygoma it is superficial, being covered only by the attrahens aurem muscle; here it is accompanied by the temporo-auricular branch of the inferior division of the fifth nerve. It gives off the following branches :—

Temporal artery.

a. Several small branches to the parotid.

b. The *transversalis faciei* (p. 77).

c. The *anterior auricular* branches ramify on the front of the pinna of the ear, inosculating with the posterior auricular.

d. The *middle temporal*, a small vessel, pierces the temporal fascia above the zygoma, and running in the substance of the temporal muscle, anastomoses with the temporal branches of the internal maxillary.

Of the two branches into which the temporal divides, the *anterior* runs tortuously towards the external angle of the frontal bone, distant from it about an inch. Its ramifications extend over the forehead, supplying the orbicularis and frontalis m., and inosculate with the supra-orbital and frontal arteries. The *posterior* runs towards the back of the head, and inosculates freely with the occipital and posterior auricular. The anterior branch is usually selected for arteriotomy, the posterior being covered by a strong and unyielding fascia.

Temporo-auricular nerve.

This nerve supplies the temples and side of the head with common sensation. It arises from the third division of the fifth pair by two roots (between which the 'middle meningeal artery' runs). From its origin it proceeds

outwards between the neck of the jaw and the internal lateral
ligament, over the root of the zygoma, where it joins the temporal
artery, and divides like it into an *anterior* and a *posterior* branch.
Its ramifications correspond with those of the artery.

Near the condyle of the jaw the temporo-auricular nerve sends
branches to the upper division of the facial nerve, endowing it
with common sensibility. It here distributes branches to the
parotid gland, meatus auditorius, and the articulation of the jaw.
Above the zygoma it gives filaments (auricular) to the outer
surface of the pinna of the ear.

Lastly, in the subcutaneous tissue of the temple, we find the
temporal branches of the facial nerve, which supply the frontalis,
the attrahens aurem, the orbicularis oculi, tensor tarsi, and corrugator supercilii.

Masseter
muscle.
This muscle *arises* from the lower edge of the zygoma,
and is *inserted* into the outer side of the ramus and
coronoid process of the jaw. The masseter is composed
of superficial and deep fibres which cross like the letter X. The
superficial fibres, constituting the principal part of the muscle,
arise from the anterior two-thirds of the zygoma by a strong
tendon which occupies the front border of the muscle, and sends
aponeurotic partitions into its substance. These fibres pass downwards and backwards, this direction giving them greater advantage,
and are inserted into the angle and part of the ramus of the jaw.
The deep fibres (which are concealed by the parotid gland) arise
from the posterior part of the zygoma, incline forwards, and are
inserted into the upper half of the ramus and the coronoid process.
Besides these, a few fibres, arising from the inner surface of the
zygoma, are inserted into the coronoid process and the tendon of
the temporal muscle. Its *action* is to masticate the food: it
closes the jaw with great force.

The following objects lie upon the masseter: 1. Glandula socia
parotidis, and parotid duct; 2. Transversalis faciei artery; 3.
Facial artery and vein; 4. Branches of the facial nerve.

Reflect the masseter from its origin. Observe the direction of
the superficial and deep fibres, and the tendinous partitions which

augment the power of the muscle by increasing its extent of origin. The masseteric nerve and artery enter the under surface of the muscle through the sigmoid notch of the jaw; the artery comes from the internal maxillary, the nerve from the motor division of the inferior maxillary.

Temporal aponeurosis. This strong shining membrane covers the temporal muscle; its chief use being to give additional origin to it. It is attached above to the temporal ridge, and increasing in thickness as it descends, divides near the zygoma into two layers, which are attached to the outer and inner surfaces of the zygomatic arch. These layers are separated by fat, in which is found a filament from the orbital branch of the superior maxillary nerve. The density of this aponeurosis explains why abscesses in the temporal fossa rarely point outwards; the matter makes its way, beneath the zygoma, into the mouth.

Reflect the aponeurosis, and notice that it is separated from the temporal muscle, near the zygoma, by fat. The absorption of this fat, and the wasting of the muscle, occasion the sinking of the temple in emaciation and old age.

Temporal muscle. This muscle *arises* from the temporal fossa and the temporal aponeurosis. It is inserted by a strong tendon into the inner surface, the apex, and anterior border of the coronoid process.

The fibres of this muscle converging from their wide origin, pass under the zygomatic arch, and terminate upon their tendon, the outer surface of which is partially concealed by the insertion of those fibres which come from the temporal aponeurosis: remove them, and see how admirably this tendon radiates into the muscle like the ribs of a fan. Thus the force of the muscle is collected into one focus.

Spheno-maxillary or pterygo-maxillary region. Remove the zygomatic arch, to expose the coronoid process of the jaw, the insertion of the temporal muscle, and the loose fat which surrounds it. Next, saw through the coronoid process in a direction downwards and forwards, so as to include the insertion of the muscle, and reflect it upwards without injuring the subjacent vessels and nerves.

To gain a good view of the muscles, nerves, and vessels of the pterygo-maxillary region, a portion of the ascending ramus of the jaw must be removed with a Hey's saw, as shown in the diagram below.

In this region we have to examine the two pterygoid muscles, the trunk and branches of the internal maxillary artery and nerve, and the internal lateral ligament of the lower jaw.

External pterygoid.   This muscle *arises* by two heads, one from the outer surface of the external pterygoid plate (a few fibres taking origin from the outer side of the tuberosity of the palate bone); the other from the great wing of the sphenoid. It is *inserted* into the neck of the jaw, and slightly into the border of the inter-articular fibro-cartilage of the joint of the jaw.

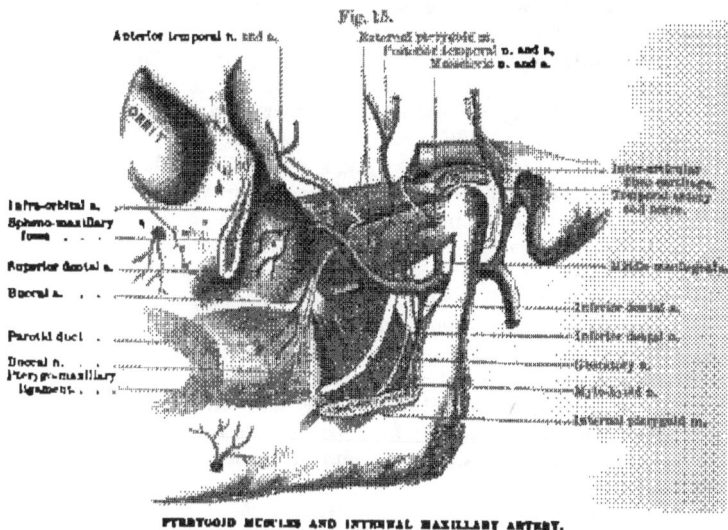

Fig. 15.

PTERYGOID MUSCLES AND INTERNAL MAXILLARY ARTERY.

The object of the insertion of some of its fibres into the inter-articular cartilage is, that the cartilage may follow the condyle in

all its movements. When the jaw is dislocated, it is chiefly by
the action of this muscle, which pulls the condyle into the zygomatic fossa; the inter-articular cartilage being dislocated with the
condyle.

Internal
pterygoid.

 This muscle *arises* from the inner surface of the external pterygoid plate, and tuberosity of the palate
bone. It is *inserted* into the inner side of the angle of
the jaw.

Notice particularly the direction of the fibres of the pterygoid
muscles. The fibres of the external run horizontally outwards and
backwards from their origin; the fibres of the internal run
downwards, backwards, and outwards from their origin. In
structure, these muscles are similar to the masseter; that is, they
are intersected by tendinous septa for the purpose of giving origin
to muscular fibres.

The action of the pterygoid muscles is to produce the lateral
movements of the jaw essential to the mastication of the food.
Consequently they are enormously developed in all ruminants,
and comparatively feebly in carnivorous animals.

Cut through the neck of the jaw, and disarticulate the condyle
with its fibro-cartilage from the glenoid cavity, and turn it
forwards with the external pterygoid, so that the condyle can be
replaced if desirable. A little dissection will bring into view the
internal lateral ligament, and the internal maxillary artery.

Internal
maxillary
artery.

 This is one of the terminal branches into which the
external carotid divides opposite the neck of the jaw.
It passes horizontally forwards between the neck of the
jaw and the internal lateral ligament, then runs tortuously, in
some cases above, in others beneath the external pterygoid,
enters the spheno-maxillary fossa between the two heads of the
external pterygoid, and terminates by dividing into several
branches.

The course of this artery is divided into three stages. In the
first, the artery lies between the neck of the jaw and the internal
lateral ligament; in the second, it lies either over or under
the external pterygoid; in the third, it lies in the spheno-maxillary
fossa.

BRANCHES OF THE INTERNAL MAXILLARY ARTERY IN THE THREE
STAGES OF ITS COURSE.

Branches in the First Stage.	Branches in the Second Stage.	Branches in the Third Stage.
Tympanic.	Six to the muscles of masti-	Superior dental.
Meningea media.	cation, namely:—	Infra-orbital.
Meningea parva.	Masseteric.	Descending palatine.
Inferior dental.	Anterior and posterior	Vidian.
	temporal.	Nasal or spheno-palatine.
	External and internal	Pterygo-palatine.
	pterygoid.	
	Buccal.	

a. The *tympanic* ascends behind the jaw, and passes through
the glenoid fissure to the tympanum. It supplies the membrana
tympani, and anastomoses with the stylo-mastoid and Vidian
arteries.

Fig. 16.

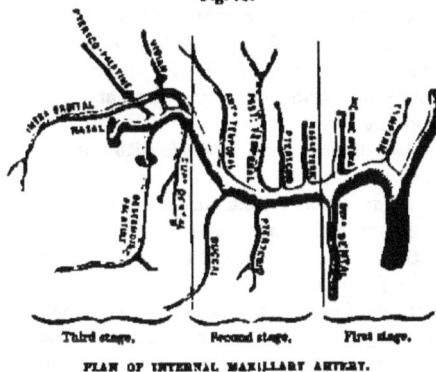

Third stage.   Second stage.   First stage.

PLAN OF INTERNAL MAXILLARY ARTERY.

b. The *middle meningeal* artery ascends between the two roots
of the temporo-auricular nerve through the foramen spinosum into
the cranium, where it ramifies between the dura mater and the
bones.

c. The *meningea parva* ascends through the foramen ovale into the skull, and supplies chiefly the ganglion of the fifth pair. It often comes from the meningea media.

d. The *inferior dental* artery descends behind the neck of the jaw to the dental foramen, which it enters with the dental nerve. It then proceeds through a canal in tho diploe to the symphysis, where it minutely inosculates with its fellow. In this canal, which runs beneath the roots of all the teeth, the artery gives branches which ascend through the little apertures in the fangs, and ramify upon the pulp in their interior. Opposite the foramen mentale arises the mental branch already described (p. 82). Before entering the jaw the dental artery furnishes a small branch—mylo-hyoid—which accompanies the nerve proceeding to the mylo-hyoid muscle.

e. The *masseteric* branch passes through the sigmoid notch of the jaw to tho under surface of the masseter, with the masseteric nerve, and inosculates with the facial artery.

f. The anterior and posterior *temporal* arteries ascend to supply the temporal muscle, ramifying close to the bone, one near the front, the other near the posterior border of the muscle.

g. The *pterygoid* branches supply the internal and external pterygoid muscles.

h. The *buccal* branch runs forwards with the buccal nerve to the buccinator.

i. The *superior-dental* branch runs along the back part of the superior maxillary bone, and sends small arteries through the foramina in the bone to the pulps of the molar and bicuspid teeth. It also supplies the gums.

j. The *infra-orbital* branch passes through the spheno-maxillary fissure, then runs forwards along the infra-orbital canal with the superior maxillary nerve, and emerges upon the face at the infra-orbital foramen. In the infra-orbital canal the artery sends branches downwards through little canals in the bone to the incisor and canine teeth.

k. The *descending palatine,* a branch of considerable size, runs down the posterior palatine canal with the palatine nerve (a branch from Meckel's ganglion), and then along the roof of the hard palate, towards the anterior palatine canal, in which, much diminished in size, it inosculates on the septum nasi with a branch of the spheno-palatine artery. It supplies the gums, the glands, and mucous membrane of this part, and furnishes branches to the soft palate.

l. The *Vidian,* an insignificant branch, runs backwards through the Vidian canal with the Vidian nerve, and is lost upon the Eustachian tube and the pharynx.

m. The *nasal* or *spheno-palatine* branch enters the nose, through the spheno-palatine foramen in company with the nasal nerve from Meckel's (spheno-palatine) ganglion, and ramifies upon the spongy bones and the septum narium.

n. The *pterygo-palatine* is a small but constant branch which runs backwards through the pterygo-palatine canal, and ramifies upon the upper part of the pharynx and the Eustachian tube.

The *internal maxillary* vein is formed by the veins corresponding to the branches of the artery. It joins the temporal in the substance of the parotid gland, and forms the external jugular.

Inferior
maxillary
nerve and
branches.
This great nerve is the largest of the three divisions of the fifth cerebral nerve. It differs from the other two divisions, i.e. the ophthalmic and the superior maxillary, in that it contains motor as well as sensitive filaments; the motor being furnished by the small non-ganglionic root of the fifth nerve. Thus much of its physiology it is necessary to know, in order to understand its extensive distribution; for the sensitive portion supplies the parts to which it is distributed with common sensation only, whilst the motor portion supplies all the muscles concerned in mastication.

The nerve, then, composed of sensitive and motor filaments, emerges from the skull through the foramen ovale as a thick trunk, under the name of the inferior maxillary. It lies directly external to the Eustachian tube, and is covered by the external pterygoid muscle, which should be turned on one side to expose it. Immediately after its exit from the skull, the nerve divides into its several branches: some, destined for the muscles, contain motor as well as sensitive filaments; others are purely sensitive, as follow :—

BRANCHES OF THE INFERIOR MAXILLARY NERVE.

BRANCHES OF COMMON SENSATION.	BRANCHES MOTOR.
Temporo-auricular.	To temporal muscle.
Inferior dental.	— masseter.
Buccal.	— external pterygoid.
Gustatory.	— internal pterygoid.
	— tensor palati.
	— mylo-hyoideus.
	— anterior belly of digastricus.

The branches to the *temporal* muscle, two in number, pass outwards close to the great wing of the sphenoid bone, and ascend with the temporal arteries to the muscle.

The branch to the *masseter* runs outwards above the external pterygoid, through the sigmoid notch of the jaw.

The branch to the *external pterygoid* comes apparently from the buccal nerve in its passage through this muscle.

The branch to the *internal pterygoid* and *tensor palati* muscles is rather difficult to find. It proceeds from the inner side of the main trunk, close to the otic ganglion, and descends between the internal pterygoid and the tensor palati, supplying them both.

The *buccal* branch passes either above or between the fibres of the external pterygoid to the buccinator, where it spreads out into filaments, which supply the skin, mucous membrane, and glands of the check with common sensation. The motor power of the buccinator, remember, is derived from the facial nerve. That this buccal branch is purely sensory is proved by the action of the muscle still continuing when the motor division of the fifth nerve is paralysed. The evidence is corroborated by a case in which this buccal branch proceeded from the second division of the fifth nerve; no communication being discovered, after very careful dissection, between it and the motor root of the third division.[*]

---

[*] Turner 'On the variation of the buccal nerve.' Journal of Anat. and Phys. No. I. 1868.

The *temporo-auricular* branch arises by two roots which embrace the middle meningeal artery before it enters the skull. The nerve runs outwards behind the external pterygoid and the neck of the jaw, ascends over the root of the zygoma with the temporal artery, and divides, like it, into an anterior and a posterior branch: these are distributed to the skin of the side of the head. Behind the

Fig. 17.

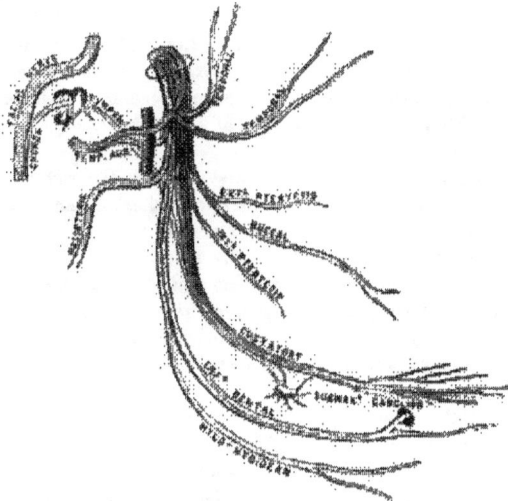

PLAN OF THE BRANCHES OF THE INFERIOR MAXILLARY NERVE.

condyle it sends filaments to the meatus auditorius, to the skin on the outer aspect of the ear and to the articulation of the jaw. It distributes also gland filaments to the parotid, and one especially to the upper division of the facial, which endows it with common sensibility.

The *inferior dental* branch emerges beneath the external pterygoid, and descends between the ramus of the jaw and the internal lateral ligament of the jaw to the dental foramen, which it enters with the dental artery. It then runs in the canal in the diploe of the jaw below the fangs of all the teeth. It furnishes filaments which ascend through the canals in the fangs of the teeth to the pulp in their interior. Opposite the foramen mentale the mental branch is given off. Observe that the same nerve which supplies the teeth supplies the gums; hence the sympathy between them.

The *mylo-hyoid* branch, apparently arising from the dental, is derived from the motor root of the fifth, and may, with careful dissection, be traced to it. It leaves the dental nerve near the foramen in the jaw, and runs in a groove on the inner side of the ramus to the lower surface of the mylo-hyoid, which muscle, together with the anterior portion of the digastricus, it supplies (p. 36).

The *gustatory* branch descends first between the ramus of the jaw and the internal pterygoid, then for a short distance between the jaw and the superior constrictor of the pharynx. Here it lies close to the mucous membrane of the mouth near the last molar tooth of the lower jaw; and division of it here has been recommended to relieve pain in cancer of the tongue. The gustatory n. then crosses obliquely the stylo-glossus, and running along the hyo-glossus to the tongue, is distributed to the papillæ of its tip and sides.

Beneath the external pterygoid the gustatory nerve is joined at an acute angle by the chorda tympani (a branch of the facial). This branch emerges from the glenoid fissure, and meeting the gustatory, runs along the lower border of that nerve to join the submaxillary ganglion. It is eventually distributed to the lingualis muscle.

Internal
lateral
ligament
of the jaw.

This 'so-called' ligament proceeds from the spinous process of the sphenoid bone, and is attached to the jaw on the inner side of the foramen dentale. Between this ligament and the neck of the jaw we find the internal maxillary artery and vein, the temporo-auricular nerve, the middle meningeal artery, the dental nerve and artery, and a portion of the parotid gland.

At this stage of the dissection you will be able to trace the course and relations of the internal carotid artery. But before doing this, examine the several objects which intervene between the external and internal carotid. These are—1. The stylo-glossus, 2. The stylo-pharyngeus, 3. The glosso-pharyngeal nerve, 4. The stylo-hyoid ligament.

Stylo-glossus. This *arises* from the styloid process near the apex, and the stylo-maxillary ligament, and is *inserted* along the side of the tongue, external to the hyo-glossus. Its action is to retract the tongue. Its nerve comes from the hypo-glossal.

Stylo-pha-ryngeus. This *arises* from the styloid process near the base, and is *inserted* into the posterior edge of the thyroid cartilage. It descends along the side of the pharynx between the superior and the middle constrictor. Curving round its lower border is seen the glosso-pharyngeal nerve. Its nerve comes from the pharyngeal plexus. Its *action* is to raise the larynx with the pharynx in deglutition.

Between the stylo-glossus and stylo-pharyngeus, and nearly parallel with both, is the *stylo-hyoid ligament.* It extends from the apex of the styloid process to the lesser cornu of the os-hyoides. It is often more or less ossified.

The *ascending palatine artery,* a branch of the external maxillary or facial (p. 38), runs up between the stylo-glossus and the stylo-pharyngeus, and divides into branches which supply these muscles, the palate, the side of the pharynx, and the tonsils. It inosculates with the descending palatine, a branch of the internal maxillary.

Glosso-pha-ryngeal nerve. The glosso-pharyngeal nerve is observed curving forwards under the lower border of the stylo-pharyngeus. It is one of the divisions of the eighth pair. It arises by four or five filaments from the medulla oblongata in the groove between the olivary body and the restiform tract. It leaves the skull through the anterior part of the foramen lacerum posterius in front of the remaining divisions of the eighth pair, and descends between the internal jugular vein and the internal carotid artery.

It then crosses in front of the artery and proceeds along the lower border of the stylo-pharyngeus. It now curves forwards over that muscle and the middle constrictor of the pharynx, and disappears beneath the hyo-glossus, where it divides into its terminal branches for the supply of the mucous membrane of the pharynx, the back of the tongue and the tonsils.

According to the present state of our knowledge, the glosso-pharyngeal is, at its origin, purely a sensitive nerve. But soon after its exit from the skull it receives communications from the facial, the pneumogastric and the sympathetic, so that it soon becomes a compound nerve—i.e. composed of both sensitive and motor filaments. At the base of the skull it is provided with two ganglia—the *jugular* and the *petrous* (ganglion of Andersch). The minute branches given off by these ganglia will be noticed hereafter ; at present we are more concerned with what is called the ' pharyngeal plexus ' of nerves.

Pharyngeal plexus. By the side of the middle constrictor of the pharynx, we find an intricate interlacement of nerves, constituting the plexus which presides over deglutition. Its dissection requires much time and care, and a pharynx prepared exclusively for the purpose. The nerves which compose it are derived from the glosso-pharyngeal, the pneumogastric, the spinal accessory, and the sympathetic. Consequently it possesses nerves of three different kinds—ganglionic, sensitive, and motor. Its minute ramifications supply the pharynx, the back of the tongue, and tonsils.

Course and relations of the internal carotid artery. The internal carotid artery, proceeding from the division of the common carotid, opposite the upper border of the thyroid cartilage, ascends to the base of the skull, *by the side of the pharynx* close to the transverse processes of the three upper cervical vertebræ. It enters the skull through the carotid canal in the temporal bone, runs very tortuously by the side of the body of the sphenoid, and terminates in branches which supply the orbit and the brain. In the first part of its course, it is situated immediately *outside* the external carotid, near the inner border of the sterno-mastoid. But it soon gets beneath the external carotid, and lies deeply seated by the side of the pharynx. In its course it is crossed successively by the hypoglossal nerve, the occipital artery, the digastricus and stylo-hyoid muscles; higher, it is crossed obliquely, by the styloid process, by the stylo-glossus and pharyngeus muscles, by the glosso-pharyngeal nerve, and the stylo-hyoid ligament, all of which last intervene between it and the external carotid.

The internal jugular vein runs along the outer side of the artery. Behind the artery are the pneumogastric nerve and the superior cervical ganglion of the sympathetic. The rectus capitis anticus major separates it from the cervical vertebræ. But after all, the most important relation of the artery in a surgical point of view is, that it ascends close by the *side of the pharynx* and *tonsils.* In opening an abscess, therefore, near the tonsils, or at the back of the pharynx, be careful to introduce the knife with its point inwards towards the mesial line; observe this caution the more, because, in some subjects, the internal carotid makes a curve, or even a complete curl upon itself, in its ascent near the pharynx. In such cases the least deviation of the instrument in an outward direction would injure the vessel.

Ascending pharyngeal artery.   This artery generally arises from the angle of the common carotid, or from the commencement of the external carotid; it ascends between the internal carotid artery and the side of the pharynx, towards the base of the skull. It gives off branches which supply the pharynx, the tonsils, the Eustachian tube, and the muscles in front of the spine. A very constant branch runs down with the levator palati, above the superior constrictor of the pharynx, and supplies the soft palate. It also sends small meningeal branches to supply the dura mater; one of which ascends through the foramen lacerum medium, and the other through the foramen jugulare with the internal jugular vein.

Pneumogastric nerve.   The pneumogastric nerve is one of the three divisions of the eighth pair of cerebral nerves. It arises from the medulla oblongata by a series of roots along the groove between the olivary body and the restiform tract. It passes out of the skull with the nervus accessorius through the foramen jugulare.

Leaving the skull at the foramen jugulare, the nerve descends in front of the cervical vertebræ, lying successively upon the rectus capitis anticus major and the longus colli. In the upper part of the neck it is situated behind the internal carotid artery; in the lower, between and behind the common carotid and the internal jugular vein. It enters the chest, on the right side crossing in front of the subclavian artery nearly at a right angle; on the left running nearly parallel with it.

In their course through the chest, the pneumogastric nerves have not similar relations. The right nerve lies beneath the subclavian vein, and then descending by the side of the trachea, is continued behind the right bronchus to the posterior part of the œsophagus. The left nerve passes behind the left brachio-cephalic vein, then crosses in front of the arch of the aorta, and behind the left bronchus to the anterior part of the œsophagus. Both nerves subdivide on this tube into a plexus; the right nerve forming the *posterior*, and the left, the *anterior œsophageal plexus*. Each plexus again collects its fibres together: thus two main nerves are formed which pass with the œsophagus through the diaphragm: of these the right is distributed over the posterior, the left over the anterior surface of the stomach.

In their long course from the medulla oblongata to the abdomen, the pneumogastric nerves supply branches to most important organs; namely, to the pharynx, the larynx, the heart, the lungs, the œsophagus, and the stomach.

Within the foramen jugulare, a small ganglion (Arnold's ganglion) is formed upon the pneumogastric nerve, which is then joined by a branch of considerable size from the nervus accessorius. Arnold's ganglion will be described hereafter. But soon after leaving the skull, the pneumogastric nerve swells out, and forms a second ganglion (inferior ganglion) of a reddish-grey colour. This ganglion occupies about an inch of the nerve, but does not involve the whole of its fibres; the branch from the spinal accessory not being included. It is united to the hypo-

glossal nerve, from which it receives filaments. It also receives
filaments from the first and second spinal nerves, and from the
superior cervical ganglion of the sympathetic.

Thus, the pneumogastric, at its origin probably a nerve of
sensation only, becomes, in consequence of the reinforcements
from these various branches, a compound nerve, and in all respects analogous to a spinal nerve. Its branches are—

1. The *auricular* (Arnold), which will be described hereafter.

2. The *pharyngeal*, which arises from the inferior ganglion, and
descends either in front of or behind the internal carotid to join
the pharyngeal plexus (p. 95).

3. The *superior laryngeal*, also derived from the inferior
ganglion, descends behind the internal carotid to the interval
between the os-hyoides and the thyroid cartilage, where it enters
the larynx through the thyro-hyoid membrane, and is distributed
to the mucous membrane of the larynx. The superior laryngeal
nerve gives off the ' *external laryngeal*,' which descends beneath
the depressors of the os-hyoides to supply the crico-thyroid
muscle.

4. The *cardiac*, two in number, which descend behind the
sheath of the carotid to the cardiac plexus. The upper branch is
small, and proceeds from the inferior ganglion; the lower comes
from the main trunk in its course down the neck. On their
passage to the heart, the right cardiac nerves run chiefly behind
the arch of the aorta to the deep cardiac plexus; the left, chiefly
in front of it, to the superficial cardiac plexus.

5. The *inferior laryngeal* or *recurrent* branch of the pneumogastric turns on the right side under the subclavian artery (p. 53),
and runs up to the larynx, between the trachea and the bodies of
the cervical vertebræ: on the left side, it turns under the arch
of the aorta, and ascends to the larynx between the trachea
and the œsophagus. On both sides it enters the larynx beneath
the lower border of the inferior constrictor, and supplies all the
intrinsic muscles of the larynx, except the crico-thyroid. The
remaining branches of the pneumogastric, to the lungs, the
œsophagus and stomach, will be examined in the dissection of
the chest.

Now examine the cervical ganglia of the sympathetic
Sympathetic system of nerves. Speaking in general terms of this
nerve.
system, it may be said that it consists of a series of
ganglia arranged on either side of the spine, from the first cervical
to the last sacral vertebra. The successive ganglia of the same
side are connected by intermediate nerves, so as to form a continuous cord on each side of the spine: this constitutes what is
called the trunk of the sympathetic system, and is connected with
all the spinal nerves. Its upper or cephalic extremity penetrates
into the cranium through the carotid canal, surrounds the internal
carotid artery, communicates with the third, fourth, fifth, and
sixth cranial nerves, and joins its fellow of the opposite side upon
the anterior communicating artery.* Its sacral extremity joins
its fellow by means of a little ' ganglion impar,' situated in the
mesial line, upon the last sacral vertebra.

The sympathetic system presides over the functions of those
organs which are withdrawn from our control. Thus it regulates
the circulation of the blood, respiration, digestion, and secretion.

Cervical gan-   In the cervical portion of the sympathetic are three
glia of sym-   ganglia, named from their position, superior, middle,
pathetic.
and inferior.

The *superior cervical ganglion*, the largest of the three, is
situated near the base of the skull, opposite the bodies of the
second and third cervical vertebræ, and lies behind the internal
carotid artery, upon the rectus capitis anticus major. It is of a
reddish-grey colour like other ganglia, of an elongated oval shape,
varying in length from one to two inches. To facilitate the
description of its several branches we divide them into—1st, those
which are presumed to connect it with other nerves ; and 2ndly,
those which originate from it.

It is then connected by branches as follow : —

a. With each of the four upper spinal nerves.

b. With the hypoglossal, pneumogastric, and glosso-pharyngeal
nerves.

* Here is situated the 'so-called' ganglion of Ribes.

H 2

c. With the third, fourth, fifth, and sixth cerebral nerves (in the cavernous sinus).

d. With the several ganglia of the sympathetic system about the head and neck ; namely, the ophthalmic, spheno-palatine, otic, and submaxillary.

The branches which it distributes are—

e. Nerves to the heart.—One or more descend behind the sheath of the carotid, and entering the chest, join the cardiac plexuses, superficial and deep.

f. Nerves to the pharynx.—These join the pharyngeal plexus on the middle constrictor of the pharynx.

g. Nerves to the blood-vessels.—These nerves, named on account of their delicacy ' nervi molles,' ramify around the external carotid artery and its branches.

The *middle cervical ganglion* is something less than a barley-corn in size. It is situated behind the carotid sheath, about the fifth or sixth cervical vertebra, near the inferior thyroid artery. It receives branches from the fifth and sixth spinal nerves, and gives off—

a. Branches to the thyroid body.—These accompany the inferior thyroid artery.

b. Branch to the heart.—This usually descends in front of the subclavian artery into the chest, and joins the deep cardiac plexus.

In cases where the middle cervical ganglion is absent, the preceding nerves are supplied by the sympathetic cord connecting the superior and inferior ganglia.

The *inferior cervical ganglion* is of considerable size, and is situated in the interval between the transverse process of the seventh cervical vertebra and the first rib, immediately behind the vertebral artery. It receives branches from the seventh and eighth spinal nerves, and others which, descending from the fourth, fifth, and sixth, through the foramina in the transverse processes of the vertebræ, form a plexus around the vertebral artery.

The branches which it gives off are—

a. Inferior cardiac nerve.—This communicates with the recurrent laryngeal, and joins the cardiac plexus beneath the arch of the aorta.

b. Nerves to the blood-vessels.—These ramify around the vertebral and subclavian arteries.

DISSECTION OF THE CHEST.

Before the several organs contained in the chest are examined, we ought to have some knowledge of its frame-work. The true ribs with their cartilages describe a series of arcs, increasing in length from above downwards, and form with the spine behind, and the sternum in front, a barrel of a conical shape, broader in the lateral than in the antero-posterior direction. The lower aperture or base of the cavity is closed in the recent state by the diaphragm, which forms a muscular partition between the chest and the abdomen. This partition is arched, so that it constitutes a vaulted floor for the chest, and by its capability of alternately falling and rising can increase or diminish the capaciousness of the chest. The spaces between the ribs are filled by the intercostal muscles. In each intercostal space there are two layers of these muscles, arranged like the letter X. The fibres of the outer layer run obliquely from above downwards, and forwards; those of the inner layer in the reverse direction.

The upper aperture of the chest gives passage to the trachea, the œsophagus, the great vessels of the head, neck, and upper extremities, the superior intercostal, and internal mammary arteries, the inferior thyroid veins, the sterno-hyoid, sterno-thyroid, and longus colli muscles, the pneumogastric, the left recurrent laryngeal, the phrenic, and the sympathetic nerves; also to the first dorsal passing up to join the brachial plexus, the thoracic duct, and, lastly, to the apices of the lungs; the interspaces between these parts being occupied by a dense fibro-cellular tissue.

Such, in outline, is the frame-work of the cavity, closed on all sides, which contains the heart and lungs. Observe that its walls are made up of different structures, bone, cartilage, and muscle,

admirably disposed to fulfil two important conditions. By their
solidity and elasticity they protect the important organs contained
in them; by their alternate dilatation and contraction they act as
mechanical powers of respiration. For they can increase the cavity
of the chest in three directions: in height, by the descent of the
diaphragm; in width, by the turning outwards of the ribs; and in
depth, by the elevation of the sternum.

The chest of the female differs from that of the male in the
following points:—Its general capacity is less; the sternum is
shorter; the upper opening is larger in proportion to the lower;
the upper ribs are more movable, and therefore permit a greater
enlargement of the chest at its upper part, in adaptation to the
condition of the abdomen during pregnancy.

In the dissection of the chest let us take the parts in the
following order:—

1. Triangularis sterni, with the internal mammary artery.
2. Anterior mediastinum.
3. Right and left brachio-cephalic veins and superior vena cava
4. Course and relations of the arch of the aorta.
5. The three great branches of the arch.
6. Course of the phrenic nerves.
7. Position and relations of the heart.
8. Pericardium.
9. Pleura.
10. Position and form of the lungs.
11. Posterior mediastinum and its contents; namely, the aorta, the thoracic duct,
    the vena azygos, the œsophagus, and pneumogastric nerves.
12. Sympathetic nerve.
13. Intercostal muscles, vessels, and nerves.
14. Cardiac plexus of nerves.

An opening must be made into the chest, by carefully removing
the upper four-fifths of the sternum, and the cartilages of all the
true ribs.* In doing this, care must be taken not to wound the
pleura, which is closely connected with the cartilages. On one

* Those who are more proficient in dissection should not remove the whole of the
sternum, but leave, say a quarter of an inch of its upper part with the first rib attached
to it. This little portion serves as a valuable landmark, although it obstructs, to a
certain extent, the view of the subjacent vessels.

side the internal mammary artery should be removed ; on the other, left.

On the under surface of the sternum and cartilages of

Triangularis sterni. the ribs is a muscle, named the 'triangularis sterni.' It arises from the ensiform cartilage and the lower part of the sternum, and is *inserted* by digitations into the cartilages of the true ribs from the sixth to the second: its fibres ascend outwards to their insertion; its action is to depress the coastal cartilages. Thus, on emergency, it acts in expiration. Its nerve comes from the intercostal nerves, its arteries from the internal mammary.

Internal mammary artery. This artery springs from the subclavian in the first part of its course. On entering the chest it is crossed by the phrenic nerve. It then descends perpendicularly, about half an inch from the sternum, between the cartilages of the ribs and the triangularis sterni : it then enters the wall of the abdomen behind the rectus abdominis, and finally inosculates with the epigastric (a branch of the external iliac). Its branches are as follow :—

a. Arteria comes nervi phrenici.—A very slender artery, which accompanies the phrenic nerve to the diaphragm, and anastomoses with the phrenic branches of the abdominal aorta.

b. Mediastinal and thymic.—These branches supply the cellular tissue of the anterior mediastinum, the pericardium, and the triangularis sterni. The *thymic* are only visible in childhood, and disappear with the thymus gland.

c. Anterior intercostal.—One, and often two, for each intercostal space are distributed to the five or six upper intercostal spaces. They lie at first between the pleura and the internal intercostal muscle, and subsequently between the two intercostals. They inosculate with the intercostal arteries from the aorta.

d. Perforating arteries, which pass through the same number of intercostal spaces as the preceding branches, and supply the pectoral muscle and skin of the chest. In the female they are of large size, for the supply of the mammary gland.

e. The *intercosto-phrenic* branch runs outwards behind the

cartilages of the false ribs, and terminates near the last intercostal
space. It supplies small arteries to the diaphragm, to the sixth,
seventh, and sometimes the eighth intercostal spaces.

Two venæ comites surround the artery, and unite into a single
trunk in the upper part of the chest, to terminate in the brachio-
cephalic vein of its own side.

There are several *absorbent glands* in the neighbourhood of the
internal mammary artery. They receive the absorbents from the
inner portion of the mammary gland, from the diaphragm, and
the upper part of the abdominal wall. In disease of the inner
portion of the mamma, these glands may enlarge without any
enlargement of those in the axilla.

Mediastina, anterior and posterior. The 'mediastina' are the spaces which the two
pleural sacs leave between them in the antero-posterior
plane of the chest. There is an anterior and a posterior mediastinum. To put these spaces in the simplest light,
let us imagine the heart and lungs to be removed from the chest,
and the two pleural sacs to be left in it by themselves. The two
sacs, if inflated, would then appear like two bladders, in contact
only in the middle, as shown by the dotted outlines in the annexed scheme (fig. 18). The interval marked a, behind the

Fig. 18.

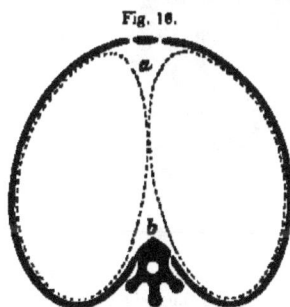

sternum, would represent the anterior mediastinum: the interval
b, the posterior mediastinum.
But now let us introduce the heart
and lungs again, between the
two pleural sacs: these must give
way to make room for them, so
that the two sacs are not in contact
anywhere in the middle line of
the chest.

Therefore, with the heart and
lungs interposed, the pleural sacs
appear as shown in the diagram, fig. 19,—which represents a transverse section through the chest. Here you see that the heart and
the lungs become invested by the pleural sacs; or, to speak more

technically, the sacs are reflected over the heart and the lungs, on each side respectively.　But the anterior and posterior mediastina remain unaltered.

Looking at the chest in front, the anterior mediastinum appears as shown in the cut (p. 117).　It is not precisely longitudinal in its direction, but inclines slightly towards the left, owing to the position of the heart.　Its area varies: thus it is extremely narrow in the middle where the edges of the lungs nearly meet; but it is wider above and below, where the lungs diverge.

What parts are contained in the anterior mediastinum?—The remains of the thymus gland, the origins of the sterno-hyoid, sterno-thyroid, and triangularis sterni muscles, the left brachio-cephalic vein (which crosses behind the first bone of the sternum), and a few absorbent glands.

Fig. 19.

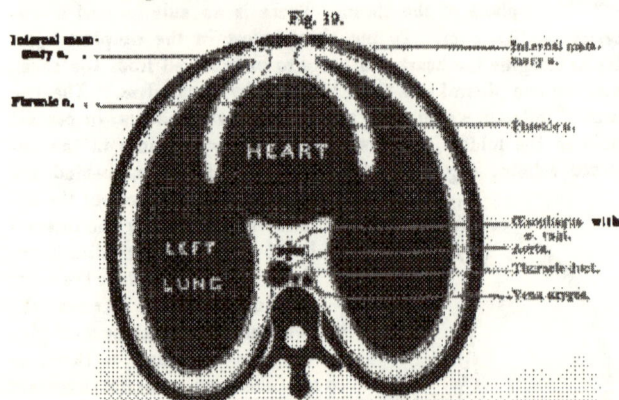

DIAGRAM OF THE REFLECTIONS OF THE PLEURAL SACS IN DOTTED LINES.

The *posterior mediastinum* (fig. 19) contains the œsophagus, the two pneumogastric nerves, the aorta, the thoracic duct, and the vena azygos.

A *middle* mediastinum is described by some anatomists.　It is the largest of the mediastina, and contains the heart with its large vessels, the phrenic nerves, and the bifurcation of the trachea.

Before we can display the brachio-cephalic veins, we must remove a layer of the deep cervical fascia, which descends over them from the neck, and is lost upon the pericardium. Their coats are closely connected to this fascia; and its chief use appears to be to keep the veins always open for the free return of blood to the heart.

Brachio-cephalic veins.
The right and left brachio-cephalic (innominate) veins are formed, near the sternal end of the clavicle, by the confluence of the internal jugular and subclavian. They differ in their course and relations, and must, therefore, be described separately.

The *left brachio-cephalic vein* passes obliquely behind the first bone of the sternum towards the right side, to join the vena cava superior. It is about two inches and a half in length, and its direction inclines a little downwards. It crosses over the trachea and the origins of the three primary branches of the arch of the aorta. We are reminded of this fact in some cases of aneurism of these vessels; for what happens? The vein becomes compressed between the aneurism and the sternum; hence the swelling and venous congestion of the parts from which it returns the blood; namely, of the left arm and left side of the neck. The upper border of the vein lies not far from the upper border of the sternum; in some instances it lies even higher, and I have seen it crossing in front of the trachea a full inch above the sternum. This occasional deviation should be borne in mind in the performance of tracheotomy.

The *right brachio-cephalic vein* descends nearly vertically to join the superior vena cava, opposite the first intercostal space. It is about one and a half inch in length, and is situated about one inch from the mesial line of the sternum. On its left side, but on a posterior plane, runs the arteria innominata; on its right side is the pleura. Between the vein and the pleura is the phrenic nerve. The brachio-cephalic veins are not provided with valves. The veins which empty themselves into the right and left brachio-cephalic are as follow :—

The Right B. C. Vein receives:—
The vertebral.
The deep cervical.
The internal mammary.
The inferior thyroid (sometimes).

The Left B. C. Vein receives:—
The vertebral.
The deep cervical.
The internal mammary.
The inferior thyroid.
The superior intercostal.
The pericardiac.

Vena cava superior.

This is the great channel through which the impure blood from the head, upper extremities, and chest, returns into the right auricle. It is formed by the confluence of the right and left brachio-cephalic veins, which unite at nearly a right angle opposite the first intercostal space on the right border of the sternum; that is, about the level of the highest point of the arch of the aorta (p. 53). The vena cava descends

Fig. 20.

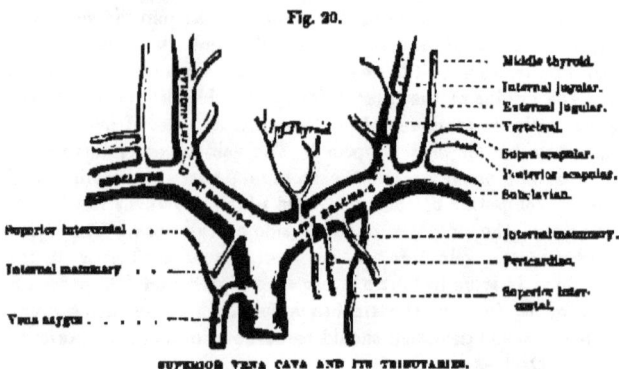

SUPERIOR VENA CAVA AND ITS TRIBUTARIES.

vertically, with a slight inclination backwards, to the upper part of the right auricle. It is from two and a half to three inches long. The lower half of it is covered by the pericardium; you must, therefore, open this sac to see that the serous layer of the pericardium is reflected over the front and sides of the vein. In respect to its relations, notice that the vein lies in front of the right bronchus and the right pulmonary vessels; and that it is

overlapped by the ascending aorta, which lies to its left side and
parallel with it. In the upper half of its course, that is, above
the pericardium, it is covered on its right side by the pleura; on
this side, in contact with it, descends the phrenic nerve.

Before it is covered by the pericardium, the vena cava receives
the right vena azygos, which comes in arching over the right
bronchus.

Course and
relations of
the arch of
the aorta.

The aorta is the great trunk from which all the
arteries of the body carrying pure blood are derived.
It arises from the upper and back part of the left ventricle of the heart. Its origin is situated behind the
pulmonary artery and on the left side of the sternum, about the
level of the third intercostal space. It ascends forwards and to
the right as high as the first intercostal space on the right side;
it then curves backwards towards the left side of the body of the
second dorsal vertebra, and turning downwards over the left side
of the third, completes the arch. The direction of the arch,
therefore, is from the sternum to the spine, and rather oblique
from right to left.

The arch of the aorta presents partial dilatations in certain
situations. One of these, called the 'sinus' or bulge of the aorta,
is observed on the right side of the arch, about the junction of
the ascending with the transverse portion: it is little marked in
the infant, but increases with age. Three other dilatations (the
sinuses of Valsalva), one corresponding to each of the valves at
the commencement of the aorta, will be examined hereafter.

For convenience of description, the arch of the aorta is divided
into an ascending, a transverse, and a descending portion.

Ascending portion.—To see this portion of the aorta, the
pericardium must be opened. You then observe that this part of
the artery is covered all round by the serous layer of the pericardium, except where it is in contact with the pulmonary artery.
It is about two inches in length, and ascends with a slight curve
to the upper border of the second costal cartilage of the right side.
Its commencement is covered by the pulmonary artery, and overlapped by the appendix of the right auricle. On its right side,

but on a posterior plane, descends the superior vena cava; on its left is the division of the pulmonary artery; behind it, are part of the auricle, the right pulmonary artery, and the right bronchus. This part of the aorta gives off the right and left coronary arteries for the supply of the heart.

Transverse portion.—This portion of the aorta arches from the front to the back of the thorax, and extends from the upper border of the second right costal cartilage to the left side of the second dorsal vertebra. In front it is covered by the left pleura, and is crossed by the left phrenic and pneumogastric nerves. Near its summit runs the left brachio-cephalic vein; within its concavity are the left bronchus, the bifurcation of the pulmonary artery, the left recurrent laryngeal nerve, and the remains of the ductus arteriosus. The artery rests upon the trachea a little above its bifurcation, the œsophagus, thoracic duct, and the left recurrent laryngeal nerve. From the transverse part of the arch arise the arteria innominata, the left carotid, and subclavian arteries.

Descending portion.—This part of the arch lies upon the left side of the body of the third dorsal vertebra. On its right side are the œsophagus and thoracic duct; on its left is the pleura.

What parts are contained within the arch of the aorta? The left bronchus, the right pulmonary artery, the left recurrent nerve, the remains of the ductus arteriosus, and the deep cardiac plexus.

Relations of the arch of the aorta to the sternum. These relations vary according to the size of the heart, the obliquity of the ribs, and the general development of the chest. In a well-formed adult the ascending aorta is, at the most prominent part of its bulge, about half of an inch behind the first bone of the sternum. The highest part of the arch is about one inch below the upper edge of the sternum.*

* The relations of the arch of the aorta to the sternum vary even in adults, more especially if there be any hypertrophy of the heart. As an instance among many, I may mention that of a young female who died of phthisis. The position of the aortic valves was opposite the middle of the sternum, on a level with the middle of the

From the upper part of the arch arise three great arteries for the head, neck, and upper limbs ; namely, the brachio-cephalic or innominate artery, the left carotid, and the left subclavian.

Brachio-ce-phalic or in-nominate artery.

This arises from the commencement of the trans-verse part of the arch. It ascends obliquely towards the right, and after a course of about one inch and a half, divides behind the right sterno-clavicular joint into two arteries of nearly equal size—the right carotid, and the right subclavian.

What are the relations of the innominate artery? It ascends obliquely in front of the trachea ; the right brachio-cephalic vein descends on its right side ; the left brachio-cephalic and inferior thyroid veins cross in front of it : parallel and close to the artery are the slender cardiac nerves.[*]

With the anatomy of the parts before you, it is easy to under-stand that an aneurism of the innominate artery might be distin-guished from an aneurism of the aorta—1. By a pulsation in the neck between the sterno-mastoid muscles, i.e. in the fossa above the sternum ; 2. By occasional dyspnœa owing to pressure on the trachea ; 3. By venous congestion in the *left* arm ; 4. By the aneurismal thrill being confined to the *right* arm.

Left carotid artery.

This artery arises from the arch of the aorta close to the arteria innominata. It ascends obliquely behind the first bone of the sternum to the neck. In the first part of its course it lies upon the trachea, but it soon passes to the left side of the trachea, and then lies for a short distance upon the œsophagus and thoracic duct. It is crossed by the left brachio-cephalic vein ; on its outer side are the left subclavian artery and

---

second costal articulation. The highest part of the arch was on a level with the upper border of the sternum ; the arteria innominata was situated entirely in front of the trachea ; and the left brachio-cephalic vein crossed the trachea so much above the sternum that it would have been directly exposed to injury in tracheotomy.

[*] In some cases the innominate artery ascends for a short distance above the clavicle before it divides, lying close to the right of the trachea. We have already alluded to the fact that it occasionally gives off a middle thyroid artery (p. 81), which ascends in front of the trachea to the thyroid body, and is therefore directly in the way in tracheotomy.

pneumogastric nerve, and on the inner side is the arteria innominata. In the rest of its course it resembles the right
carotid (p. 27).

This is the third branch of the arch. It ascends out of the
Left sub- chest to the inner border of the first rib, and then
clavian curves outwards behind the scalenus anticus. In the
artery. first part of its course it is deeply seated, and is
covered on its left side by the pleura. Close to its right side
are the trachea and œsophagus; between the artery and the
œsophagus we find the thoracic duct. Like the other primary
branches of the arch, it is crossed by the left brachio-cephalic vein.
It is covered in front by the left lung, and it rests upon the
longus colli. The upper part of its course, where the vessel
passes in front of the apex of the lung, has been described with
the anatomy of the neck (p. 54).

Course of the The phrenic nerve comes from the third, fourth, and
phrenic nerves fifth cervical nerves. It descends over the scalenus
through the anticus, and enters the chest between the subclavian
chest. vein and artery. It then runs in front of the root
of the lung between the pleura and the pericardium to the diaphragm (fig. 21), to the under surface of which it is distributed.

In what respects do the phrenic nerves differ from each other in
their course?—The right phrenic runs along the outer side of the
brachio-cephalic vein and superior vena cava; the left crosses
in front of the transverse part of the arch of the aorta; besides
which, the left is rather longer than the right, because it has to go
round the apex of the heart.[*]

Before the phrenic nerve divides into branches to supply the
diaphragm, it sends off minute filaments to the pleura and the
pericardium.

Having studied these anatomical details, consider for a moment
what kind of symptoms are likely to be produced by an aneurism
of the arch of the aorta, or any of the primary branches. A glance
at the important parts in the neighbourhood will answer the

[*] In the upper part of the chest the phrenic is sometimes joined by a branch from
the brachial plexus, less frequently by a branch from the descendens noni.

question. The effects will vary according to the part of the artery
which is the seat of the aneurism, and, according to the volume,
the form, and the position of the tumour. One can understand

Fig. 21.

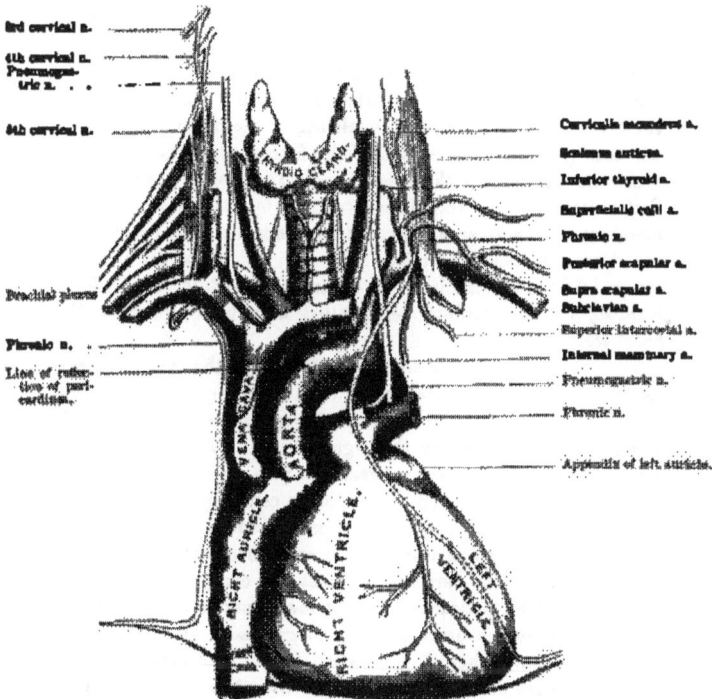

that compression of the vena cava superior, or either of the brachio-
cephalic veins, would occasion swelling and congestion of the parts
from which it returns the blood; that compression of the trachea
or one of the bronchi might occasion dyspnœa, and thus simulate

disease of the larynx;[*] that compression of the œsophagus would give rise to symptoms of stricture. Nor must we forget the immediate vicinity of the thoracic duct and the recurrent nerve,[†] and the effects which would be produced by their compression. Can one, then, be surprised that a disease which may give rise to so many different symptoms should be a fertile source of fallacy in diagnosis?

You can easily see how aneurisms of the aorta prove fatal, by bursting into the contiguous tubes or cavities; for instance, into the trachea, the œsophagus, the pleura, or the pericardium. You will see, too, why an aneurism of the first part of the arch is so much more dangerous than elsewhere. The reason is, that in this part of its course the aorta is covered only by a thin layer of serous membrane: now if an aneurism take place here, the coats of the vessel soon become distended, give way, and allow the blood to escape into the pericardium; an occurrence which is speedily fatal, because, the pericardium being filled with blood, prevents the heart from acting.

Position and form of the heart. The heart is situated obliquely in the chest, between the lungs. Its base, i.e. the part by which it is attached, and from which its great vessels proceed, is directed upwards towards the right shoulder; its apex points downwards and to the left, between the fifth and sixth costal cartilages. It is supported by the tendinous centre of the diaphragm. It is maintained in its position by a membranous bag termed the 'pericardium,' which is lined by a serous membrane to facilitate its movements. The pericardium must first claim our attention.

Pericardium. The pericardium is the membranous bag which encloses the heart and the large vessels at its base. It is broadest below, where it is attached to the tendinous centre of the diaphragm; above it is prolonged over the great vessels of the heart, and is connected with the deep cervical fascia. On each

---

[*] In the Museum of Guy's Hospital there is a preparation, No. 1487, in which laryngotomy was performed under the circumstances described in the text.

[†] See Med. Gaz., Dec. 22nd, 1843. A case in which loss of voice was produced by the pressure of an aneurismal tumour upon the left recurrent nerve.

I

side it is covered by the pleura; the phrenic nerve running down
between them. In front of it, is the anterior mediastinum; behind

Fig. 22.

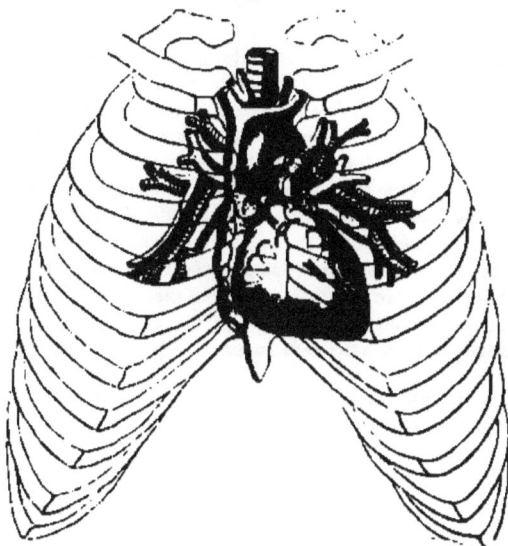

RELATIVE POSITION OF THE HEART AND ITS VALVES WITH REGARD TO THE WALLS OF
THE CHEST.

The valves are denoted by curved lines. The aortic valves are opposite the third intercostal space on the left side, close to the sternum. The pulmonary valves are
just above the aortic, opposite the junction of the third rib with the sternum. The
mitral valves are opposite the third intercostal space, about one inch to the left of
the sternum. The tricuspid valves lie behind the middle of the sternum, about the
level of the fourth rib. Aortic murmurs, as shown by the arrow, are propagated
up the aorta: mitral murmurs, as shown by the arrow, are propagated towards the
apex of the heart.

it, the posterior. Of all the objects in the posterior mediastinum,
that which is nearest to the pericardium is the œsophagus. It is

worth remembering that the œsophagus is in close contact with the back of the pericardium for nearly two inches; this fact accounts for what one sometimes observes in cases of pericarditis where there is much effusion ; I mean pain and difficulty in swallowing.

The pericardium is what is called a '*fibro serous*' membrane. Its fibrous layer, which constitutes its chief strength, is external. This layer is attached below to the central tendon of the diaphragm. Above, it forms eight sheaths for the vessels at the base of the heart; namely, one for the vena cava superior, four for the pulmonary veins, two for the pulmonary arteries, and one for the aorta. The *serous* layer forms a shut sac. It lines the fibrous layer, and is reflected over the great vessels and the heart. To see where the serous layer is reflected over the vessels, distend the pericardium with air. Thus you will find that this layer is reflected over the aorta as high as the origin of the arteria innominata. It is reflected over the vena cava superior, after the entrance of the vena azygos.[*]

In the healthy state the capacity of the pericardium pretty nearly corresponds to the size of the heart when distended to its utmost. The healthy pericardium, with the heart *in situ*, may be made to hold in the adult about ten ounces of fluid. The pericardium is not extensible. When an aneurism bursts into it, death

---

[*] Those who choose to follow the reflections of the serous layer of the pericardium, will find that it covers the great vessels to an extent greater than is generally imagined; though in truth the extent is not precisely similar in all bodies. The aorta and pulmonary artery are wrapped in a complete sheath, two inches in length, so that these vessels are covered all round by the serous layer, except where they are in contact. Indeed you can pass your finger behind them both, through a foramen bounded in front by the two great vessels themselves, behind, by the upper part of the auricles, and above by the right pulmonary artery. Again, the back of the aorta, where it lies on the auricles, is covered by the serous pericardium. The superior cava is covered all round, except behind where it crosses the right pulmonary artery. What little there is of the inferior cava within the pericardium is also covered all round. The left pulmonary veins are covered nearly all round; the right less so. Behind the auricles, chiefly the left, the serous layer extends upwards in the form of a pouch, rising above their upper border, so as to be loosely connected to the left bronchus.

I 2

is caused not by loss of blood, but by compression of the heart in consequence of the inextensibility of the pericardium.

The pericardium derives its blood from the internal mammary, bronchial, and œsophageal arteries.

Cut open the pericardium, and observe that the heart is conical in form, and convex everywhere except upon its lower surface, which is flat, and rests upon the tendinous centre of the diaphragm. When the pericardium is thus laid open, the following objects are exposed: viz. 1. Part of the right ventricle; 2. Part of the left ventricle; 3. Part of the right auricle with its appendix overlapping the root of the aorta; 4. The appendix of the left auricle overlapping the root of the pulmonary artery; 5. The aorta; 6. The pulmonary artery; 7. The vena cava superior; 8. The right and left coronary arteries.

The heart then is placed behind the lower half of the sternum, occupies more of the left than the right half of the chest, and rests upon the central tendon of the diaphragm, which is nearly on a plane with the lowest part of the fifth rib. At each contraction the apex of the heart may be felt beating between the cartilages of the fifth and sixth ribs, about two inches below the nipple, and one inch on its sternal side. Its base extends as high as the upper border of the third costal cartilage, and about half an inch to the right of the sternum.

The ' *præcordial region* ' is the outline of the heart
Præcordial   traced upon the front wall of the chest. We ought to
region.   be able to define this region with something like precision. We should know how much of it is covered and separated from the wall of the chest by intervening lung (fig. 23). This then is the rule:—Let the middle of the fifth costal cartilage be the centre of a circle two inches in diameter: this circle will define well enough, for all practical purposes, that part of the præcordial region which is naturally less resonant to percussion; here the heart is uncovered except by pericardium and loose cellular tissue, and is very near the wall of the chest. In the rest of the præcordial region the heart is covered and separated from the chest by intervening lung.

Where should we put the stethoscope when we listen to the valves of the heart? For practical purposes it is enough to remember that the mouth of an ordinary-sized stethoscope will cover a portion of them all, if it be placed a little to the left of the mesial line of the sternum opposite the third intercostal space (fig. 23). They are all covered by a thin portion of lung: therefore we ask a patient to stop breathing while we listen to his heart.

Fig. 23.

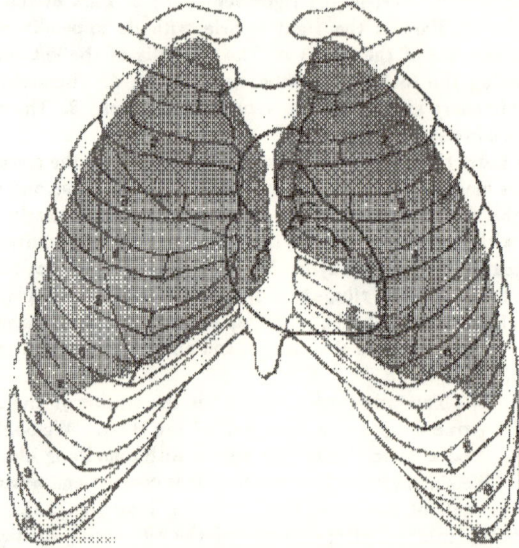

FORM OF THE LUNGS, AND THE EXTENT TO WHICH THEY OVERLAP THE HEART AND ITS VALVES.

The position of the heart alters a little with the position of the body. Of this any one may convince himself by leaning alternately forwards and backwards, by lying on this side and on that, placing at the same time the hand upon the præcordial region. He will find that he can, in a slight degree, alter the place and the extent

of the impulse of the heart. Inspiration and expiration also alter
the position of the heart. In inspiration the heart descends with
the tendinous centre of the diaphragm about half an inch.

Pleura.   As the lungs are continually gliding to and fro, within
the chest, they are provided with a serous membrane
to facilitate their motion. This membrane is termed the pleura.
There is one for each lung. Each pleura forms a completely
closed sac, and is disposed like all other serous sacs; that is, one
part of the sac lines the containing cavity, the other is reflected
over the contained organ. Its several parts are named after the
surface to which they adhere: that which lines the ribs is called
' pleura costalis;' that which forms the mediastinum, ' pleura
mediastinalis;' that which covers the lung, ' pleura pulmonalis.'
Unlike the peritoneum, the pleura forms no folds except a small
one called ' *ligamentum latum pulmonis,*' which extends from
the root of the lung to the diaphragm.

If asked to describe the reflections of the pleural sac (fig. 19,
p.105), I should say, that it lines the ribs and part of the sternum ;
from the sternum it is reflected backwards over the pericardium ;
from thence it passes over the front of the root of the lung, and so
on over the entire lung to the back part of its root, whence it is
reflected over the sides of the vertebræ, and thus reaches the ribs
again.

The spaces called ' anterior' and ' posterior' mediastina, formed
by the pleuræ, have been already described, p. 104.

In health the internal surface of the pleura is smooth, polished,
and lubricated by moisture sufficient to facilitate the sliding of
the lung. When this surface is thickened and roughened by
inflammation, the moving lung produces a ' friction' sound.
When the pleural sac is distended by serum, it constitutes hydro-
thorax; when by pus, ' empyema;' and when by air, ' pneumo-
thorax.'

Introduce your hand into the pleural sac, and ascertain that the
reflection of the pleura on to the diaphragm corresponds with an
imaginary line commencing at the lower part of the sternum, and
sloping along the cartilages of the successive ribs down to the

lower border of the last rib. Suppose a musket ball to lodge in
the pleural sac, it would fall upon the dome of the diaphragm,
and roll down to the lowest part of the pleural cavity. The place,
therefore, to extract it would be in the back, at the eleventh
intercostal space. This operation has been done during life with
success.

Position and   The lungs are situated in the chest, one on each side
form of the   of the heart. Each fits accurately into the cavity which
lungs.   contains it. Each, therefore, is conical in form; the
base rests on the diaphragm; the apex projects in the neck a little
more than an inch above the sternal end of the clavicle. Its outer
surface is adapted to the ribs; its inner surface is excavated to
make room for the heart. But the best way to see the shape of
the lungs is to inject the trachea with wax, which is tantamount to
taking a cast of each thoracic cavity. In such a preparation,
besides the general convexities and concavities alluded to, you
would find in the right lung a little indentation for the right
brachio-cephalic vein, in the left an indentation for the arch of the
aorta and the left subclavian artery.

Each lung is divided into an upper and a lower lobe by a deep
fissure, which commences behind about three inches from the
apex, and proceeds obliquely downwards to the front a little lower
than the fifth costal cartilage. Speaking broadly, the whole of the
anterior portion of the lung is formed by the upper lobe; the whole
of the posterior portion by the lower lobe. It should be noticed,
however, that the upper lobe of the right lung is divided by a
second fissure which slices off a triangular portion called the
'middle lobe.'

The dimensions of the right lung are greater than those of the
left in all directions except the vertical; the reason of this exception is the greater elevation of the diaphragm on the right side
by the liver. On an average, the right lung is to the left, in point
of size, as 11 to 10.

To understand rightly the shape and play of the lungs in inspiration and expiration, take an opportunity of making the following experiment:—Cut away the intercostal muscles and the pleura,

without wounding the lungs, and then distend the lungs by blowing
into the trachea with bellows. Thus, you will ascertain how far
the front edge of the lung overlaps the pericardium; how low the
lung descends between the ribs and the diaphragm on the side and
at the back of the chest. You will see the great gap in the left
lung for the point of the heart. By making the lung expand and
contract, you will observe how it slides along the pleural lining of
the chest. This sliding takes place in health in silence. But
when the naturally polished surface of the pleura becomes roughened by inflammatory deposit, a sound of greater or less distinctness
(friction sound) may be heard.

The practical result of this investigation should be to enable us
to trace upon a living chest the outline of the lungs, that we may
know what parts are naturally resonant on percussion.

Commencing, then, from above (fig. 23, p. 117), we find that the
apex of the lung rises into the neck a little more than an inch
above the sternal end of the clavicle. This part of the lung
mounts up behind the subclavian artery and the anterior scalene
muscle, and deserves especial attention, because it is, more than
any other, the seat of tubercular disease. From the sternal end
of the clavicles the lungs converge towards the mesial line, where
their edges almost meet opposite the junction of the second rib.
There is little or no lung behind the first bone of the sternum.

From the level of the second costal cartilage to the level of the
fourth, the inner margins of each lung run parallel and almost
close behind the middle of the sternum; consequently they overlap the great vessels at the root of the heart.

Below the level of the fourth costal cartilage the margins of the
lungs diverge from each other, but not in an equal degree. The
left presents the notch for the heart, and curves nearly in the
course of the fourth costal cartilage; at the lower part of its curve
it projects more or less over the apex of the heart. The *right*
descends almost perpendicularly behind the sternum as low as the
attachment of the ensiform cartilage, and then, turning outwards,
corresponds with the direction of the sixth costal cartilage. Hypertrophy of the heart, or effusion into the pericardium, will not

only raise above the ordinary level the point where the lungs diverge, but also increase their divergence; hence the greater dulness on percussion.

Posterior mediastinum and its contents. The posterior mediastinum (p. 105) is formed by the reflection of the pleural sac on each side, from the root of the lung to the sides of the bodies of the dorsal vertebræ. It is bounded in front by the pericardium. To obtain a view of it, draw out the right lung, and fasten it to the left side. This mediastinum contains the aorta ; in front of the aorta, the œsophagus, with the pneumogastric nerves; on the right of the aorta is the vena azygos; between this vein and the aorta is the thoracic duct; inferiorly are the splanchnic nerves and some lymphatic glands. To expose these last, we have to remove the pleura, and a layer of firm fascia which lines the chest outside it.

Thoracic aorta. We have already traced the arch of the aorta to the lower border of the body of the third dorsal vertebra. From this point, the aorta descends on the left side of the spine, gradually approaching towards the middle line. Opposite the last dorsal vertebra it passes between the crura of the diaphragm and enters the abdomen. Its left side is covered by pleura; on its right run the vena azygos and thoracic duct; in front of it are, the root of the left lung, the pericardium, and nearer to the mesial line is the œsophagus. Its branches will be described presently.

Vena azygos. This vein commences in the abdomen by small branches from one of the lumbar veins, and generally communicates with the renal, or the vena cava itself. This, indeed, is the main point about the origin of the vena azygos, that it communicates directly or indirectly with the vena cava inferior. It enters the chest through the aortic opening of the diaphragm, and ascends on the right side of the aorta through the posterior mediastinum, in front of the bodies of the lower dorsal vertebræ and over the right intercostal arteries. When the vein reaches the level of the third dorsal vertebra, it arches over the right bronchus, and terminates in the superior vena cava, just before this vessel is covered by pericardium. In its course it receives all the right intercostal veins, the spinal veins, the œsophageal and commonly the right bronchial vein. Opposite the sixth dorsal vertebra it is joined by the left vena azygos.

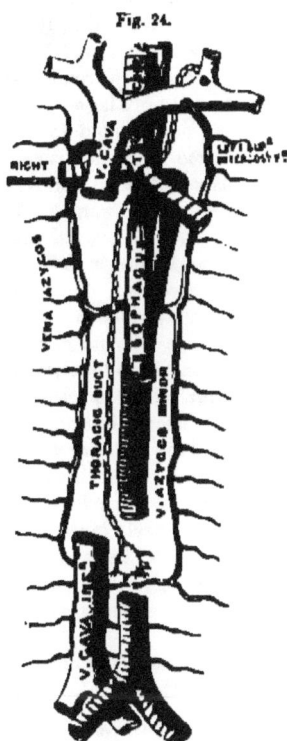

Fig. 24.

The left vena azygos, 'vena azygos minor,' runs up the left side of the spine. This vein commences in the abdomen by small branches communicating with the inferior vena cava, and ascends on the left side of the aorta, through the aortic opening in the diaphragm. On a level with the sixth or seventh dorsal vertebra, it passes beneath the aorta and joins the azygos major. Before passing beneath the aorta it usually communicates with the left superior intercostal vein. It receives five or six of the lower intercostal veins of the left side. None of these veins are provided with valves. The purpose of the azygos vein is to be supplemental to the inferior vena cava.

Thoracic duct. The thoracic duct (fig. 24) is a canal about eighteen inches long, through which the contents of the lacteal vessels from the intestines and the absorbents from the lower limbs are conveyed into the blood. These vessels converge to a general receptacle, termed 'receptaculum chyli,' situated in front of the body of the second lumbar vertebra. From this receptacle, the duct passes

DIAGRAM TO SHOW THE COURSE OF THE VENA AZYGOS AND THE THORACIC DUCT.

through the aortic opening of the diaphragm into the chest, and
runs up the posterior mediastinum along the right side of the
aorta. Near the *third* dorsal vertebra, it passes under the œsophagus, and ascends on the left side of this tube, between it and
the left subclavian artery, as high as the seventh cervical vertebra,
where it describes a curve with the convexity upwards, and opens
in front of the scalenus anticus into the back part of the confluence
of the left internal jugular and subclavian veins. The orifice of
the duct is guarded by two valves which permit fluid to pass
from the duct into the vein, but not *vice versâ*. Valves, disposed
like those in the venous system, are placed at short intervals
along the duct, so that its contents can only pass upwards. The
duct is not much larger than a crow-quill; its walls are thin and
transparent.* The calibre of the duct varies in size in different
parts of its course; it is large at the commencement, diminishes
in the middle, and again enlarges towards the termination.

Œsophagus.   The 'œsophagus' is that part of the alimentary canal
which conveys the food from the pharynx to the stomach.
It commences about the fifth cervical vertebra, nearly opposite the
cricoid cartilage; runs down first to the right side of the transverse
portion of the arch of the aorta, then through the posterior mediastinum in front of the descending aorta, and passes through a
special opening in the diaphragm to the stomach. It is from nine
to ten inches long. Its course is not exactly vertical: in the neck,
it lies to the left of the trachea; in the chest, i.e. about the
fourth dorsal vertebra, it inclines towards the right side, to make
way for the aorta; but it again inclines to the left before it perforates
the diaphragm.

The œsophagus, in the first part of its course, rests upon the
longus colli muscle, then upon the third, fourth, and fifth inter-

* It is right to state that the thoracic duct varies in size in different individuals.
I have seen it of all sizes intermediate between a crow-quill and a goose-quill. It
may divide in its course into two branches, which subsequently reunite; instead of
one, there may be several terminal orifices. Instances have been observed in which
the duct has terminated on the right instead of the left side (Fleischman, Leichen-
öffnungen, 1815). It has been seen to terminate in the vena azygos (Müller's Archives,
1834).

costal vessels of the right side, and, lastly, lies in front, and slightly
to the left side of the aorta.   In front of it is the left bronchus;
and before it passes through the diaphragm it lies in close contact
with the pericardium for nearly two inches: this fact accounts for
the pain which is sometimes experienced in cases of pericarditis,
during the passage of food.   The œsophagus is surrounded by a
nervous plexus, formed by the pneumogastric nerves, the left being
in front and the right behind it.

The œsophagus is supplied with blood by the inferior thyroid,
the œsophageal branches of the aorta, and the coronaria ventriculi.
It is supplied with nerves by the pneumogastric and the sympathetic.   The œsophagus is composed of three coats, an external or
muscular, a middle or cellular, and an internal or mucous.   The
muscular coat consists of an outer longitudinal and an inner
circular layer of fibres.   Both are of the non-striped variety.
The longitudinal layer is particularly strong, and arranged all
round the œsophagus so as to support the circular.   The middle
coat is composed of cellular tissue, and connects very loosely the
muscular and mucous coats.   The mucous membrane is of a pale
colour, and considerable thickness, and in the contracted state of
the œsophagus is arranged in longitudinal folds.   It is lined by a
very thick layer of scaly epithelium.   In the submucous tissue are
many small compound glands—œsophageal glands—especially
towards the lower end of the œsophagus.

Course and   The *right* pneumogastric nerve enters the chest between
branches of   the subclavian artery and vein, descends by the side of
the pneu-   the trachea, then behind the root of the right lung to
mogastric
nerves.   the posterior surface of the œsophagus, upon which it
divides into branches, which form a plexus (posterior œsophageal)
upon the tube.   The plexus then reunites into a single trunk,
which passes into the abdomen through the œsophageal opening in
the diaphragm.   The *left* pneumogastric descends into the chest
between the left subclavian and carotid arteries, and behind the
left brachio-cephalic vein.   It then crosses in front of the arch
of the aorta, and passes behind the root of the left lung to the
anterior surface of the œsophagus, upon which it also forms a

plexus (anterior œsophageal). The branches of the pneumogastric nerve in the chest are as follow:—

a. The inferior laryngeal or recurrent.—This nerve on the right side turns under the subclavian and the common carotid artery (p. 53); on the left, under the arch of the aorta, and ascends to the larynx. It enters the larynx beneath the lower border of the inferior constrictor of the pharynx. It supplies with motor power all the muscles which act upon the rima glottidis, except the crico-thyroid (supplied by the external laryngeal branch of the superior laryngeal nerve).

b. Cardiac branches.—These are very small, and join the cardiac plexuses; the right arise from the right recurrent laryngeal and the right pneumogastric, close to the trachea; the left come from the left recurrent laryngeal nerve.

c. Pulmonary branches.—These accompany the bronchial tubes. The greater number run behind the root of the lung, forming the *posterior* pulmonary plexus. A few, forming the *anterior* pulmonary plexus, proceed over the front of the lung's root. Both these plexuses are joined by filaments from the sympathetic system. But the nerves of the lungs are very small, and cannot be traced far into their substance.*

d. Œsophageal plexus.—Below the root of the lung each pneumogastric nerve is subdivided so as to form an interlacement of nerves round the œsophagus (plexus gulæ). From this plexus numerous filaments supply the coats of the tube; but the majority of them are collected into two nerves—the continuation of the left pneumogastric nerve lying in front of the œsophagus; the continuation of the right lying behind it. Both nerves pass through the diaphragm for the supply of the stomach.

Having examined the contents of the posterior mediastinum from the right side, now do so from the left. The left lung is to be turned out of its cavity and fastened by hooks towards the right side. After removing the pleura, we see the descending thoracic aorta, the pneumogastric nerve crossing the arch and sending the recurrent branch through it; also the first part of the

* Upon this subject, see the beautiful plates of Scarpa.

course of the left subclavian, covered externally by pleura. The
pneumogastric nerve must be traced behind the root of the left
lung to the œsophagus, and the œsophageal plexus of this side
dissected. Lastly, notice the lesser vena azygos which crosses
under the aorta about the sixth or seventh dorsal vertebra to join
the vena azygos major.

Thoracic por-   This portion of the sympathetic system is generally
tion of the   composed of twelve ganglia covered by the pleura; one
sympathetic.   ganglion being found over the head of each rib. Often
there are only ten ganglia, in consequence of one or two of them

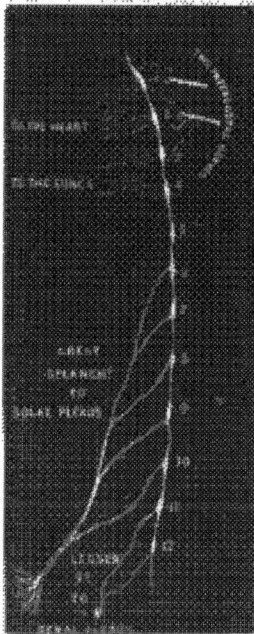

fusing together. The first thoracic
ganglion is the largest.

Each ganglion is connected by two
branches with the corresponding spinal
nerve. The nerves proceeding from
the ganglia pass inwards to supply
the thoracic and part of the abdominal
viscera. The branches which proceed
from the upper six ganglia are small
and are distributed as follow (see the
diagram):—

a. Minute nerves from the first and
second ganglia to the deep *cardiac
plexus*.

b. Minute nerves from the third
and fourth ganglia to the *posterior
pulmonary plexus*.

The branches arising from the six
lower ganglia unite to form three nerves
—the *great splanchnic*, the *lesser*, and
the *smallest splanchnic nerves*.

a. The *great splanchnic* nerve is
generally formed by branches from
the sixth to the tenth ganglia. They
descend obliquely along the sides of
the bodies of the dorsal vertebræ, and

DIAGRAM OF THE THORACIC PORTION
OF THE SYMPATHETIC.

unite into a single nerve, which passes through the corresponding
crus of the diaphragm, and joins the semilunar ganglion of the
abdomen, sending also branches to the renal plexus.

b. The *lesser splanchnic* nerve is commonly formed by branches
from the tenth and the eleventh ganglia. It passes through the
crus of the diaphragm to the renal plexus.*

c. The *smallest splanchnic* nerve comes from the twelfth
ganglion, passes through the crus of the diaphragm, and terminates
in the renal plexus. (This is not seen in the diagram.)

Intercostal muscles.
The intercostal muscles occupy the intervals between
the ribs. Between each rib there are two layers of
muscles which cross like the letter X. The external
layer runs obliquely from behind, forwards, like the external
oblique muscle of the abdomen. The internal layer runs from
before backwards like the internal oblique. Observe that a few
fibres of the inner layer pass over one or even two ribs, and terminate upon a rib lower down.

But neither of these layers extends all the way between the
sternum and the spine: the outer layer, beginning at the spine,
ceases at the cartilages of the ribs; the inner, commencing at the
sternum, ceases at the angles of the ribs.

The intercostal muscles present a curious intermixture of tendinous and fleshy fibres; and they are covered inside and outside
the chest by a glistening fascia, to give greater protection to the
intercostal spaces.

The external intercostal muscles elevate the ribs, and are therefore muscles of inspiration. The internal intercostal muscles depress the ribs, and are therefore muscles of expiration.

Intercostal arteries.
There are twelve intercostal arteries on each side.
The two upper are supplied by the intercostal branch
of the subclavian; the remaining ten are furnished by
the aorta: and since this vessel lies rather on the left side of the
spine, the right intercostal arteries are longer than the left. The

* In a few instances we have traced a minute filament from one of the ganglia into
the body of a vertebra. According to a celebrated French anatomist (Cruveilhier),
each vertebra receives one.

upper intercostal arteries from the aorta ascend obliquely to reach
their intercostal spaces; the lower run more transversely.   As
they pass outwards, they are covered by the pleura and the sympathetic nerves; the right, in addition, pass behind the œsophagus,
thoracic duct, and the vena azygos major. Having reached the
intercostal space, each artery divides into an *anterior* and a
posterior branch.   The *anterior* branch in direction and size
appears to be the continuation of the common trunk. At first it
runs *along the middle of the intercostal space*, lying upon the
external intercostal muscle, and is separated from the cavity of
the chest by the pleura and intercostal fascia. Here, therefore,
it is liable to be injured by a wound in the back. But near the
angle of the rib it passes between the intercostal muscles, and
occupies the groove in the lower border of the rib above. Here it
gives off a small branch, which runs for some distance along the
upper border of the rib below, and is lost in the muscles. In
some cases I have seen this branch as large as the intercostal
itself, and situated so as to be directly exposed to injury in the
operation of tapping the chest.

In its course along the intercostal space, each artery sends
branches to the intercostal muscles and the ribs. About midway
between the sternum and the spine, each gives off a small branch,
which accompanies the lateral cutaneous branch of the intercostal
nerve.   The continued trunk, gradually decreasing in size, becomes very small-towards the anterior part of the space, and is
placed more in the middle of it. Those of the true intercostal
spaces inosculate with branches of the internal mammary, and
thoracic branches of the axillary; those of the false run between
the layers of the abdominal muscles, and anastomose with the
epigastric and lumbar arteries.

The posterior branch passes backwards between the transverse
processes of the vertebræ, to the muscles and skin of the back.
Each sends an artery through the intervertebral foramen to the
spinal cord and its membranes.

On the right side the intercostal veins terminate in the vena
azygos major; on the left, the lower seven or eight terminate

in the vena azygos minor, the remainder in the left superior intercostal vein.

Intercostal nerves.

These are twelve in number, and are the anterior divisions of the dorsal spinal nerves. Each dorsal nerve (like all the spinal nerves) arises from the spinal cord by two roots, an anterior or motor, and a posterior or sensitive. The sensitive root has a ganglion upon it. The two roots unite in the intervertebral foramen and form a *compound* nerve.

After passing through the foramen, it divides into an *anterior* and a *posterior* branch. The *posterior* branches pass backwards between the transverse processes of the dorsal vertebræ, and supply the muscles of the back. The *anterior* branches or the proper *intercostal* nerves proceed along the intercostal spaces in company with, and immediately below, their corresponding arteries. Midway between the spine and the sternum, they give off lateral cutaneous branches, which supply the skin over the scapula and the thorax.

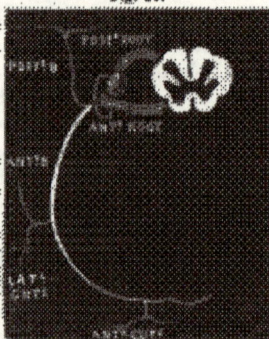

Fig. 26.

DIAGRAM OF A SPINAL NERVE.

The intercostal nerves terminate in front, in the anterior cutaneous nerves; the upper six, coming through their respective intercostal spaces, supply the skin over the chest; the six lower terminate in the front wall of the abdomen, near the linea alba.

Notice, that the first dorsal nerve ascends nearly perpendicularly over the neck of the first rib to form part of the brachial plexus. Before doing so, it sends a nerve to the first intercostal space. This, as a rule, has no lateral cutaneous branch.

Intercostal absorbent glands.—These are situated near the heads of the ribs; there are some between the layers of the intercostal muscles. They are of small size, and send their absorbent vessels into the thoracic duct. I have seen these intercostal glands enlarged and diseased in phthisis.

K

Bronchial and   Small arteries, arising on the right side most fre-
œsophageal   quently from the first aortic intercostal artery, and on
arteries.   the left from the concavity of the arch of the aorta,
accompany the bronchial tube on its posterior aspect into the
substance of the lung. Their distribution and office will be considered with the anatomy of the lung. Other arteries proceed from
the front of the descending aorta to ramify on the œsophagus, when
they inosculate with the œsophageal branches of the inferior thyroid
and phrenic arteries.

Having finished the posterior mediastinum, replace the lung, and
turn your attention once more to the great vessels at the root of
the heart.

Pulmonary   This vessel is about two inches in length, and conveys
artery   the impure blood from the heart to the lungs. It pro-
                ceeds from the right ventricle, crosses obliquely in front
of the root of the aorta, and on the left side of that vessel divides
into two branches, one for each lung. The right branch passes
through the arch of the aorta to the lung; the left is easily followed to its lung by removing its investing layer of pericardium.

Search should be made for a short fibrous cord which connects
the commencement of the left pulmonary artery with the concavity
of the arch of the aorta. This cord is the remains of the *ductus
arteriosus*, a canal which in fœtal life conveyed blood from the
pulmonary artery to the aorta.

Draw towards the left side the first part of the arch of the aorta,
and dissect the pericardium from the great vessels at the base of
the heart. Thus a good view will be obtained of the trachea and
its bifurcation into the two bronchi. Below the division of the
trachea the right pulmonary artery is seen passing in front of the
right bronchus. The superior vena cava is seen descending in
front of, and nearly at right angles to, the right pulmonary artery.
The vena azygos is also seen arching over the right bronchus and
terminating in the vena cava. Notice, especially, a number of
absorbent glands called '*bronchial*,' at the angle of bifurcation
of the trachea. The situation of these glands in the midst of so
many tubes explains the variety of symptoms which may be produced by their enlargement.

Cardiac plexus of nerves.

The nerves of the heart are derived from the pneumogastric and from the cervical ganglia of the sympathetic. A general description of them will suffice. The cardiac nerves of the right side descend chiefly *behind* the arch of

Fig. 27.

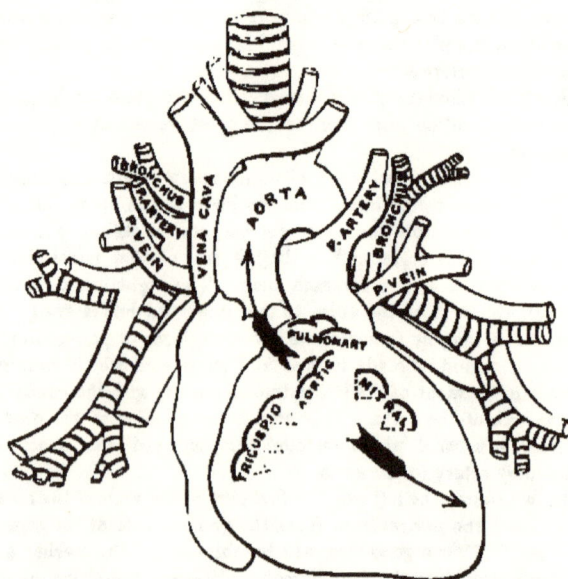

DIAGRAM SHOWING THE CONSTITUENTS OF THE ROOT OF EACH LUNG, AND THEIR RELATIVE POSITION : ALSO THE POSITION OF THE VALVES OF THE HEART. THE ARROWS INDICATE THE DIRECTION IN WHICH AORTIC AND MITRAL MURMURS ARE PROPAGATED.

the aorta; those of the left chiefly in *front* of the arch. The nerves from both sides, however, converge to form a plexus called the '*cardiac*.' From this two secondary plexuses proceed; the *superficial* and the *deep* cardiac plexus. The superficial one lies

K 2

more in front of the aorta: the deep plexus is between the arch
of the aorta and the bifurcation of the pulmonary artery.

From these plexuses the nerves proceed, in company with the
coronary arteries, to the heart. Those which accompany the
anterior coronary artery form the ' anterior coronary plexus.' The
' posterior coronary plexus ' proceeds with its artery to the posterior
part of the heart.

But it is not an easy matter to trace the nerves into the substance of the heart. For this purpose a horse's heart is the best,
and previous maceration in water is desirable. The nerves in the
substance of the heart are peculiar in this respect ; that they present minute ganglia in their course, which are presumed to preside
over the rhythmical contractions of the heart.*

Constituents
of the root of
each lung.
Draw aside the margin of the right lung; divide the
superior vena cava above the vena azygos, and turn
down the lower part. Remove the layer of pericardium
which covers the pulmonary veins, and the constituent parts of the
root of the right lung will be exposed. It is composed of the
pulmonary artery, the pulmonary veins, bronchus, bronchial vessels,
anterior and posterior pulmonic plexus, and some lymphatics. The
following is the disposition of the large vessels forming the root of
the lung. In front are the two pulmonary veins: behind the
veins are the subdivisions of the pulmonary artery ; behind the
artery are the divisions of the bronchus. From above downwards
they are disposed thus:—On the right side we find—1st, the
bronchus ; 2nd, the artery; 3rd, the veins. On the left, we find:—
1st, the artery; 2nd, the bronchus ; 3rd, the veins, as shown in
fig. 27.

DISSECTION OF THE HEART.

The heart is conical in form, and more or less convex on its
external aspect. It is situated obliquely in the chest, having its
base directed upwards and to the right; its apex downwards and
to the left. Notice the longitudinal grooves on the upper and

* For the demonstration of the nerves of the heart, the student should see the
beautiful dissections by Pettigrew in the Museum of the Royal College of Surgeons.

lower surfaces of the heart, indicating the divisions of the ventricles, and the circular groove near the base, indicating the separation between the ventricles and auricles. These grooves are occupied by the coronary vessels and by more or less fat.

Weight.   The average weight of the heart is from ten to twelve ounces in the male, and from eight to ten in the female ; but much depends upon the size and condition of the body generally. As a rule, it may be stated that the heart gradually increases in length, breadth, and thickness, from childhood to age.[*]

The heart is a double muscular organ; that is, it is composed of two hearts, a right and a left, separated by a septum. Each consists of an auricle and a ventricle, which communicate by a wide orifice : the right heart propels the blood through the lungs, and is called the *pulmonic* ; the left propels the blood through the body, and is called the *systemic*. These two hearts are not placed apart, because important advantages result from their union : by being enclosed in a single bag they occupy less room in the chest ; and the action of their corresponding cavities being precisely synchronous, their fibres, mutually intermixing, contribute to their mutual support. The cavities of the heart should now be examined in the order in which the blood circulates through them.

Right auricle.   This is situated at the right side of the base of the heart, and forms a quadrangular cavity between the two venæ cavæ, from which it receives the blood. From its front a small pouch projects towards the left, and overlaps the root of the aorta; this part is termed the *appendix* of the auricle, and resembles a dog's ear in shape ; *unde nomen.*

To see the interior, make a horizontal incision through the anterior wall from the apex of the appendix, transversely across the cavity : from this make another upwards at right angles into the superior vena cava. Observe that the interior is lined by a polished membrane called the '*endocardium*,' and that it is everywhere smooth except in the appendix, where the muscular fibres are collected into bundles, called, from their resemblance to the teeth of a comb, '*musculi pectinati*.' They radiate from the

[*] Consult Bizot, Mém. de la Soc. Méd. d'Obser. de Paris, tom. i. 1836.

auricles to the edges of the auriculo-ventricular opening. Examine carefully the openings of the two venæ cavæ: they are not directly opposite to each other; the superior is situated on a plane rather in front of the inferior, that the streams of blood may not meet.

Fig. 28.

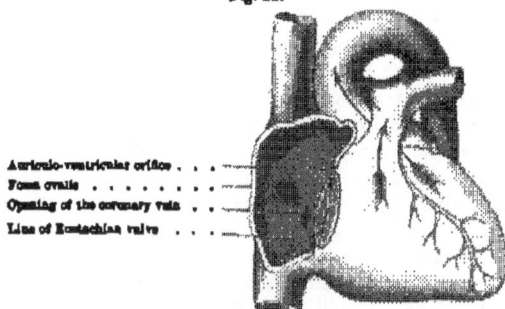

Auriculo-ventricular orifice . . .
Fossa ovalis . . . .
Opening of the coronary vein . . .
Line of Eustachian valve . . . .

DIAGRAM OF THE INTERIOR OF THE RIGHT AURICLE.

The inferior cava, after passing through the tendinous centre of the diaphragm, makes a slight curve to the left before it opens into the auricle, that the stream of its blood may be directed towards the auriculo-ventricular opening. The orifice of each vena cava is nearly circular, and surrounded by muscular fibres continuous with those of the auricle.

The internal wall of the auricle is formed by the 'septum auricularum.' Upon this septum, above the orifice of the vena cava inferior, is an oval depression (fossa ovalis), bounded by a prominent border (annulus ovalis). This depression indicates the remains of the opening (foramen ovale) through which the auricles communicated in fœtal life. After birth this opening closes; but if the closure is imperfect, the stream of dark blood in the right auricle mixes with the florid blood in the left, and occasions what is called 'morbus cœruleus.' A valvular communication, however, not unfrequently exists between the auricles in this situation which is not attended with indications of this disease.

Extending from the anterior margin of the vena cava inferior to the anterior border of the fossa ovalis, is seen a thin fold of the lining membrane of the heart: it is the remains of what was, in foetal life, the *Eustachian* * *valve.* The direction of this valve is such that it directs the current of blood from the inferior cava towards the foramen ovale. It is a valve of considerable size in the foetus, and contains a few muscular fibres; but after birth it diminishes, being no longer required.

To the left of the Eustachian valve, that is, between its remains and the auriculo-ventricular opening, is the orifice of the *coronary vein*; it is covered by a semicircular valve, called '*valvula Thebesii*,' to prevent regurgitation of the blood during the auricular contraction. Here and there upon the posterior wall of the auricle may be observed minute openings called '*foramina Thebesii*:' they are the orifices of small veins returning blood from the substance of the heart. Lastly, to the left, and rather in front of the orifice of the vena cava inferior, is the *auriculo-ventricular* opening. It is oval in form, and will admit the passage of three fingers.

Right ven-
tricle.

This forms the right border and about two-thirds of the front surface of the heart. To examine its interior, a triangular flap should be raised from its anterior wall. The apex of this flap should be below: one cut along the right edge of the ventricle, the other along the line of the ventricular septum. Observe that the wall of the ventricle is much thicker than that of the auricle. The cavity of the ventricle is conical, with its base upwards and to the right. From its walls project bands of muscular fibres (columnæ carneæ) of various length and thickness, which cross each other in every direction; this muscular network is generally filled with coagulated blood. Of these columnæ carneæ there are three kinds: one stands out in relief from the ventricle; another is attached to the ventricle by their extremities only, the intermediate portion being free; a third, and by far the most important set, called '*musculi papillares*,' is fixed by one extremity to the wall of the ventricle, while the other extremity gives attachment to the fine tendinous cords (*cordæ tendineæ*) which regulate the action of the tricuspid valve. The

* Eustachius, Libell. de vena sine pari.

number of these musculi papillares is equal to the number of the
chief divisions of the valve; consequently there are three in the
right and two in the left ventricle. Of those in the right ventricle,
one proceeds from the septum.

There are two openings in the right ventricle. One, the *auriculo-
ventricular*, through which the blood passes from the auricle, is
oval in form and placed at the base of the ventricle. It is surrounded by a ring of fibrous tissue, to which is attached the tricuspid valve. From the upper and front part of the ventricle, a
smooth passage ('*infundibulum*' or '*conus arteriosus*') leads to
the opening of the pulmonary artery. It is situated to the left
and in front of the auriculo-ventricular, and about three-fourths of
an inch higher.

Tricuspid valve. This is situated at the right auriculo-ventricular
opening, and consists of three principal triangular flaps,
and besides these of intermediate flaps of smaller size.
Like all the valves of the heart, it is formed by a fold of the lining
membrane ('*endocardium*') of the heart, strengthened by fibrous
tissue, in which muscular fibres may be demonstrated. The base
of the valve is attached to the tendinous ring round the opening;
its segments lying in the cavity of the right ventricle. Of its
three principal flaps, the largest is so placed that when not in
action, it partially covers the orifice of the pulmonary artery:
another lies behind the anterior wall of the ventricle, and the third
rests upon the septum ventriculorum.

Observe the arrangement of the tendinous cords which regulate
the action of the valve. First, they are all attached to the ventricular surface of the valve. Secondly, the tendinous cords proceeding from a given papillary muscle are attached to the adjacent
halves of two of the larger flaps, and to a smaller intermediate
one; consequently, when the ventricle contracts, and the papillary
muscle also, the adjacent borders of the flaps will be approximated.
Thirdly, to insure the strength of every part of the valve, the
tendinous cords are inserted at three different points of it in
straight lines; accordingly, they are divisible into three sets.
Those of the first, which are three or four in number, are attached

to the base of the valve; those of the second, from four to six, proceed to the middle of it; those of the third, which are the most numerous, are attached to its free margin.*

Pulmonary or semilunar valves These are three membranous folds, situated at the orifice of the pulmonary artery. Their convex borders are attached to the fibrous ring at the root of the artery; their free edges, which look upwards, present a festooned border, in the centre of which is a small cartilaginous body called the '*nodulus*' or '*corpus Arantii*.' The use of these bodies is obvious. Since the valves are semilunar, when they fall together they would not exactly close the artery; there would be a space of a triangular form left between them in the centre, just as there is when we put the thumb, fore, and middle fingers together. This space is filled up by these nodules, so that the closure becomes complete.

The valves are composed of a fold of the '*endocardium*,' or lining membrane of the heart, and contained between the folds is a thin layer of fibrous tissue, which is prolonged from the tendinous ring at the orifice of the artery. This layer of fibrous tissue, however, reaches the free edge of the valve at three points only; namely, at the centre, or corpus Arantii, and at each extremity. Between these points it stops short, and leaves a crescent-shaped portion of the valve thinner than the rest, and consisting simply of endocardium. This crescent-shaped portion (called the '*lunula*') is not wholly without fibrous tissue, for a thin tendinous cord runs along its free edge, to give it additional strength to resist the impulse of the blood. Behind each of the valves the artery bulges and forms three slight dilatations called

---

* The best mode of showing the action of the valve is to introduce a glass tube into the pulmonary artery, and then to pour water through it into the ventricle until the cavity is quite distended. By gently squeezing the ventricle in the hand, so as artificially to imitate its natural contraction, the tricuspid valve will flap back like a flood-gate, and close the auriculo-ventricular opening. In this way one can understand how, when the ventricle contracts, the blood catches the margin of the valve, and by its pressure gives it the proper distention and figure requisite to block up the aperture into the auricle. It is obvious that the tendinous cords will prevent the valve from being pushed too far back into the auricle; and this purpose is assisted by the papillary muscles, which nicely adjust the degree of tension of the cords at a time when they would otherwise be too much slackened by the contraction of the ventricle.

the 'sinuses of Valsalva.' These, we shall presently see, are
more marked at the orifice of the aorta.

The action of these valves is obvious. During the contraction
of the ventricle the valves lie against the side of the artery, and
offer no impediment to the current of blood; during its dilatation,
the elasticity of the distended artery would force back the column
of blood, but that the valves, being caught by the refluent blood,
bag, and fall together so as to close the tube. The greater the
pressure, the more accurate is the closure. The coats of the
artery are very elastic and yielding, while the valve, like the
circumference to which it is attached, is quite unyielding; consequently, when the artery is distended by the impulse of the blood,
its wall is removed from the contact of the free margin of the
valves, and these are the more readily caught by the retrograde
motion of the blood. The force of the reflux is sustained by the
tendinous part of the valves, and by the muscular wall of the
ventricle (probably in a state of contraction), as shown by Mr.
Savory. According to Haller, the valves are capable of sustaining
a weight of sixty-three pounds before they give way. The thinner
portions (lunulæ) become placed so as to lie side by side, each one
with that of the adjacent valve. This may be demonstrated by
filling the artery with water.

Left auricle.   This is situated at the left side and posterior part of
the base of the heart, and is somewhat smaller than
the right auricle. It is quadrilateral and receives the four pulmonary veins, two on either side, which return the purified blood
from the lungs. From its upper and left side, the auricular appendage projects towards the right, curling over the root of the
pulmonary artery. The auricle should be opened by a horizontal
incision from one pulmonary vein to another: from this a second
should be made into the appendix. Its interior is smooth and flat,
excepting in the appendix, which contains the 'musculi pectinati.'
Notice the openings of the four pulmonary veins. Upon the septum between the auricles is a depression indicating the remains of
the foramen ovale. At the lower and front part of the auricle is the
auriculo-ventricular opening. It is oval, with its long axis nearly
transverse, and in the adult will admit the passage of two fingers.

Left ventricle. This occupies the left border, and forms the apex of the heart. One third of it only is seen on the anterior surface, the rest being on its posterior. To examine the interior, raise a triangular flap, with the apex below, from its front wall. Observe that it is about three times as thick as that of the right ventricle, and that this thickness gradually diminishes towards the apex. The interior of the left ventricle so closely resembles that of the right that there is no necessity to describe it in detail. The *auriculo-ventricular valve* consists of only two principal flaps: hence its name '*mitral*' or '*bicuspid.*' The larger of these flaps is placed between the aortic and auriculo-ventricular orifices. There are only two '*musculi* papillares;' one attached to the anterior, the other to the posterior wall of the ventricle. They are thicker and their '*cordæ tendineæ*' stronger than those of the right ventricle, but their arrangement is precisely similar. From the upper and back part of the ventricle, a smooth passage leads to the orifice of the aorta. This orifice is placed rather in front, and to the right side of the auriculo-ventricular opening; but the two orifices are close together, and only separated by the larger flap of the mitral valve. The aortic orifice is guarded by three semilunar valves, of which the arrangement, structure, and mode of action are similar to those of the pulmonary artery. Their framework is proportionately stronger, consistently with the greater strength of the left ventricle, and the greater impulse of the blood. In the '*sinuses of Valsalva*' are observed the orifices of the two coronary arteries.

Fibrous rings. At the openings between the auricles and ventricles, and also at the commencement of the aorta and pulmonary artery, we find fibrous rings. These rings serve as fixed points for the attachment of the muscular fibres of the heart, the tricuspid and the mitral valves. The rings on the left side are stronger than those on the right.

Attachment of the great arteries to the ventricles. The fibrous rings at the arterial orifices present three festoons with concavities directed upwards. These festoons give attachment to the middle coat of the artery above, to the muscular fibres of the heart below, and internally to the tendinous fibres of the valves. The vessels

are also connected to the heart by the serous layer of the pericardium, and by a continuation of the lining membrane (endocardium) of the ventricle.

Coronary
arteries.
The heart is supplied with blood by the two coronary
arteries, a *right* or posterior, and a *left* or anterior.

Both arise from the aorta just above the semilunar
valves, and at such a distance as always to admit the passage of
blood : both run in the furrows between the ventricles and
auricles : both are accompanied by branches of the coronary vein,
and by the cardiac nerves.

The *anterior*, or left coronary artery, the smaller of the two,
arises from the left side of the aorta. It appears on the left of
the pulmonary artery, and then runs down the inter-ventricular
furrow on the anterior surface of the heart to the apex, where it
inosculates with the posterior coronary. In this course, its principal branch turns to the left, along the furrow between the left
ventricle and auricle, and then communicates at the back of the
heart with a branch of the posterior coronary.

The *posterior* or right coronary artery arises from the right
side of the aorta, and passes down between the pulmonary artery
and the appendix of the right auricle. It turns to the right along
the furrow between the right ventricle and auricle to the back of
the heart, whence it inosculates with the horizontal branch of the
left coronary. Besides this, it sends a branch down the inter-
ventricular furrow at the back of the heart to the apex, where it
communicates with the left coronary.

Thus the coronary arteries form two circles about the heart:
the one, horizontal, runs round the base of the heart, in the
furrow between the auricles and ventricles. The other, perpendicular, runs in the furrow between the ventricles.

Coronary
veins.
The veins corresponding to the coronary arteries
terminate in a single trunk—'*the coronary sinus*'—
which opens into the right auricle between the remains
of the Eustachian valve and the auriculo-ventricular opening. The
orifice of the vein is guarded by a valve, to prevent regurgitation
of the blood.

The muscular fibres of the heart are of the striped variety, but differ from ordinary striped muscular tissue, in being somewhat smaller, destitute of sarcolemma, and branched. Most of the fibres are attached by both extremities to the fibrous rings of the heart. The fibres of the auricles are distinct from those of the ventricles. They consist of a *superficial* layer common to both cavities, and a *deeper* layer proper to each. The *superficial* fibres run transversely across the auricles, and are most marked on the anterior surface; some pass into the septum. Of the *deeper* fibres, some run in circles chiefly round the auricular appendages and the entrance of the great veins, upon which a few may be traced for a short distance; others run over the auricles, and are attached in front and behind to the auriculo-ventricular rings.

(margin: Arrangement of the muscular fibres of the heart.)

Of the ventricular fibres, some are common to both ventricles, others proper to each. The septum is formed principally by the fibres of the left. The *superficial* fibres take a more or less spiral course from the base towards the apex of the heart, where they coil round, pass into the interior of the ventricle, and form either the 'carneæ columnæ' or 'musculi papillares.' Most of these fibres are eventually inserted into the auriculo-ventricular rings. The *circular* fibres are chiefly found near the base of the ventricles, and passing round become attached to the rings at the base of the heart.*

Reduced to their simplest expression, the ventricles consist of two muscular sacs, enclosed in a third equally muscular. The same may be said of the auricles.

The average thickness of the right auricle is about one line; that of the left, one and a half. The measure must not be taken during the 'rigor mortis.'

(margin: Thickness of the cavities.)

The average thickness of the right ventricle at its thickest part —i.e. the base—is about two lines: that of the left ventricle at its thickest part—i.e. the middle—is about half an inch. In the female the average is less.

* For further information upon this subject, see the article in Todd's Cyclopædia. Examine also the beautiful and elaborate dissections by Pettigrew, in the Museum of the College of Surgeons.

Peculiarities of fœtal heart.   The heart of the fœtus differs from that of the adult in the following points:—1. The Eustachian valve is well developed in order to guide the current of blood from the vena cava inferior into the foramen ovale. 2. The

Fig. 39.

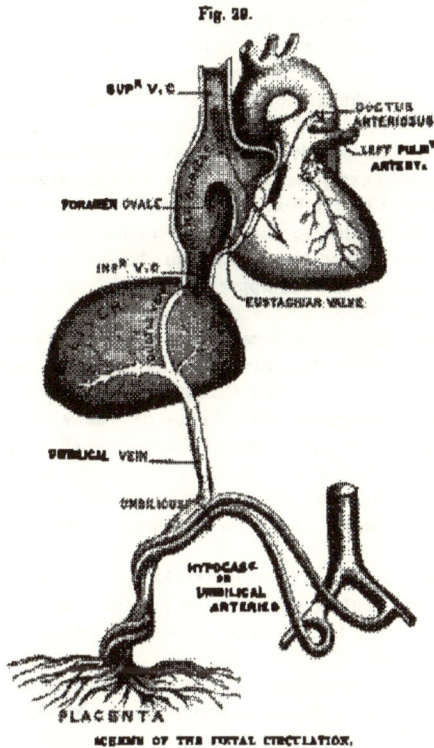

SCHEME OF THE FŒTAL CIRCULATION.

foramen ovale is widely open. 3. The right and left pulmonary arteries are very much contracted, so as to admit very little blood to the lungs. 4. The ductus arteriosus (from the pulmonary artery to the aorta) is open. 5. The right and left ventricles are of equal thickness because they have equal work to do.

Circulation of the blood in the fœtus. The umbilical vein, fig. 29, bringing pure blood from the placenta, enters at the umbilicus, and passes to the under surface of the liver, where it sends off some small branches to the left lobe. At the transverse fissure it divides into two branches: one, the smaller, termed the 'ductus venosus,' passes straight to the inferior vena cava; the other or right division joins the vena porta, and after ramifying in the liver, returns its blood through the hepatic veins into the inferior vena cava. From the inferior vena cava, the blood enters the right auricle, and this stream (directed by the Eustachian valve) flows through the foramen ovale into the left auricle. From the left auricle it runs into the left ventricle, and thence through the aorta, into the great vessels of the head and the upper limbs, which are thus supplied by almost pure blood.

From the head and the upper limbs, the blood returns (impure) through the superior vena cava into the right auricle, and flows into the right ventricle. From the right ventricle it passes through the pulmonary artery, and the 'ductus arteriosus,' into the third part of the arch of the aorta; only a very small quantity of it going to the lungs. From the aorta part of the blood is distributed to the pelvis and lower extremities; and part is conveyed through the umbilical arteries to the placenta, where it becomes purified.

The following changes take place in the circulation after birth:—

1. The umbilical vein becomes obliterated from the second to the fifth day after birth, and subsequently forms the round ligament of the liver.

2. The ductus venosus also becomes closed about the same period.

3. The foramen ovale and ductus arteriosus become completely closed from the sixth to the tenth day.

4. The pulmonary arteries enlarge and convey impure blood to the lungs. These organs during fœtal life receive only a small quantity of blood from these arteries.

5. The *hypogastric arteries* become obliterated from the fourth or fifth day after birth.

STRUCTURE OF THE LUNGS.

The lungs are very vascular, spongy organs, in which the blood is purified by exposure to atmospheric air. Their situation and shape have been already described (p. 119). We have now to examine their general structure.

The lungs are composed of cartilaginous and membranous tubes, of which the successive subdivisions convey the air into closely-packed minute cells, called the 'air vesicles;' of the ramifications of the pulmonary artery and veins; of the bronchial vessels concerned in their nutrition; of lymphatics and nerves. These component parts are united by areolar tissue, and covered externally by pleura. The point at which they respectively pass in and out is called the 'root' of the lung.

The lungs are the lightest organs in the body, and float in water. When entirely deprived of air, they sink. This is observed in certain pathological conditions; e.g. when one lung is compressed by effusion into the chest, or rendered solid by inflammation.

Contractility of the lung. When an opening is made into the chest, the lung, which was in contact with the ribs, immediately recedes from them, and, provided there be no adhesions, gradually contracts. If the lungs be artificially inflated, either in or out of the chest, we observe that, left to themselves, they spontaneously expel a part of the air. This constant disposition to contract, in the living and the dead lung, is owing to the elastic tissue in the bronchial tubes and the air-cells; but more especially to a layer of delicate elastic tissue on the surface of the lung, which has been described by some anatomists as a distinct coat, under the name of the second or inner layer of the pleura.*

Colour. The lungs are of a livid red or violet colour; they often present a mixture of tints, giving them a marble-

* In some animals, the seal especially, the elasticity of this tissue is very strongly marked.

like appearance. This is not the natural colour of the organ, since it is produced in the act of dying. It depends upon the stagnation of the venous blood, which the right ventricle still propels into the lungs, though respiration is failing. The tint varies in particular situations in proportion to the accumulation of the blood, and is always the deepest at the back of the lung. But the colour of the proper tissue of the lung apart from the blood which it contains is pale and light grey. This colour is seldom seen except in the lungs of infants who have never breathed, or after death from profuse hæmorrhage.

Upon or near the surface of the lungs, numerous dark spots are observed, which do not depend upon the blood, since they are seen in the palest lungs. They vary in number and size, and increase with age. The source of these discolourations is not exactly known; but they are probably deposits of minute particles of carbonaceous matter which have been inhaled with the air.

Trachea. This is a partly membranous, partly cartilaginous tube, which proceeds from the larynx opposite the fifth cervical vertebra, and divides about the third dorsal vertebra into two tubes, called the right and left bronchi, one for each lung. Its length is from four to four and a half inches. Its transverse diameter is about eight or ten lines in the adult, but it varies according to the age of the individual, and the natural volume of the lungs. It is kept permanently open by a series of cartilaginous rings, from sixteen to twenty in number, which extend round the anterior two-thirds of its circumference. These rings are deficient at the posterior part of the tube, where it is completed by fibrous membrane. This deficiency is for the purpose of allowing the trachea to expand or contract; and the membranous part of the tube is provided with transverse muscular fibres which can approximate the ends of the rings.

Bronchi. The two bronchi differ in length, direction and diameter. The *right*, shorter than the left, is about an inch in length, and passes more horizontally to the root of its lung. It is larger in all its diameters than the left; hence, foreign bodies which have accidentally dropped into the trachea are more

L

likely to be carried into the right bronchus by the stream of the air. The *left* bronchus is about two inches in length, and descends more obliquely to its lung than the right.

The *cartilages* of the trachea vary in number from sixteen to twenty; those of the right bronchus from six to eight; those of the left from nine to twelve. They form about two-thirds of a circle, and resemble a horse-shoe in form. The cartilage at the bifurcation of the trachea is shaped like the letter V; its angle projects into the centre of the main tube, and its sides belong one to each bronchus.

The cartilages are connected, and covered on their outer and inner surfaces by a tough membrane, consisting of fibrous and yellow elastic tissue. This membrane is attached to the circumference of the cricoid cartilage, and is continued through the whole extent of the trachea and the bronchial tubes. Posteriorly, where the cartilages are deficient, it maintains the integrity of the tube; in this situation, it consists of parallel and closely arranged longitudinal fibres, which are seated immediately beneath the mucous membrane, and raise it into folds. The elasticity of this structure admits of the elongation and contraction of the trachea.

Between the fibrous and muscular layers of the trachea are a large number of small mucous glands, which are most numerous on the posterior part of the tube. In health, their secretion is clear, not tenacious, and just sufficient to lubricate the air-passages. In bronchitis, they are the sources of the abundant viscid expectoration.

Tracheal glands.

After removing the fibrous membrane and the tracheal glands from the back of the trachea, we expose a thin stratum of non-striped muscular fibres, some of which extend transversely between the posterior free ends of the cartilages, while others are arranged in longitudinal bundles. By their contraction, they approximate the ends of the cartilages, and diminish the calibre of the tube.

Muscular fibres.

The *mucous membrane* lining the air-passages is a continuation from that of the larynx. Its colour in the natural state is nearly white, but in catarrhal affections it becomes bright red, in consequence of the accumulation of blood in the capillary vessels. It is continued into the ultimate air-cells, where it becomes thinner and more transparent. Its surface is lined by a layer of epithelium of the ciliated kind, of which the vibratile movement is directed in such a way as to favour the expectoration of the mucus. The ciliated epithelium lining the mucous membrane ceases at the commencement of the air-cells, where it is replaced by the squamous variety.

At the root of the lung each bronchus divides into two branches, an upper and a lower, corresponding to the lobes of the lung; on the right side the lower branch sends a small division to the third lobe. The tubes diverge through the lung, and divide into branches, successively smaller and smaller, until they lead to the air-cells. These ramifications do not communicate with each other, they are like the branches of a tree; hence when a bronchial tube is obstructed, all supply of air is cut off from the cells to which it leads.

The several tissues, cartilaginous, fibrous, muscular, mucous, and glandular, which collectively compose the air-passages, are not present in equal proportions throughout all their ramifications, but each is placed in greater or less amount where it is required. The cartilaginous rings, necessary to keep the larger bronchi permanently open, become in the smaller tubes fewer and less regular in form: as the subdivisions of the tubes multiply, the cartilages consist of small pieces placed here and there,—they become less and less firm, and finally disappear altogether. The walls of the air-passages, when no longer traceable by the naked eye, are entirely membranous, being formed of fibrous, elastic, and muscular tissues.

Lobules of the lung. The surface of the healthy lung is marked by faint white lines, which map it out into a number of angular spaces of various size. These spaces indicate the lobules of the lung. Each lobule is a lung in miniature. Whoever understands the structure of a single lobule, understands the structure of the entire lung. The lobules are connected by fine areolar tissue, called 'interlobular,' which is everywhere soft and elastic to allow the free expansion of the organ. The cells of this tissue have no communication with the air-vesicles unless the latter be ruptured by excessive straining, and then this intermediate tissue becomes inflated with air, and gives rise to 'interlobular emphysema.' When infiltrated with serum it constitutes 'œdema' of the lungs.

Each lobule receives a small bronchial tube, which subdivides into smaller branches. Thus reduced in size, the walls of the tubes

Fig. 30.   Fig. 31.

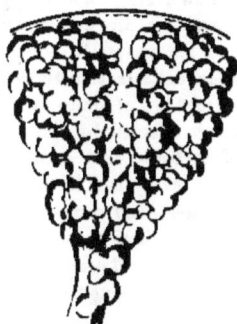   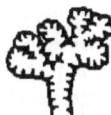

ULTIMATE AIR-CELLS OF THE LUNG (FROM KOLLIKER). MAGNIFIED TWENTY-FIVE TIMES

no longer present traces of cartilaginous tissue, but are composed of a delicate elastic membrane upon which the capillaries ramify in a very minute network.[*] Each tube finally leads into an irregular passage (*intercellular passage*), from which proceed on all sides numerous dilatations : these are the air-cells, which vary from the $\frac{1}{700}$th to the $\frac{1}{70}$th of an inch in diameter (fig. 31). The air-cells themselves present a number of shallow depressions, separated by somewhat prominent partitions, so that their interior has a

[*] In phthisis the expectoration contains some of the debris of this elastic framework of the air-vesicles; they can be seen under the microscope. This is not a bad test of the character of the sputa.

honeycomb appearance, as shown in fig 31. The purpose of this is to increase the extent of surface upon which the capillaries may ramify. The structure of the minute air-cell of the human lung is in all respects similar to the large respiratory sac of the reptile.

Pulmonary vessels. The branches of the pulmonary artery subdivide with the bronchial tubes. Their ultimate ramifications spread out in such profusion over the air-cells, that a successfully injected lung appears a mass of the finest network of capillaries. This network is so close that the interstices are even narrower than the vessels, which are on an average about $\frac{1}{5000}$th of an inch in diameter. The blood and air are not in actual contact. Nothing, however, intervenes but the wall of the cell and the capillary vessel, which are such delicate structures that they oppose no obstacle to the free interchange of gases by which the blood is purified. This purification is effected by the taking in of oxygen, and the elimination of carbonic acid and watery vapour. The most complete purification takes place in the single layer of capillaries between the folds of membrane projecting into the cell; for in this situation both sides of these vessels are exposed to the action of the air. The blood, circulating in steady streams through this capillary plexus, returns through the pulmonary veins. These, at first extremely minute, gradually coalesce into larger and larger branches, which accompany those of the arteries, and finally emerge from the root of the lung by two large trunks which carry the pure florid blood to the left auricle of the heart.

From this outline of the anatomy of the lung, we see that the organ is so constructed as, in a given space, to allow the largest possible quantity of impure blood to be brought in communication with the largest possible quantity of atmospheric air. It is difficult to conceive how any apparatus could be better adapted to the object in view. A stratum of blood of great superficial extent is exposed to an equal stratum of air, and these strata of contiguous fluids are contained in the interior of an organ so small as to lie within the compass of the chest.

These are small arteries, two or more in number for
Bronchial arteries. each lung. The right arises either from the first aortic
intercostal or, conjointly with the left bronchial, from the
concavity of the arch of the aorta. They enter the lung behind
the divisions of the bronchi, which they accompany. They are
the proper nutritive vessels of the organ. The old anatomists
called them the '*vasa privata pulmonum*,' to distinguish them
from the '*vasa publica pulmonum*'—namely, the pulmonary
arteries. The former provide '*pro existentia privata pulmonum;*' the latter '*pro bono publico totius organismi.*' The
bronchial vessels are distributed in various ways; some of their
branches supply the coats of the air-passages and the large blood-
vessels, others the interlobular tissue, and a few reach the surface
of the lung, and ramify beneath the pleura. The right *bronchial
veins* terminate in the vena azygos; the left, in the superior intercostal vein.

The *nerves* of the lung are derived from the pneumogastric and
the sympathetic. They enter with the bronchial tubes, forming a
plexus in front and behind them (anterior and posterior pulmonary
plexus).

The *absorbents* of the lung form a network upon its surface
and in the interlobular spaces. They all pass through the bronchial glands. Of these, the larger are situated about the bronchi
near the root of the lung, particularly under the bifurcation of the
trachea.

DISSECTION OF THE PHARYNX.

To obtain a view of the pharynx, cut through the trachea, œsophagus, and the great vessels of the neck, and then separate them
from the bodies of the cervical vertebræ, to which they are loosely
connected. The base of the skull should be sawn through between
the vertebral column and the styloid processes of the temporal
bones, so as to leave the pharynx and larynx attached to the anterior
half of the section. Horsehair should be introduced through the
mouth and œsophagus to distend the pharynx.

The term '*pharynx*' is applied to that part of the alimentary canal which receives the food after it has been masticated, and propels it downwards into the œsophagus. It is a funnel-shaped muscular bag, about four and a half inches in length. Its broadest portion is situated opposite the os-hyoides. Its upper part is attached to the basilar process of the occipital bone; from thence it extends perpendicularly as low as the cricoid cartilage, or the level of the fifth cervical vertebra, where the continuation of it takes the name of 'œsophagus.' The bag is connected behind to the bodies of the cervical vertebræ by loose areolar tissue which never contains fat. In abscesses at the back of the pharynx, the matter is seated in this tissue. *Parallel with and close to its sides run the internal carotid arteries.* Its dimensions are not equal throughout. Its breadth at the upper part is just equal to that of the posterior openings of the nose; here it is only required to transmit air; but it becomes much wider in the situation where it transmits the food—that is, at the back of the mouth: thence it gradually contracts to the œsophagus. The pharynx, therefore, may be compared to a funnel communicating in front by wide apertures with the nose, the mouth, and the larynx; while the œsophagus represents the tube leading from its lower end. The upper part of the funnel forms a cul-de-sac at the basilar process of the occipital bone. At this part there is, on each side, the opening of a narrow canal, called the 'Eustachian tube,' through which air passes to the tympanum of the ear.*

Before the muscles of the pharynx can be examined, we must remove a layer of condensed cellular membrane, called by some anatomists the '*pharyngeal fascia*.' It is a layer of deep cervical

---

* Observe that the pharynx conducts to the œsophagus by a gradual contraction of its channel. This transition, however, is in some cases sufficiently abrupt to detain a foreign body, such as a morsel of food more bulky than usual, at the top of the œsophagus. If such a substance become firmly impacted in this situation, one can readily understand that it will not only prevent the descent of food into the stomach, but that it may occasion, by its pressure on the trachea, alarming symptoms of suffocation. Supposing that the obstacle can neither be removed by the forceps, nor pushed into the stomach by the probang, it may then become necessary to extract it by making an incision into the œsophagus on the left side of the neck.

fascia behind the pharynx, and must not be confounded with the proper pharyngeal 'aponeurosis,' which intervenes between its muscular and mucous walls.

At the back of the pharynx, near the base of the skull, we find

Fig. 32.

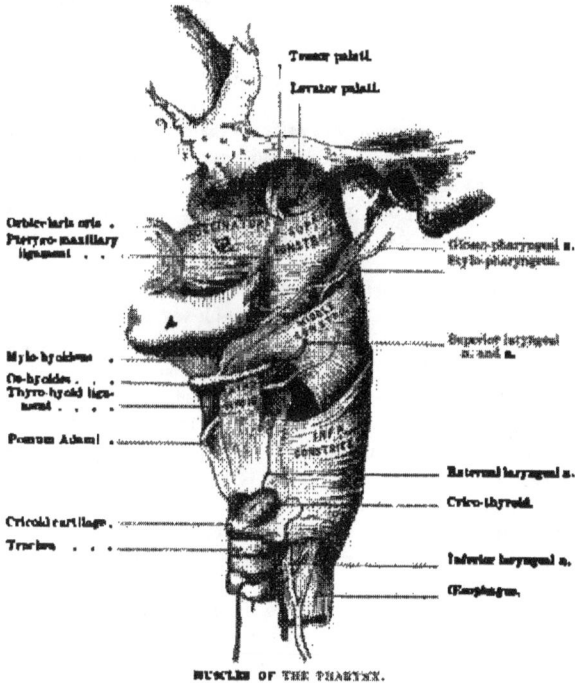

MUSCLES OF THE PHARYNX.

some *absorbent glands*. They sometimes enlarge, and form a perceptible tumour in the pharynx.

In removing the fascia from the pharyngeal muscles, notice

that a number of veins ramify and communicate in all directions.
They constitute the '*pharyngeal venous plexus*,' and terminate
in the internal jugular.

Constrictor muscles of the pharynx. They are three in number, and arranged so that they
overlap each other—i.e. the inferior overlaps the
middle, and the middle the superior (fig. 32). They
have the same attachments on both sides of the body; and the
fibres from the right and left meet together, and are inserted in
the mesial line, the insertion being marked by a white longitudinal
line called the ' raphé.'

The *inferior constrictor arises* from the side of the cricoid and
thyroid cartilages. Its fibres expand over the lower part of the
pharynx. The superior fibres ascend; the middle run transversely;
the inferior descend, and are identified with the œsophagus. Beneath its lower border the recurrent laryngeal nerve enters the
larynx.

The *middle constrictor arises* from the upper edge of the
greater cornu of the os-hyoides, from its lesser cornu, and part of
the stylo-hyoid ligament. Its fibres take different directions, so
that with those of the opposite muscle they form a lozenge. The
lower angle of the lozenge is covered by the inferior constrictor;
the upper angle ascends nearly to the basilar process of the occipital bone, and terminates upon the pharyngeal aponeurosis.
The external surface of the muscle is covered at its origin by the
hyo-glossus.

Between the middle and inferior constrictors, the superior
laryngeal artery and nerve perforate the thyro-hyoid membrane to
supply the larynx.

The *superior constrictor arises* from the hamular process of
the sphenoid bone, and from the lower part of its internal pterygoid plate; from the pterygo-maxillary ligament (which connects
it with the buccinator); from the mylo-hyoid ridge of the lower
jaw, and from the side of the tongue. The fibres pass backwards
to the mesial line: some of them are inserted through the medium
of the pharyngeal aponeurosis into the basilar process.

The upper border of the superior constrictor presents on either

side a free semilunar edge with its concavity upwards, so that
between it and the base of the skull a space is left in which the
muscle is deficient (fig. 32). Here the pharynx is strengthened
and walled in by its own aponeurosis. The space is called the
'sinus of Morgagni;' and in it, with a little dissection, we expose
the muscles which raise and tighten the soft palate : i.e. the levator
palati, and the tensor palati. The Eustachian tube opens into the
pharynx just here. Observe that the fibres of the stylo-pharyngeus
pass in between the superior and middle constrictors, and expand
upon the side of the pharynx ; some of them mingle with those of
the constrictors, but most of them are inserted into the posterior
margin of the thyroid cartilage.

Pharyngeal membrane or aponeurosis. The pharyngeal aponeurosis intervenes between the
muscles and the mucous membrane of the pharynx. It
is attached to the basilar process of the occipital bone,
and to the points of the petrous portions of the temporal bones.
It maintains the strength and integrity of the pharynx at its
upper part, where the muscular fibres are deficient; but it
gradually diminishes in thickness as it descends, and is finally lost
on the œsophagus. Notice the number of mucous glands upon
this aponeurosis, especially near the base of the skull and the
Eustachian tube. These glands sometimes enlarge and occasion
deafness from pressure on the tube.

Opening into the pharynx. Lay open the pharynx by a longitudinal incision, and
observe the seven openings leading into it (fig. 33):—
1. The two posterior openings of the nares.   2. On
either side of them, near the lower turbinated bones, are the
openings of the Eustachian tubes : below the nares is the soft
palate, with the uvula. 3. Below the soft palate is the communication with the mouth, called the 'isthmus faucium.' On either
side of this are two folds of mucous membrane, constituting the
anterior and posterior half-arches of the palate; between them are
the tonsils. Below the isthmus faucium is the epiglottis, which is
connected to the base of the tongue by three folds of mucous
membrane. 4. Below the epiglottis is the aperture of the larynx.
5. Lastly, is the opening into the œsophagus.

All these parts are lined by mucous membrane common to the entire tract of the respiratory passages and the alimentary canal. But this membrane presents characteristic differences in the dif-

Fig. 33.

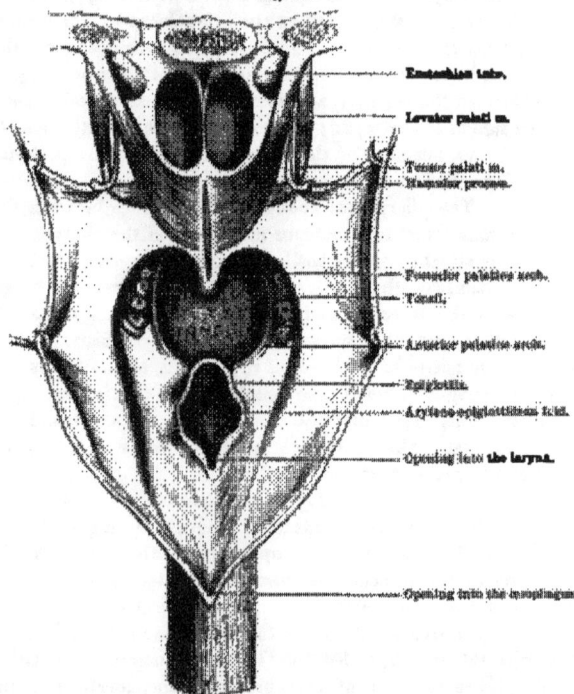

Eustachian tube.

Levator palati m.

Tensor palati m.
Hamulus process.

Posterior palatine arch.

Tonsil.

Anterior palatine arch.

Epiglottis.

Aryteno-epiglottidean fold.

Opening into the larynx.

Opening into the œsophagus.

VIEW OF THE PHARYNX LAID OPEN FROM BEHIND.

ferent parts of these channels, according as they are intended as passages for air or for food. The mucous membrane of the pharynx above the velum palati, being intended to transmit air only, is very

delicate in its texture, and lined by ciliated epithelium like the rest
of the air-passages. But opposite the fauces, the mucous membrane
in every respect resembles that of the mouth, and is provided with
squamous epithelium. At the back of the larynx the membrane is
corrugated into folds, to allow the expansion of the pharynx during
the passage of the food.

The membrane is lubricated by a plentiful secretion from the
numerous mucous glands which are situated in the submucous
tissue throughout the whole extent of the pharynx, more particularly
in the neighbourhood of the Eustachian tubes.

Posterior
openings of
the nose.
These are two oval openings, each of which is about
an inch long, and half an inch in the short diameter.
They are bounded above by the body of the sphenoid
bone, externally by its pterygoid plate, below by the horizontal
portion of the palate bone; they are separated from each other by
the vomer.

If you remove the mucous membrane from the posterior part of
the roof of the nose, and the top of the pharynx, you will find beneath
it much fibrous tissue. Hence polypi growing from these parts
are generally of a fibrous nature.

Isthmus
faucium.
This name is given to the opening by which the
mouth communicates with the pharynx. It is bounded,
above by the soft palate and uvula, below by the root of
the tongue, and on either side by the arches of the palate, enclosing
the tonsils between them.

Soft palate.
This movable prolongation of the roof of the mouth
is attached to the posterior border of the hard palate.
Inferiorly it is free, and from the middle hangs a pointed process
called the ' uvula.' It constitutes an imperfect partition between
the mouth and the posterior nares. Its upper or nasal surface is
convex and continuous with the floor of the nose; its lower surface
is concave, in adaptation to the back of the tongue, and is marked
in the middle by a ridge, indicating its original formation by two
lateral halves. When the soft palate is at rest, it hangs obliquely
downwards and backwards; but in swallowing, it is raised to the
horizontal position by the levatores palati, comes into apposition

with the back of the pharynx, and thus prevents the food from returning through the nose.

On making a perpendicular section through the soft palate, you see that the great bulk of it is made up of mucous glands, which lie thick on its under surface to lubricate the passage of the food. Above these glands we come upon the aponeurosis of the palate, still higher, upon the two portions of the palato-pharyngeus, separated by the fibres of the levator palati, and, lastly, upon the azygos uvulæ covered by the nasal mucous membrane. The soft palate is supplied with blood by the descending palatine branch of the internal maxillary, and the ascending palatine branch of the external maxillary. Its nerves are derived from the palatine branches of the second division of the fifth and from the glosso-pharyngeal.

Uvula. The uvula projects from the middle of the soft palate, and gives the free edge of it the appearance of a double arch. It contains a number of mucous glands, and a small muscle, the 'azygos uvulæ.' Its length varies in different individuals, and in the same person at different times, according to the state of its muscle. It occasionally becomes permanently elongated, and causes considerable irritation, a tickle in the throat, and harassing cough. When you have to remove a portion of it, cut off only the redundant mucous membrane.

Arches of the palate. The soft palate is continued into the tongue and pharynx by two folds of mucous membrane on each side, enclosing muscular fibres. These are the *anterior* and *posterior half arches* or *pillars* of the palate. The anterior arch describes a curve from the base of the uvula to the side of the tongue. It is well seen when the tongue is put out. The posterior arch, commencing at the side of the uvula, curves along the free margin of the palate, and terminates on the side of the pharynx. The posterior arches, when the tongue is depressed, can be seen through the span of the anterior. The pillars of each side diverge from their origin, and in the triangular space thus formed is situated the tonsil. The chief use of the arches of the palate is to assist in the mechanism of deglutition. The anterior (enclosing the *palato-glossi* muscles) contract so as to prevent the food

from coming back into the mouth: the posterior (enclosing the
'*palato-pharyngei*') contract like side curtains, and co-operate in
preventing the food from passing into the nose. In vomiting, food
does sometimes escape through the nostrils, but one cannot wonder
at this, considering the violence with which it is driven into the
pharynx.

Muscles of the soft palate. The muscles of the soft palate lie immediately under
the mucous membrane. There are five pairs—namely,
the 'levatores palati,' the 'circumflexi or tensores palati,'
the 'palato-glossi,' the 'palato-pharyngei,' and the 'azygos uvulæ.'
This last pair is sometimes described as a single muscle.

Levator palati. This muscle *arises* from the apex of the petrous
portion of the temporal bone and from the cartilage of
the Eustachian tube. Its fibres spread out, and are
inserted along the upper surface of the soft palate, meeting those
of its fellow in the middle line (fig. 33). Its action is to raise the
soft palate, so as to make it horizontal in deglutition.

Circumflexus or tensor palati. This muscle is situated between the internal pterygoid m. and the internal pterygoid plate of the sphenoid
bone. It *arises* from the scaphoid fossa, and from the
outer side of the cartilage of the Eustachian tube. Thence it descends perpendicularly, ends in a tendon which turns round the
hamular process, and expands into a broad aponeurosis, which is
inserted into the horizontal plate of the palate bone, and is also
connected to its fellow of the opposite side. It gives strength to
the soft palate. A synovial membrane facilitates the play of the
tendon round the hamular process. Its *action* is to draw down
and tighten the soft palate, and, owing to its insertion into the
palate bone, also to keep the Eustachian tube open.

Azygos or levator uvulæ. This consists of two thin bundles of muscular fibres
situated one on each side of the middle line. They
arise from the aponeurosis of the palate and descend
along the uvula nearly down to its extremity.

Palato-glossus and palato-pharyngeus. These muscles are contained within the arches of
the soft palate. The *palato-glossus*, within the an-
terior arch, proceeds from the anterior surface of the

soft palate to the side of the tongue, and is lost in the stylo-glossus muscle. The *palato-pharyngeus*, within the posterior arch, arises from the posterior border of the soft palate by two origins separated by the levator palati. It descends to the side of the pharynx, and mixes with the fibres of the inferior constrictor and the stylo-pharyngeus.

Tonsils. The tonsils are situated at the entrance of the fauces, between the arches of the palate. Their use is to lubricate the fauces during the passage of the food. On their inner surface are visible from twelve to fifteen orifices leading into depressions which give the tonsil an appearance like the shell of an almond. Hence, as well as from their oval figure, they are called the '*amygdulæ*.'

These openings lead into small follicles in the substance of the tonsil, lined by mucous membrane. Their walls are thick, and formed by a layer of closed cells situated in the submucous tissue. The cells secrete a glairy fluid, and closely resemble 'Peyers'' glands found in the intestines. The fluid, viscid and transparent, in the healthy state, is apt to become white and opaque in inflammatory affections of the tonsils, and occasionally accumulates in these superficial depressions, giving rise to the deceptive appearance of a small ulcer, or even a slough in the part.

Concerning the relations of the tonsil, remember that it lies close to the inner side of the internal carotid artery. It is only separated from this vessel by the superior constrictor and the aponeurosis of the pharynx. Therefore, in removing a portion of the tonsil, or in opening an abscess near it, the point of the instrument should never be directed outwards, but *inwards* towards the mesial line.* The tonsils are supplied with blood by the tonsillar branch of the external maxillary, and the descending palatine branch of the internal maxillary.

Eustachian tube. This canal conveys air from the pharynx to the tympanum of the ear. Its orifice is situated opposite the back part of the inferior spongy bone. The direc-

---

* Cases are related by Portal and Béclard, in which the carotid artery was punctured in opening an abscess in the tonsil. The result was immediately fatal hæmorrhage.

tion of the tube from the pharynx is upwards, backwards, and
outwards; it is an inch and a half long. The narrowest part is
about the middle, and here its walls are in contact. Near the
tympanum its walls are osseous, but towards the pharynx they are
composed of fibro-cartilage and fibrous membrane. The cartilaginous end projects between the origins of the levator and the
tensor palati, and gives attachment to some of their fibres. It is
situated at the base of the skull, in the furrow between the petrous
portion of the temporal and the great wing of the sphenoid bone.
It adheres closely to the bony furrow, as well as to the fibro-
cartilage filling up the 'foramen lacerum medium.' The orifice
is not trumpet-shaped, as usually described, but an elliptical slit
about half an inch long and nearly perpendicular. The fibro-
cartilage bounds it only on the inner and the upper part of the
circumference; the integrity of the canal externally is maintained
by tough fibrous membrane.

The Eustachian tube is lined by a continuation of the mucous
membrane of the pharynx, and covered by ciliated epithelium.
Hence, inflammatory affections of the throat or tonsils are liable
to be attended with deafness, from temporary obstruction of the
tube.

Mucous glands surround the orifice of the tube like a second
tonsil. They are similar in nature and function to the glands
beneath the mucous membrane of the mouth, the palate, and the
pharynx.

The hard palate, formed by the superior maxillary and palate
bones, serves as a fulcrum for the tongue in the act of tasting, in
mastication, in deglutition, and in the articulation of sounds. The
tissue covering the bones is thick and close in texture, and firmly
united to the asperities on the bones. But it is not everywhere of
equal thickness. Along the raphé in the mesial line, it is much
thinner than at the sides; for this reason, the hard palate is
in this situation more prone to be perforated by syphilitic disease.

A thick layer of glands (*glandulæ palatinæ*) is arranged in
rows on either side of the hard palate. These glands become more
numerous and larger towards the soft palate. Their orifices are

visible to the naked eye. The mucous membrane has a very thick epithelial coat, which gives the white colour to the palate. The descending palatine branch of the internal maxillary artery, and the palatine nerves from the superior maxillary, may be traced along each side of the roof of the mouth. The ramifications of these arteries and nerves supply the soft as well as the hard palate.

Mechanism of deglutition. With the anatomy of the parts fresh in your mind, consider for a moment the mechanism of deglutition. The food duly masticated, is collected into a mass upon the back of the tongue; the lower jaw is then closed to give a fixed point for the action of the muscles which raise the os-hyoides and larynx, and the food is carried back into the pharynx by the pressure of the tongue against the palate, at the same time that the pharynx is elevated and expanded to receive it.* Having reached the pharynx, the food is prevented from ascending into the nasal passages by the approximation of the posterior palatine arches, and the elevation of the soft palate, which thus forms a horizontal temporary roof to the pharynx; it is prevented from returning into the mouth by the pressure of the retracted tongue, and the contraction of the anterior palatine arches: it cannot enter the larynx, because its upper opening is closed and protected by the falling of the epiglottis:† consequently, being forcibly compressed by the constrictors of the pharynx, the food passes into the œsophagus.

The food passes with different degrees of rapidity through the different parts of its course; but most rapidly through the pharynx. The necessity of this is obvious, when we reflect that the air-tube must be closed while the food passes over it, and that the closure produces a temporary interruption to respiration. The progress of the food through the œsophagus is slow and gradual.

* The larynx being also elevated and drawn forward, a greater space is thus left between it and the vertebræ for the distention of the pharynx.

† This falling of the epiglottis is effected, not by special muscular agency, but by the simultaneous elevation of the larynx and the retraction of the tongue. A perpendicular section through all the parts concerned is necessary to show the working of this beautiful mechanism.

M

DISSECTION OF THE LARYNX.

Before commencing the dissection of the larynx, make yourself familiar with the cartilages which compose it, and the ligaments which connect them, as seen in a dry preparation.

Os-hyoides. This bone, named from its resemblance to the Greek letter Upsilon, is situated between the larynx and the tongue, and serves for the attachment of the muscles of the tongue. It may be felt immediately below, and one inch and a half behind the symphysis of the jaw. It is divided into a body, two greater and two lesser cornua. The *body* is the thick central portion. Its anterior surface is convex, and has a median vertical ridge; on each side of which are depressions for the attachment of muscles; its posterior surface is smooth, concave, and corresponds to the epiglottis. The *greater cornua* (right and left) project backwards for about an inch and a half, with a slight inclination upwards, and terminate in blunt ends tipped with cartilage. In young subjects they are connected to the body of the bone by fibro-cartilage; this in process of years becomes ossified. The *lesser cornua* are connected, one on each side, to the point of junction between the body and the greater cornua, by means of a little joint lined by synovial membrane, which admits of free motion. They are about the size of a barley-corn, and the stylo-hyoid ligaments are attached to them.

The os-hyoides is connected to the thyroid cartilage by several ligaments, which contain a quantity of elastic tissue. There is:—

1. The *thyro-hyoid membrane*, which proceeds from the superior border of the thyroid cartilage to the upper and posterior part of the body of the hyoid bone. In front of this membrane there is, in the perfect larynx, a *bursa*, of which the use is to facilitate the play of the thyroid cartilage behind the os-hyoides. The central portion is stronger than the lateral, hence it is sometimes called the *anterior thyro-hyoid* ligament. Through the lateral part of this membrane the superior laryngeal nerve and artery enter the larynx. 2. The right and left lateral *thyro-hyoid ligaments*

extend between the extremities of the greater cornua of the os-hyoides and the ascending cornua of the thyroid cartilage. They often contain a little nodule of cartilage.

Cartilages of the larynx. The frame-work of the larynx is composed of five cartilages connected by joints and elastic ligaments, so that they can be moved upon each other by appropriate muscles; the object of this motion being to act upon two elastic ligaments called the 'vocal cords,' upon which the voice essentially depends.

Thyroid cartilage. This cartilage, so called because it shields the beautiful mechanism behind it,* consists of two lateral halves (ala) united at an acute angle in front, which forms the prominence termed '*Pomum Adami.*' This prominence presents a notch at its upper part, to allow it to play behind the os-hyoides in deglutition. There is a bursa in front of it. I have seen this bursa as large as a pigeon's egg. The *outer* surface of each ala is marked by an oblique line passing downwards and forwards from the upper cornu, which gives attachment to the sterno-thyroid and thyro-hyoid muscles. The *inferior* border is slightly arched in the middle, and on either side presents a convex prominence, which gives attachment to the crico-thyroid muscle. The *superior* border is nearly horizontal. The *posterior* border is nearly vertical, and gives insertion to the stylo-pharyngeus and palato-pharyngeus muscles. This border terminates above and below in round projections called the *upper* and *lower cornua.* The upper is the longer; the lower articulates with the side of the cricoid cartilage.

Cricoid cartilage. This cartilage, named from its resemblance to a ring,† is situated below the thyroid. It is not of equal depth all round. It is narrow in front, where it may be felt about one quarter of an inch below the thyroid: from this part, the upper border gradually rises, so that, posteriorly, the ring is a full inch in vertical depth, and occupies part of the interval left between the alæ of the thyroid. In the middle of

---

* Θυρεὸς, a shield.   † Κρίκος, a ring.

this broad posterior surface is a vertical ridge, on either side of
which observe a superficial excavation for the origin of the crico-
arytenoidei postici. On its upper part are two oval slightly convex
surfaces for the articulation of the arytenoid cartilages. In front,
its upper border presents a broad excavation to which the crico-
thyroid ligament is attached. On its *lower* border, external to
the depression for the crico-arytenoideus posticus, is an elevated
facet which articulates with the inferior cornu of the thyroid cartilage. The lower border is connected by elastic membrane to the
first ring of the trachea.

The thyroid is connected to the cricoid cartilage in front by
the crico-thyroid membrane, which consists chiefly of elastic tissue,
and laterally by its two inferior horns. Between these two cartilages there is a perfect joint on either side, provided with a synovial membrane, and secured by capsular ligaments. The object of
this joint is to permit the approximation of the cartilages.

Arytenoid cartilages. These cartilages are situated, one on either side, at
the back of the cricoid. In the recent state, before the
membranes and muscles have been removed, the space
between them resembles the lip of a ewer;[*] hence their name.
Each is pyramidal with the apex upwards. The *posterior* surface
of each is concave, and gives attachment to the arytenoid muscle:
the *anterior* surface is convex and gives attachment to the thyro-
arytenoideus and the false vocal cord: the *internal* surface is
covered with mucous membrane and faces the corresponding surface of the opposite cartilage: the *base* presents an oval surface,
which articulates with the cricoid cartilage. This joint has a very
loose capsular and synovial membrane, which permits motion in
all directions, like the first joint of the thumb. In front of the
base is a tubercle (*anterior tubercle*), which gives attachment to
the true vocal cord, and contributes to form part of the boundary
of the rima glottidis. At the outer and back part of the base is
another tubercle (*external tubercle*), into which certain muscles
moving the cartilage are inserted; namely, the crico-arytenoideus

[*] 'Αρύταινα, a ewer.

posticus and crico-arytenoideus lateralis. The apex of the cartilage is surmounted by one or two cartilaginous nodules, called '*cornicula laryngis*.'

Epiglottis. This is a piece of yellow fibro-cartilage, which projects over the larynx like a valve. It is like a leaf in shape, with its stalk directed downwards. Its ordinary position is perpendicular, leaving the glottis free for respiration ; but during the elevation of the larynx in deglutition it becomes horizontal, falls over the glottis, and prevents the entrance of food into the larynx. Understand that this falling of the epiglottis is accomplished, not by special muscular agency, but by the simultaneous elevation of the larynx and the retraction of the tongue. Its apex or lower part is attached by the *thyro-epiglottidean* ligament to the angle of the thyroid cartilage ; it is also connected by another ligament (*hyo-epiglottidean*) to the os-hyoides.

The cartilages of the larynx resemble those of the ribs in structure. In the young they are dense and elastic, but they have a tendency to ossify with age. In very old subjects, the thyroid and cricoid cartilages are often completely ossified, and their interior presents an areolar tissue, containing oily matter, analogous to the spongy texture of the bones. The epiglottis is never ossified on account of its peculiar organisation, which resembles that of the ear and the nose.

The larynx is now to be examined in its perfect condition.

Mucous membrane of the larynx. Except on the true vocal cords and the epiglottis, the mucous membrane of the larynx presents a wrinkled appearance, and is loosely connected to the subjacent structures by an abundance of fibro-cellular tissue, which admits of its being pinched up into large folds. This tissue deserves notice from the rapidity with which it becomes the seat of serous effusion in acute inflammation of the larynx, and thus produces sudden and alarming symptoms of suffocation. From the root of the tongue to the anterior surface of the epiglottis, the membrane forms three folds (glosso-epiglottidean), one median, and two lateral, containing elastic tissue. From the epiglottis it is continued backwards on either side to the apices of the arytenoid

cartilages, forming the 'aryteno-epiglottidean' folds which bound
the entrance into the larynx. In the natural state it is of a pale
rose colour, and covered by ciliated epithelium below the false
vocal cords, above these by squamous epithelium.

The mucous membrane of the larynx is remarkable for its acute
sensibility. This is requisite to guard the glottis during the
passage of the food over it. The glottis is closed during the act of
deglutition; but, if during this process, any one attempt to speak
or laugh, the glottis opens, and allows the food to go, as it is
termed, the wrong way. As soon as the foreign body touches the
mucous membrane of the larynx, a spasmodic fit of coughing
expels it.

The sub-mucous tissue of the larynx is studded with mucous
glands. An oblong mass of them lies in the aryteno-epiglottidean
fold, and they are particularly numerous about the 'ventricles' of
the larynx. The surface of the epiglottis towards the tongue is
abundantly provided with them. Their ducts pass through the
epiglottis, and may be recognised as minute openings on its laryngeal aspect.

Superior   This is the opening by which the larynx communi-
opening of   cates with the pharynx. Its outline is triangular, with
the larynx.   its base directed forwards. Anteriorly it is bounded by
the epiglottis, laterally by the aryteno-epiglottidean folds, posteriorly by the arytenoid cartilages. The apex presents the funnel-
shape appearance from which the arytenoid cartilages derive their
name.

Inferior   Look down into the larynx and observe the trian-
opening of   gular horizontal opening in the middle line; this is the
the larynx,   'rima glottidis,' or 'glottis.' Its apex is directed
or rima
glottidis.   forwards, its base backwards. The anterior two-thirds
of this opening is bounded by the inferior or true vocal cords, the
posterior third by the arytenoid cartilages. Above the true vocal
cords are situated the superior or false vocal cords. On each side
of the larynx, between the true and false vocal cords, is a small
recess, the ventricle of the larynx, which leads into a pouch called
'sacculus laryngis.' Pass the handle of the scalpel into one of

these cavities, and observe that it leads into a cul-de-sac, which ascends for a short distance by the side of the thyroid cartilage. These pouches contain a large number of muciparous glands. The probable use of these cavities is to allow free space for the vibration of the vocal cords. The mucous membrane lining them is so sensitive that if a foreign body accidentally lodges there, the patient has no rest until it is expelled.

False vocal cords.
These are the prominent folds which form the upper boundaries of the ventricles. They are called the 'false vocal cords' because they have little or nothing to do with the production of the voice. They are composed of elastic tissue, like the true vocal cords; but they also contain fatty tissue, which the true ones do not.

Cords vocales.
These are two cords, composed of elastic tissue, extending horizontally from the angle of the thyroid cartilage to the base of each of the arytenoid. They diverge as they pass backwards; the space between them is called the 'rima glottidis.' We shall presently see that, through the muscles which act upon the arytenoid cartilages, these cords can be approximated or removed from each other; in other words, the rima glottidis can be closed or dilated. When sufficiently tightened, and brought parallel by means of certain muscles, the cords are made to vibrate by the stream of the expired air, and thus is produced the voice.

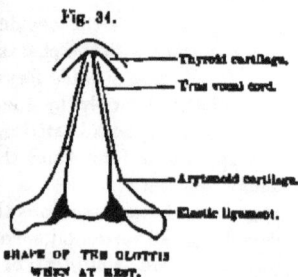

Fig. 34.

Thyroid cartilage.
True vocal cord.
Arytenoid cartilage.
Elastic ligament.

SHAPE OF THE GLOTTIS WHEN AT REST.

What is the length of the true vocal cords? In the adult male they measure about five-eighths of an inch; in the female about four-eighths. In boys they are shorter; hence their peculiar voice. At puberty, the cords lengthen, and the voice breaks.

The glottis admits of being dilated, contracted, and even completely closed by its appropriate muscles. When at rest, its shape

is triangular, as shown in fig. 34, where the arytenoid cartilages are
cut through on a level with the vocal cords. During every inspiration, the glottis is dilated by the crico-arytenoidei postici; it
then becomes spear-shaped (fig. 36). During expiration, it re-
sumes its triangular shape: and this return to a state of rest is
effected, not by muscular agency, but by two elastic ligaments
shown in fig. 34, which draw the arytenoid cartilages together.
Thus then the glottis, like the chest, is dilated by *muscular*
tissue; like the chest, also, it is contracted by *elastic* tissue. In

Fig. 35.

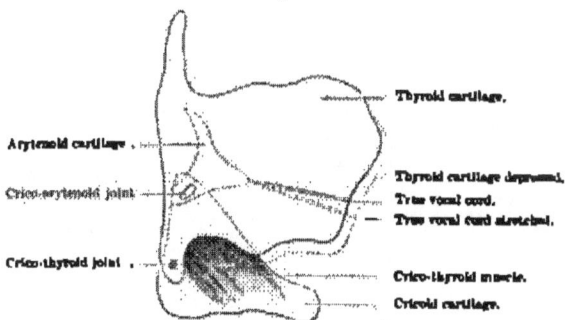

DIAGRAM SHOWING THE ACTION OF THE CRICO-THYROID MUSCLE.

speaking or singing, the glottis assumes what is called the vocalising position—that is, the opening becomes narrower and its
edges nearly parallel.

Intrinsic   There are nine muscles which act upon the 'rima
muscles of   glottidis:' four on each side and one in the middle.
the larynx.   The four pairs are—the crico-thyroidei, the crico-arytenoidei postici, the crico-arytenoidei laterales, and the thyro-aryte-
noidei. The single one is the arytenoideus.

                    This muscle is situated on the front of the larynx.
M. crico-   It *arises* from the side of the cricoid cartilage, ascends
thyroideus.   obliquely outwards, and is *inserted* into the inferior

border of the thyroid. Its *action* is to tighten the vocal cords. It does this by depressing the thyroid cartilage: for this cartilage cannot be depressed without lengthening these cords, as shown by the dotted line, fig. 35. Its nerve is the *external laryngeal* branch of the superior laryngeal.

M. crico-arytenoideus posticus.   This muscle *arises* from the posterior part of the cricoid cartilage: its fibres pass outwards and upwards, and are *inserted* into the external tubercle of the arytenoid. Its *action* is to dilate the glottis. It does this by drawing the posterior tubercle of the arytenoid cartilage *towards* the

Fig. 36.

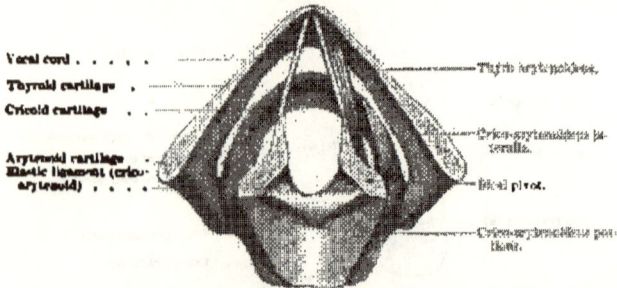

Vocal cord . . . . .
Thyroid cartilage . . .
Cricoid cartilage . . .
Arytenoid cartilage
Elastic ligament (crico-arytenoid) . . . .

Thyro-arytenoideus.
Crico-arytenoideus lateralis.
Ideal pivot.
Crico-arytenoideus posticus.

GLOTTIS DILATED. MUSCLES DILATING IT REPRESENTED WAVY.

mesial line, and therefore the anterior tubercle (to which the vocal cord is attached) *from* the mesial line (fig. 36). In this movement the arytenoid cartilage rotates as upon a pivot, and acts as a lever of the first order; the fulcrum or ideal pivot being intermediate between the power and the weight. This muscle dilates the glottis every time we inspire. Its nerve comes from the inferior laryngeal.

M. aryte-noideus.   This single muscle occupies the interval between the back of the arytenoid cartilages. The fibres pass across from one cartilage to the other. Most of them are transverse, but some cross like the letter X, running from the base of the one to the apex of the other cartilage. *Action.*—By clasping tho arytenoid cartilages, they assist in contracting the glottis.

M. crico-
arytenoideus
lateralis.   To expose this muscle, cut away the ala of the thyroid cartilage. It *arises* from the side of the cricoid cartilage, and is *inserted* into the external tubercle of the base of the arytenoid. *Action.*—By drawing the arytenoid cartilages inwards, the muscles of opposite sides contract

Fig. 37.

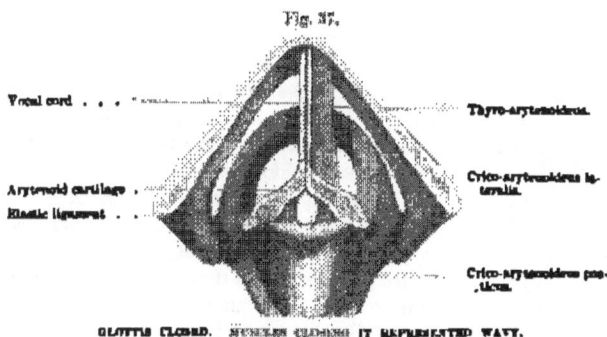

Vocal cord . . .   Thyro-arytenoideus.

Arytenoid cartilage .   Crico-arytenoideus la-
Elastic ligament . .   teralis.

                                                    Crico-arytenoideus pos-
                                                       ticus.

GLOTTIS CLOSED.   MUSCLES CLOSING IT REPRESENTED WAVY.

the glottis (fig. 37). Its nerve comes from the inferior laryngeal.

M. thyro-
arytenoi-
deus.   This muscle *arises* from the angle of the thyroid cartilage and the crico-thyroid membrane, runs horizontally backwards, and is *inserted* into the base and anterior border of the arytenoid. Its fibres run parallel with the vocal cord, and some of them are directly inserted into it. Part of the muscle spreads out so as to form a floor for the ventricle of the larynx, and is inserted into the outer border of the arytenoid cartilage. Nerve from the inferior laryngeal.

This muscle relaxes the vocal cord. More than this, it puts the lip of the glottis in the 'vocalising' position; in this position, the lips of the glottis are parallel, and the chink is reduced to the breadth of a shilling.*

* *M. aryteno-epiglottideus.*—This consists of a few pale muscular fibres enclosed in the aryteno-epiglottidean fold. Some of them run near the free margin of the fold.

The following table shows the action of the several muscles which act upon the glottis:—

Crico-thyroidei . . .	Stretch the Vocal Cords,
Thyro-arytenoidei . .	Relax the Vocal Cords, and place them in the vocalising position.
Crico-arytenoidei postici .	Dilate the glottis.
Crico-arytenoidei laterales .	Draw together the arytenoid cartilages
Arytenoideus . . .	Ditto Ditto Ditto

close the glottis.

The *blood-vessels of the larynx* are derived from the *superior* and *inferior thyroid arteries.* The laryngeal branch of the superior thyroid passes through the thyro-hyoid membrane with the corresponding nerve, and divides into branches, which supply the muscles and the mucous membrane. The laryngeal branches of the inferior thyroid ascend behind the cricoid cartilage. A constant artery passes through the crico-thyroid membrane.

The *nerves* of the larynx are the *superior* and *inferior* (recurrent) *laryngeal* branches of the pneumogastric.

The *superior laryngeal,* having passed through the thyro-hyoid membrane, divides into branches, distributed to the mucous membrane of the larynx. Its filaments spread out in various directions; some to the anterior and posterior surfaces of the epiglottis, and to the aryteno-epiglottidean folds, others to the interior of the larynx and the vocal cords. A constant filament descends behind the ala of the thyroid cartilage, and communicates with the recurrent. Its external laryngeal branch supplies the crico-thyroid muscle (p. 98).

The *inferior (recurrent) laryngeal nerve* enters the larynx beneath the Inferior constrictor, and ascends behind the joint between the thyroid and cricoid cartilages. It supplies all the intrinsic muscles of the larynx, except the crico-thyroid. If the recurrent nerve be divided, or in any way injured, the muscles

others are found lower down. These, being distributed over the ventricle of the larynx, can approximate its walls so as almost to obliterate the cavity. Hence the name 'compressor sacculi laryngis,' given to this part of the muscle by Mr. Hilton (Guy's Hospital Reports, vol. ii.), who first drew attention to it.

moving the glottis become paralysed, but its sensibility remains
unimpaired. When the nerve is compressed by a tumour—for
instance, an aneurism of the arch of the aorta—the voice is
changed to a whisper,* or even lost.

Difference
between the
male and
the female
larynx.

Until the approach of puberty, there is no great difference in the relative size of the male and female
larynx. The male larynx, within two years after this
time, becomes nearly doubled in size; the female grows
larger, but to a less extent.

The larynx of the adult male is in all proportions about one
third larger than that of the adult female.

The alæ of the thyroid cartilage form a more acute angle in the
male; hence the greater projection of the 'pomum Adami,' and
the greater length of the vocal cords, in the male.

The average length of the vocal cords is in the { Male . . . 8 lines. / Female . . 6 „

The average length of the glottis is in the . { Male . . . 12 lines. / Female . . 10 „

The size of the larynx does not necessarily follow the proportions
of the general stature; it may be as large in a little person as in a
tall one: this corresponds with what we know of the voice.

Crico-thy-
roid articu-
lation.

This joint is provided with a capsule and synovial
membrane. There are, besides, two strong ligaments.
Both proceed from the cornu of the thyroid cartilage;
the one upwards and backwards, the other downwards and forwards
to the cricoid. Remember that the only kind of motion permitted
is vertical: and that this motion regulates the tension of the
vocal cords.

DISSECTION OF THE TONGUE.

The tongue is a complex muscular organ, subservient to taste,
speech, suction, mastication, and deglutition. It is connected by
muscles (genio-hyo-glossus, hyo-glossus, and stylo-glossus) to the

* Medical Gazette, Dec. 1843.

symphysis of the jaw, to the os-hyoides, and to the styloid process of the temporal bone. To the soft palate it is connected by the anterior palatine arch (p. 157); and to the epiglottis by three folds of mucous membrane: in the middle fold is enclosed a layer of elastic tissue, called the 'glosso-epiglottidean' ligament. This pulls up the epiglottis when the tongue is put out of the mouth: hence the rule of never attempting to pass a tube into the œsophagus without pushing back the tongue; otherwise the tube would pass into the larynx.

The posterior part or root of the tongue is connected to the hyoid bone by the hyo-glossi and the genio-hyo-glossi muscles; its anterior part or tip is free, and lies behind the lower incisor teeth. Its upper surface or *dorsum* is convex with a median groove which terminates posteriorly in a mucous follicle, the '*foramen cæcum.*' On its under surface is a fold of mucous membrane, called the '*frænum linguæ,*' which connects the tongue to the floor of the mouth.

The surface of the tongue is covered with mucous membrane which consists of structures similar to those of the skin generally; that is to say, it consists of a 'cutis,' or true skin with numerous projections, called '*papillæ,*' and of a thick layer of squamous epithelium. The cutis is much thinner than that of the skin; it affords insertion to some of the superficial muscular fibres of the tongue, and the blood-vessels form a close network in it before they pass into the papillæ.

The papillæ on the tongue are distinguished, according to their size and form, into three kinds, viz. '*papillæ maximæ* or *circumvallatæ,*' '*papillæ fungiformæ,*' '*papillæ filiformæ.*' (Fig. 38.)

Papillæ of the tongue.

The *papillæ circumvallatæ* vary in number from eight to twelve. They are arranged at the back of the tongue in two rows, which converge like the branches of the letter V, with the apex backwards, towards the so-called 'foramen cæcum.' Each of these papillæ is circular, from the $\frac{1}{15}$th to $\frac{1}{17}$th of an inch wide, with a central depression, and surrounded by a fossa: the fossa itself is circumscribed by an elevated ring.

The *papillæ fungiformæ*, smaller and more numerous than the *circumvallata*, are scattered chiefly over the sides and tip of the tongue, and sparingly over its upper surface. They vary in shape, some being cylindrical, others having heads like mushrooms; whence their name. Near the apex of the tongue they may be distinguished during life from the other papillæ by their redder colour. In scarlatina, and some exanthematous fevers, these papillæ become elongated, and of a bright red colour: as the fever subsides, their points acquire a brownish tint; giving rise to what is called 'the strawberry tongue.'

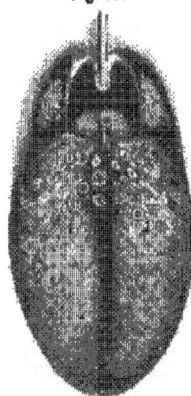

Fig. 38.

1. Papillæ circumvallatæ.
2. Papillæ fungiformæ.

The *papillæ filiformæ* are the smallest and most numerous. They are so closely aggregated that they give the tongue a velvet-like appearance. Their points are directed backwards, so that the tongue feels smooth, if the finger be passed over it from apex to base; but rough, if in the contrary direction. These papillæ consist of small conical processes arranged for the most part in a series of lines running parallel to the two rows of the papillæ circumvallatæ. Each papilla is covered with a thick layer of epithelium, which is prolonged into a number of free hair-like processes.

If the papillæ be injected, and examined under the microscope, it is found that they are not simple elevations, like those of the skin, but that from them arise secondary papillæ. The 'papillæ circumvallatæ' consist of an aggregation of smaller papillæ arranged parallel to each other; and the papillæ fungiformæ consist of central stems from which minute secondary papillæ shoot off. This elaborate structure escapes observation because it is buried beneath the epithelium.* Each secondary papilla receives a blood-vessel, which passes nearly to its apex, and returns in a loop-like manner,

* See Bowman and Todd's 'Physiological Anatomy.'

Filaments of the gustatory nerve have been traced in the papillæ circumvallatæ and fungiformæ, where they terminate in a minute plexus. Their mode of termination in the papillæ filiformæ has not been satisfactorily determined.

All the papillæ are covered with a layer of squamous or tessellated epithelium. That which covers the filiform is thicker than the rest, and with a microscope is seen to project from their sides like hair. The various kinds of 'fur' on the tongue consist of thickened and sodden epithelium.

Respecting the use of the papillæ, it is probable that they enable the tongue to detect impressions with greater delicacy; and that they are instrumental in detecting different kinds of sensation, whether of taste or touch. From the density and arrangement of their epithelial coat, the filiform papillæ give the surface of the tongue a roughness which is useful in its action upon the food. An apparatus of this kind, proportionately stronger and more developed, makes the tongue of ruminant animals an instrument by which they lay hold of their food. In the feline tribe, e.g. the lion and tiger, these papillæ are so sharp and strong that they act like rasps, and enable the animal to lick the periosteum from the bones by a single stroke of his tongue. In some mammalia, they act like combs for cleaning the skin and the hair.

Numerous small glands are found in the submucous tissue at the root of the tongue. They are similar in structure and secretion to the tonsillar and palatine glands, so that there is a complete ring of glands round the isthmus faucium. Small round orifices upon their surface indicate the termination of their ducts. Other mucous glands, with ducts from one quarter to half an inch long, are situated in the muscular substance of the tongue.

Glands beneath the apex of the tongue. On the under surface of the apex of the tongue is placed, on either side, a group of glands presumed to be salivary. Considering each group as one gland, observe that it is oblong, with the long diameter from seven to ten lines, parallel with the axis of the tongue. It lies near the mesial line, a little below the ranine artery, on the outer side of the branches of the gustatory nerve, under some of the fibres of the stylo-glossus. Four or five ducts proceed from each group, and terminate by separate orifices on the under surface of the tongue.

Muscular fibres of the tongue. The interior of the tongue is composed of muscular fibre and of a small quantity of fat. The *extrinsic* muscles of the tongue have been described in the dissection of the submaxillary region (p. 41). We have now to examine its *intrinsic* muscles. For this purpose the mucous membrane must be removed from the top of the tongue. On dissection it will be found that the great bulk of the organ consists of fibres which proceed in a longitudinal direction, constituting the ' *linguales* ' muscles. The lingualis of each half of the tongue is separated into a *superior* and *inferior* layer by some transverse fibres which pass nearly horizontally outwards from the ' *fibrous septum* ' of the tongue. The *superior* fibres run in a longitudinal direction under the mucous membrane of the dorsum, and are inserted into the submucous tissue. The ' *inferior* fibres ' (or ' *true lingualis* '), more numerous than the preceding, are situated between the genio-hyo-glossus and the hyo-glossus, and proceed from the base to the apex of the tongue : these are readily exposed by dissecting on the under surface of the tongue immediately on the outer surface of the genio-hyo-glossus. By the action of this mass of longitudinal fibres the tongue can be moved so as to reach any part of the mouth. Besides these longitudinal fibres, there are *transverse* fibres which arise from the fibrous septum. These pass outwards, running between the superior and inferior lingualis, and are inserted into the sides of the tongue. A considerable quantity of fat is found among these fibres.

If we trace the genio-hyo-glossi of opposite sides into the tongue, we find that some of their fibres ascend directly to the surface ; others cross each other in the middle line, intersect the longitudinal fibres, and finally terminate upon the sides of the tongue. Lastly, the fibres of the stylo-glossus should be traced along the side of the tongue to the apex.

Fibrous septum of the tongue. In the mesial line, extending from the base to the apex of the tongue, is found a vertical plane of fibrous tissue, ' *the fibrous septum* ; ' connected behind to the body of the hyoid bone, and lost in front between the muscles. In it is sometimes found a piece of fibro-cartilage, called '*nucleus fibrosus linguæ*,' a feeble representative of the lingual bone in some of the lower animals.

The *nerves supplying the tongue* should be followed into its substance. The hypoglossal nerve supplies all the muscles with motor power. The gustatory or lingual branch of the fifth pair is distributed to the mucous membrane about the apex and sides of the tongue, and endows it with most acute sensibility. Upon this nerve depends the sensation of all ordinary impressions, such as that of hardness, softness, heat, cold, and the like. The glosso-pharyngeal nerve supplies the mucous membrane at the back and sides of the tongue. It is especially a nerve of taste.

DISSECTION OF THE ORBIT.

To expose the contents of the orbit, saw through the roof of the orbit as far back as the optic foramen, making one section on the outer side and the other on the inner side of the roof. In doing this, be careful not to injure the little pulley on the inner side for the superior oblique. The anterior fourth of the roof should be left *in situ*, the remainder removed by bone forceps. The eyeball should be made tense by blowing air through a blow-pipe, passed well into the globe through the end of the optic nerve.

Periosteum of the orbit. The roof being removed, we expose the fibrous membrane, which lines the walls of the orbit. It is a continuation of the dura mater through the sphenoidal fissure. Traced forwards, we find that at the margin of the orbit it divides into two layers, one of which is continuous with the periosteum of the forehead, the other forms the broad tarsal ligament which fixes the tarsal cartilage.

Fascia of the orbit. The fascia of the orbit serves the same purpose that fascia does in other parts. It provides the lachrymal gland, and each of the muscles, with a loose sheath, thin and delicate at the back of the orbit, but stronger near the eye. In this situation it passes from one rectus muscle to the other, so that their tendinous insertions into the globe are connected by it. From the insertion of the muscles it is reflected backwards over the globe of the eye, and the optic nerve, and separates the eye from the fat at the bottom of the orbit.

Muscles and nerves of the orbit.   There are six muscles to move the eye; four of which, running in a straight direction, are called the 'recti,' and are arranged one above, one below, and one on each side of the globe. The remaining two are called from their direction, 'obliqui,' one superior, the other inferior. There is also a muscle to raise the upper eyelid, termed 'levator palpebræ.'

Fig. 39.

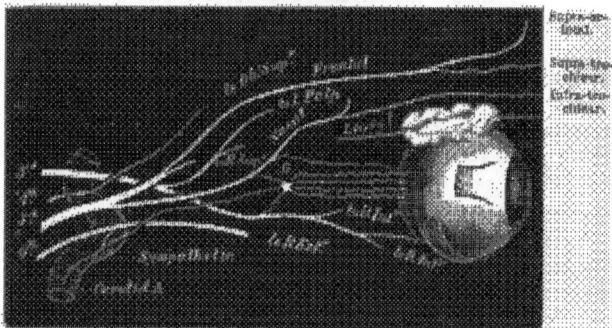

DIAGRAM OF THE NERVES OF THE ORBIT.

The *nerves* are: the optic, which passes through the optic foramen; the third, the fourth, the first division of the fifth, and the sixth, all of which pass through the sphenoidal fissure. The third supplies all the muscles with motor power, except the superior oblique, which is supplied by the fourth, and the external rectus, which is supplied by the sixth. The ophthalmic division of the fifth divides into a frontal, lachrymal, and nasal branch. The orbit contains, also, a considerable quantity of soft fat, which forms a bed for the eye and prevents it from being pulled too far back by its muscles. Upon the quantity of this fat depends, in some measure, the difference in the prominence of the eyes. Its absorp-

tion in disease or old age occasions the sinking of the eyes. The
eye is separated from the fat by a fold of the orbital fascia, which,
like a 'tunica vaginalis,' enables the globe to roll with the greatest
rapidity and precision. Lastly, the orbit contains the lachrymal
gland.

After the removal of the periosteum, and the fascia of the orbit,
the following objects are seen. In the middle we observe the
frontal nerve and artery, lying upon the levator palpebræ; on the
inner side is the superior oblique muscle with its nerve (the 4th);
on the outer side is the lachrymal gland with the *lachrymal* nerve
and artery.

Frontal nerve. This is the largest of the three branches of the ophthalmic division of the fifth. It runs forwards upon
the upper surface of the levator palpebræ, on which it
divides into two branches :—

a. The *supra-trochlear* runs above the pulley of the superior
oblique to the inner angle of the orbit, and divides into branches,
which supply the skin of the upper eyelid, forehead, and nose.
One or two very delicate filaments may be traced through the
bone to the mucous membrane of the frontal sinuses.*

b. The *supra-orbital* runs forwards to the supra-orbital notch,
through which it ascends. It supplies the skin of the upper eyelid, forehead, and scalp.

Lachrymal nerve. This is the smallest of the three divisions of the
ophthalmic. It runs along the outer side of the orbit
with the lachrymal artery, through the lachrymal gland,
and is distributed to the upper eyelid. Its branches within the
orbit are: 1, filaments to the *lachrymal gland*; 2, a *malar*,
which traverses a canal in the malar bone, and supplies the skin
of the cheek; 3, one or two nerves, which pass down to communicate with the orbital branch of the superior maxillary division of
the fifth.

Fourth, or nervus patheticus. This nerve enters the orbit above the other nerves
which pass through the sphenoidal fissure. It runs
along the inner side of the frontal nerve, and enters

* These filaments have been noticed by Blumenbach, ' De Sinibus Frontal.'
x 2

the orbital surface of the superior oblique, to which it is exclusively distributed.

Lacbrymal gland. This gland is situated within the external angular process of the frontal bone. It is about the size and shape of an almond. Its upper surface is convex, in adaptation to the roof of the orbit; its lower is concave, in adaptation to the eyeball. The anterior part of the gland lies sometimes detached from the rest, close to the back part of the upper eyelid, and is covered by the conjunctiva. The whole gland is kept in place by a capsule * formed by the fascia of the orbit. In structure it resembles the salivary glands.

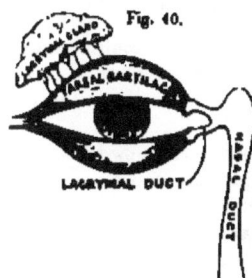

Fig. 40.

It consists of an aggregation of small lobes composed of smaller lobules, connected by fibro-cellular tissue. The excretory ducts, seven to ten in number, run parallel, and perforate the conjunctiva about a quarter of an inch above the edge of the tarsal cartilage (fig. 40). They are not easily discovered in the human eye, but in that of the horse or bullock they are large enough to admit a small probe. The secretion of the gland keeps the surface of the cornea constantly moist and polished; but if dust, or any foreign substance, irritate the eye, the tears flow in abundance, and wash it off.

All the muscles of the orbit, with the exception of the inferior oblique, arise from the margin of the foramen opticum, and pass forwards, like ribands, to their insertions.

Levator palpebræ superioris. This muscle *arises* from the roof of the orbit, immediately in front of the optic foramen. It gradually increases in breadth, and terminates in a broad, thin aponeurosis, which is *inserted* into the upper surface of the tarsal cartilage beneath the palpebral ligament. It is constantly in

---

* This capsule, being a little stronger on the under surface of the gland, is described and figured by Sœmmerring as a distinct ligament, ' Icones Oculi Humani,' tab. vii.

action when the eyes are open, in order to counteract the tendency of the lids to fall. As sleep approaches, the muscle relaxes,
the eyes feel heavy, and the lids close. Its nerve comes from the
superior division of the third nerve, and enters it on its under
aspect.

Obliquus
superior.

This muscle *arises* from the inner side of the foramen opticum. It runs along the inner side of the
orbit, and terminates in a round tendon, which passes
through a cartilaginous pulley attached to the anterior and inner
part of the roof of the orbit. From this pulley the tendon is
reflected outwards and backwards to the globe of the eye. It
gradually expands, and is inserted into the outer and back part of
the sclerotica, between the external and superior recti. The
pulley is lined by a synovial membrane, which is continued upon
the tendon. The *action* of this muscle is to roll the eye on its own
axis. It is supplied by the fourth nerve, which enters the back
part of its upper surface.

The frontal nerve and levator palpebræ should now be reflected
from their middle, to expose the superior rectus muscle.

Recti
muscles.

These four muscles have a tendinous origin round
the foramen opticum, so that collectively they embrace
the optic nerve. They diverge from each other, one
above, one below, and one on either side of the optic nerve; and
are named, accordingly, *rectus superior, inferior, externus,* and
internus. Their broad thin tendons are inserted into the opposite
sides of the sclerotic coat of the eye, about a quarter of an inch
from the margin of the cornea (fig. 41).

The *external* rectus not only arises from the circumference of
the optic foramen, but has another origin from the lower margin
of the sphenoid fissure. Between these origins pass the third nerve,
the nasal branch of the fifth, the sixth, and the ophthalmic vein.

The recti muscles enable us to direct the eye towards different
points; hence the names given to them by Albinus—attollens,
depressor, adductor, and abductor oculi. It is obvious that by
the single action of one, or the combined action of two, the eye
can be turned towards any direction.

The rectus superior is supplied by the upper division of the third nerve; the rectus internus, the rectus inferior and obliquus inferior, by the lower division. The rectus externus is supplied by the sixth.

Follow the recti to the eye, in order to see the tendons by which they are inserted. Notice also the 'anterior ciliary arteries,' which run to the eye along the tendons. The congestion of these little

Fig. 41.

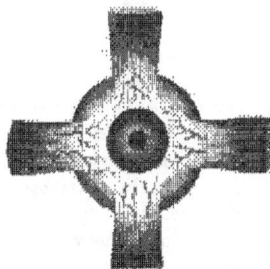

INSERTION OF THE RECTI MUSCLES WITH ANTERIOR CILIARY ARTERIES.

vessels occasions the red zone round the cornea in iritis. It has been already mentioned that the tendons are invested by a fascia, which passes from one to the other, forming a loose tunic over the back of the eye. It is this fascia which resists the passage of the hook in the operation for the cure of squinting. Even after the complete division of the tendon, the eye may still be held in its faulty position, if this tissue, instead of possessing its proper softness and pliancy, happen to have become contracted and unyielding. Under such circumstances it is necessary to divide it freely with the scissors.

By removing the conjunctival coat of the eye, the tendons of the recti are soon exposed. The breadth and the precise situation of their insertion deserve attention in reference to the operation for strabismus. The breadth of their insertion is about three eighths of an inch, but the line of this insertion is not at all points equidistant from the cornea. The centre of the insertion is nearer to the cornea by about one line than either end. Taking the internal rectus, which has most frequently to be divided in strabismus, we find that the centre of its tendon is, upon an average, three lines only from the cornea, the lower part nearly five lines, and the upper four. It is, therefore, very possible that the lower part may be left undivided in the operation, being more in the background than the rest. The tendon of the internal rectus is nearer to the cornea than either of the others.

The superior rectus must now be reflected : in doing so, observe the branch from the upper division of the third nerve, which supplies it and the levator palpebræ. After the removal of a quantity of fat, we expose the following objects:—1, the optic nerve ; 2, the nasal nerve, the ophthalmic artery and vein, all of which cross over the optic nerve from without inwards; 3, the inferior part of the third nerve; 4, deeper towards the back of the orbit, between the optic nerve and the external rectus, is situated the ' ophthalmic or lenticular ' ganglion ; and 5, the sixth nerve entering the ocular aspect of the rectus externus.

Nasal nerve. This is one of the three divisions of the ophthalmic branch of the fifth pair (p. 178). It enters the orbit through the sphenoidal fissure between the two origins of the external rectus, and then crosses obliquely over the optic nerve towards the inner wall of the orbit. After giving off the *infra-trochlear* branch, the nerve runs out of the orbit between the superior oblique and internal rectus, through the foramen orbitale anterius, into the cranium, where it lies beneath the dura mater, upon the cribriform plate of the ethmoid bone. However, it soon leaves the cranium through a slit near the ' crista galli,' and enters the nose. Here it sends filaments to the mucous membrane of the upper part of the septum, and superior spongy bone ; but the main continuation of the nerve runs behind the nasal bone, becomes superficial between the bone and the cartilage, and, under the name of naso-lobular, is distributed to the skin of the ala and tip of the nose.

The nasal nerve gives off the following branches in the orbit:—

a. One or two slender filaments to the *lenticular ganglion,* forming its upper or long root.

b. One or two *long ciliary* nerves. They run to the back of the globe of the eye, and pass through the sclerotic coat to supply the iris.

c. *Infra-trochlear* nerve.—This runs below the pulley of the superior oblique, where it communicates with the supra-trochlear

branch of the frontal nerve. It then divides into filaments, which
supply the skin of the eyelids, the lachrymal sac, and the side of
the nose.

Optic nerve.   Having passed through the optic foramen, this nerve
proceeds forwards and a little outwards to the globe of
the eye, which it enters on the nasal side of its axis. It then
expands to form the retina. The nerve is invested by a fibrous
coat derived from the dura mater. At the optic foramen it is surrounded by the tendinous origins of the recti; in the rest of its
course, by loose fat and by the ciliary nerves and arteries.

Ophthalmic artery.   This artery arises from the internal carotid. It
enters the orbit through the optic foramen, outside the
optic nerve; occasionally through the sphenoidal fissure. Its course is remarkably tortuous. Situated at first on the
outer side of the optic nerve, it soon crosses over it, and runs along
the inner side of the orbit, to inosculate with the internal angular
artery (the terminal branch of the facial). Its branches arise in
the following order :—

a. *Lachrymal artery.*—This branch proceeds along the outer
side of the orbit to the lachrymal gland. After supplying the
gland, it terminates in the upper eyelid. It anastomoses with the
deep temporal arteries, and also with a branch from the arteria
meningea media.

b. *Supra-orbital artery.*—This branch runs forwards with the
frontal nerve along the roof of the orbit, and emerges on the forehead through the supra-orbital notch.

c. *Arteria centralis retinæ.*—This small branch enters the
optic nerve, and runs in the centre of this nerve to the interior of
the eye.

d. *Ciliary arteries.*—These branches proceed tortuously forwards
with the optic nerve. They vary from fifteen to twenty in number,
and perforate the sclerotic coat at the back of the eye, to supply
the choroid coat and the iris. They are sometimes called '*posterior ciliary*,' to distinguish them from others named '*anterior
ciliary*' (branches of the muscular arteries), which proceed with
the tendons of the recti muscles, and enter the front part of the

sclerotica. In inflammation of the iris the vascular zone round the cornea arises from enlargement and congestion of the anterior ciliary arteries.

e. Ethmoidal arteries.—These branches are two in number, the *anterior*, the larger, passes through the anterior orbital foramen with the nasal nerve; the *posterior* enters the posterior orbital foramen. Both give off anterior meningeal branches to the dura mater, and also supply the mucous membrane of the nose.

f. Muscular arteries.—These are uncertain in their origin, and give off the anterior ciliary branches.

g. Pulpebral arteries.—These branches proceed from the lachrymal, nasal, and supra-orbital arteries.

h. Nasal artery.—This branch may be considered one of the terminal divisions of the ophthalmic. It leaves the orbit on the nasal side of the eye, and inosculates with the angular artery (termination of the facial). It supplies the side of the nose and the lachrymal sac.

i. Frontal artery.—This is the other terminal branch of the ophthalmic. It emerges at the inner angle of the eye, runs upwards, and inosculates with the supra-orbital artery.

Ophthalmic vein. This commences at the inner angle of the eye, by a communication with the frontal and angular veins. It runs backwards above the optic nerve in a straighter course than the artery, receives corresponding branches, and finally passes between the two origins of the external rectus, to terminate in the cavernous sinus.

Ophthalmic or lenticular ganglion. This little ganglion (*o*, p. 178), about the size of a pin's head, is situated at the back of the orbit, between the optic nerve and the external rectus. It receives a *sensitive* branch (long root) from the nasal nerve, which joins its posterior superior angle; a *motor* branch (short root) from the lower division of the third, which enters its posterior inferior angle; and it also receives (*sympathetic*) filaments from the plexus round the internal carotid artery, which enter the ganglion between its long and short roots. The ganglion thus furnished with motor, sensitive, and sympathetic roots, gives off the ciliary nerves.

These, from ten to twelve in number, run forward very tortuously with the optic nerve, pass through the back of the sclerotica, and are distributed to the iris. Since the ciliary nerves derive their motor influence from the third nerve, we see that the iris must lose its power of motion when this nerve is paralysed.

Third nerve, motor oculi.   Just before it enters the sphenoidal fissure, the third nerve divides into two branches, both of which pass between the origins of the external rectus. The upper division has been already traced into the superior rectus and levator palpebræ. The lower division supplies a branch to the internal rectus, another to the inferior rectus, and then runs along the floor of the orbit to the inferior oblique muscle.

What is the result of paralysis of the third nerve? falling of the upper eyelid (ptosis), external squint, dilatation and immobility of the pupil.

Sixth nerve, motor externus.   This nerve enters the orbit between the origins of the external rectus, and terminates in fine filaments, which are exclusively distributed to the ocular surface of this muscle.

Respecting the motor nerves in the orbit, observe that they all enter the ocular surface of the muscles, with the exception of the fourth.

Inferior oblique muscle.   This muscle arises by a flat tendon from the superior maxillary bone, near the lower part of the lachrymal groove. It runs outwards and backwards between the rectus inferior and the orbit, then curves upwards between the globe and the external rectus, and is inserted by a broad thin tendon into the outer and back part of the sclerotic coat, close to the tendon of the superior oblique. It is supplied by the lower division of the third n.

Action of the oblique muscles of the eye.   The use of the oblique muscles is to rotate the eye upon its antero-posterior axis, so that, however much the head be moved obliquely to one side or the other, the image of the object may be always kept stationary upon one and the same point of the retina. This was first explained by Hunter. He says—' When the head is moved towards

the right shoulder, the superior oblique muscle of the right side
acts and keeps the right eye fixed on the object, and a similar
effect is produced upon the left eye by the action of its inferior
oblique muscle. When the head moves in a contrary direction,
the other oblique muscles produce the same effect.' *

Tensor tarsi.   This muscle has been particularly described by
Horner,† an American anatomist. To expose it, cut
perpendicularly through the middle of the upper and lower lids,
and evert the inner halves towards the nose. After removing the
mucous membrane, the muscle will be seen *arising* from the ridge
on the lachrymal bone. It passes outwards and divides into two
portions, which are *inserted* into the upper and lower tarsal
cartilages, close to the orifices of the lachrymal ducts. It is
probable that the tensor tarsi draws backwards the open mouths
of the ducts, so that they may absorb the tears at the inner angle
of the eye. It is supplied by a small branch of the facial nerve.

Orbital
branch of
the superior
maxillary
nerve.   This is always very small, and is sometimes absent.
It comes from the trunk of the superior maxillary in
the spheno-maxillary fossa (see diagram), enters the
orbit through the spheno-maxillary fissure, and divides
into two branches. Of these, one, the *temporal*, after sending a
branch of communication to the lachrymal nerve in the orbit,
passes through a foramen in the malar bone to the temporal fossa.
It then pierces the temporal aponeurosis an inch above the
zygoma, and supplies the skin of the temple, joining the temporo-
auricular branch of the inferior maxillary. The other branch, *the
malar* ('*subcutaneus malæ*'), also passes through a foramen in
the malar bone, and supplies the skin of the cheek.

Superior
maxillary
nerve, and
spheno-pala-
tine ganglion.   To trace this nerve and its branches, we must remove
the outer wall of the orbit, so as to expose the spheno-
maxillary fossa.
The superior maxillary nerve is the second division
of the fifth cerebral nerve. Proceeding from the Gasserian gan-

---

* Observations on Certain Parts of the Animal Economy.

† Philadelphia Journal, Nov. 1824. But this muscle was accurately described by
Rosenmüller in his Handbuch der Anatomie. Leipzig, 1819.

glion (fig. 42), it leaves the skull through the foramen rotundum, passes horizontally forwards across the spheno-maxillary fossa, enters the infra-orbital canal with the corresponding artery, and finally emerges upon the face, through the infra-orbital foramen, beneath the levator labii superioris. The branches given off are:—

a. The *orbital* branch already described (p. 187).

b. Two branches to the *spheno-palatine ganglion* (Meckel's), situated in the spheno-maxillary fossa.

c. *Posterior dental* branches, two or three. They descend along the back part of the superior maxillary bone, and divide into

Fig. 42.

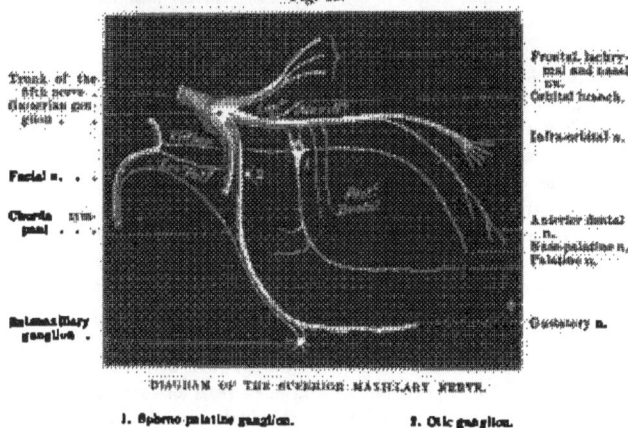

DIAGRAM OF THE SUPERIOR MAXILLARY NERVE.

1. Spheno-palatine ganglion.   2. Otic ganglion.

smaller branches, which pass through holes in the bone in company with minute arteries, and then run up the fangs of the molar teeth to supply the pulp. They also supply the gums, and the lining membrane of the antrum.

d. *Anterior dental* branch.—This arises just before the nerve emerges from the infra-orbital foramen. It descends in a special canal in the anterior wall of the upper jaw, and gives filaments to

the fangs of the first molar, canine, and incisor teeth. It also
supplies the gums and the mucous lining of the antrum.

· *e.* The terminal branch, namely, the *infra-orbital*, was dissected
with the face (p. 82).

At this stage of the dissection, make a vertical incision rather on
one side of the middle line of the skull, to expose the cavity of
the nose. We shall thus be able to dissect the 'spheno-palatine
ganglion' and its branches.

Spheno-pala-
tine ganglion.

This little body (fig. 42), called, after its discoverer,
'*Meckel's ganglion,*' is deeply situated in the spheno-
maxillary fossa, close to the outer side of the spheno-
palatine foramen, immediately below the superior maxillary nerve.
Its *sensitive* roots proceed from the superior maxillary; Its *motor*
root from the vidian branch of the facial; its *sympathetic* from the
carotid plexus, which joins the vidian nerve before it enters the
ganglion. Thus supplied, it furnishes branches to the mucous
membrane and glands of the hard and soft palate, and to the back
part of the nose.

Meckel's ganglion gives off the following branches:—

a. Branches to the palate.—To see these the mucous membrane
must be removed from the back part of the nose; we shall then be
able to trace the nerves through their bony canals. Their course
is indicated by corresponding arteries. There are generally three
of these nerves, called by names originally given to them by
Meckel, *anterior, middle,* and *posterior* palatine. The *anterior,*
the large palatine nerve, descends through the posterior palatine
canal to the roof of the mouth, and then runs forwards along the
hard palate nearly to the gums of the incisor teeth; but one or
two branches proceed backwards to supply the soft palate. The
middle palatine descends either in the same canal with the preceding, or in a smaller one of its own, and terminates exclusively
in the mucous membrane and glands of the soft palate. The *posterior* palatine nerve may be traced in a special bony canal down
to the soft palate, where it terminates in the mucous membrane
and glands. One or two filaments pass into the uvula.[*]

[*] According to Longet (Anat. et Physiol. du Système Nerveux: Paris, 1842), the
posterior palatine nerve supplies the levator palati and the azygos uvulæ with motor

b. *Spheno-palatine* or *nasal branches.*—These, three or four
in number, pass through the spheno-palatine foramen to the
mucous membrane of the nose. To see them clearly, the parts
should have been steeped for some time in dilute nitric acid:
afterwards, when well washed, these minute nerves may be easily
recognised beneath the mucous membrane covering the spongy
bones. Most of them ramify upon the outer wall of the nose and
the spongy bones. One branch (fig. 42), originally called by
Scarpa ' *naso-palatine*,' traverses the roof of the nose, distributes
filaments to the back part of the septum narium, and then proceeds obliquely forwards along the septum to the foramen incisivum, through which it passes, and finally terminates in the
palate behind the incisor teeth.

According to Cloquet, the corresponding nerves of opposite
sides unite at the foramen incisivum in a small ganglion which he
calls the ' naso-palatine.' *

c. *Branches to the pharynx and Eustachian tube.*—In parts
prepared for the purpose we may sometimes trace minute filaments to the mucous membrane of the back of the nares, the
Eustachian tube, and sphenoidal sinus.

d. *Vidian branch.*—This proceeds, from the posterior part of
the ganglion, backwards through the vidian canal of the sphenoid
bone, traverses the fibro-cartilage at the base of the skull, and
here divides into two branches, fig. 43. One (*the carotid*) joins
the sympathetic plexus about the internal carotid artery; the
other (sometimes called the *great petrosal*) enters the cranium,
runs under the Gasserian ganglion and the dura mater, in a small
groove on the petrous portion of the temporal bone, enters the
' hiatus Fallopii,' and joins the facial nerve. It is probable that
the vidian nerve proceeds, not from, but to the ganglion, and that

power. In this view of the subject the nerve is considered to be the continuation or
terminal branch of the motor root of the ganglion, that, namely, derived from the
facial. This opinion is supported by cases in which the uvula is stated to have been
drawn on one side in consequence of paralysis of the opposite facial nerve. However,
we have not succeeded in tracing the nerve into these muscles.

* Dissert. sur les Odeurs et les Organes de l'Olfaction: Paris, 1815.

it is the medium through which motor filaments are conveyed
to it.

Otic ganglion. The otic ganglion was discovered and described by
Arnold, a German anatomist, in 1826.[*] 'It is situated,' he says, 'on the inner side of the inferior maxillary division of the fifth pair, immediately below its exit through
the foramen ovale. (See diagram, page 188.) Its inner surface is
in contact with the circumflexus palati muscle and the cartilage
of the Eustachian tube, and immediately behind it is the middle
meningeal artery.' It is always of very small size.

Respecting its connections with other nerves, Arnold states that
the otic ganglion derives filaments (of sensation) from the inferior
maxillary, and also from the branch of this nerve, which goes to
the internal pterygoid muscle. It also derives a slender filament
from the temporo-auricular nerve. Its communication with the
sympathetic is established by filaments which proceed from the
'nervi molles' round the middle meningeal artery. It communicates also with the facial and glosso-pharyngeal nerves by a
branch commonly called the lesser *petrosal* nerve. This nerve
passes backwards either through the foramen ovale or the foramen
spinosum, or through a small hole between the two, and runs
beneath the dura mater along a minute groove on the petrous
bone (outside the great petrosal nerve). Here it divides into two
filaments, one of which joins the facial nerve in the aqueductus
Fallopii, the other joins the tympanic branch of the glosso-pharyngeal. These nerves are exceedingly difficult to trace, not only
on account of their minute size, but also because they frequently
run in canals in the petrous portion of the temporal bone.

The otic ganglion sends a branch to the tensor tympani and to
the circumflexus palati muscles.

[*] J. Arnold, Diss. inaug. med. &c.; Heidelbergæ, 1820.

DISSECTION OF THE EIGHTH PAIR OF NERVES AT THE BASE OF THE SKULL.

In this dissection we propose to examine the glosso-pharyngeal, pneumogastric, and spinal accessory nerves in the jugular fossa, and the ganglia and nerves belonging to them in this part of their

Fig. 43.

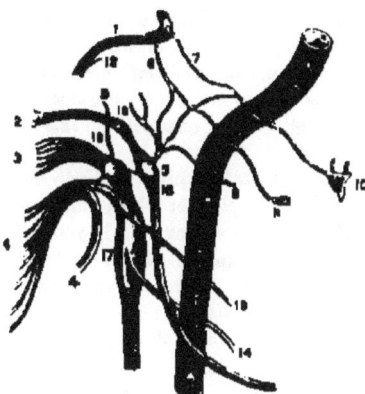

DIAGRAM OF THE EIGHTH PAIR OF NERVES AT THE BASE OF THE SKULL.

1. Facial nerve.
2. Glosso-pharyngeal n.
3. Pneumogastric.
4. Spinal accessory.
5. Jacobson's or tympanic nerve.
6. Lesser petrosal.
7. Great petrosal branch, or Vidian.
8. Branch to Eustachian tube.
9. Arnold's or auricular n.

10. Spheno-palatine or Mechel's ganglion.
11. Otic ganglion.
12. Chorda tympani.
13. Pharyngeal n.
14. Superior laryngeal n.
15. Jugular ganglion } of glosso-pharyngeal.
16. Petrous ganglion }
17. Inferior ganglion } of pneumogastric.
18. Superior ganglion }

course.   These are difficult to trace, and cannot be followed out with success unless the nerves have been previously hardened by spirit, and the bones softened by acid. The first thing to be done is to remove the outer wall of the jugular fossa.

Glosso-pha-ryngeal.   This nerve passes through a separate tube of dura mater in front of that for the other two nerves. Looking at it from the interior of the skull, we observe that it is situated immediately in front and rather to the inner side of the jugular fossa.

In its passage through the fossa, the nerve presents two ganglionic enlargements, named respectively the *jugular* and the *petrous*.

The *jugular ganglion* (ganglion superius) has been particularly described by Müller.* It is found upon the nerve immediately after its entrance into the canal of the dura mater, and is so small that its size does not in any direction exceed $\frac{1}{12}$th of an inch. It occupies the outer side of the nerve, and does not implicate all its fibres. According to our observation, this ganglion is frequently absent.

The *petrous ganglion* (called, after its discoverer, the ganglion of Andersch†) is situated upon the glosso-pharyngeal nerve, near the lower part of the jugular fossa. It is oval, and about $\frac{1}{4}$th of an inch long. It is connected by filaments to the pneumogastric and sympathetic nerves, and it gives off the *tympanic* or Jacobson's nerve.‡ This *tympanic* branch of the glosso-pharyngeal ascends through a minute canal in the bony ridge which separates the carotid from the jugular fossa, to the inner wall of the tympanum, and terminates in several filaments. One traverses a bony canal to the plexus of sympathetic nerves round the carotid artery; a second goes to the fenestra ovalis; a third to the fenestra rotunda; a fourth is distributed to the mucous membrane of the Eustachian tube; a fifth ascends in front of the fenestra ovalis, and joins the great petrosal nerve in the hiatus Fallopii; a sixth takes nearly a similar course, and under the name of the lesser petrosal nerve proceeds along the front surface of the

* Medicin. Zeitung, Berlin, 1833, No. 32.
† Andersch, Fragm. descript. nerv. cardiac., 1791.
‡ This nerve, though commonly called Jacobson's, was fully described by Andersch.

petrous bone to the otic ganglion. This tympanic branch is thus distributed to the mucous membrane of the tympanum and the Eustachian tube, and it communicates with the spheno-palatine ganglion through the great petrosal nerve, and with the otic ganglion through the lesser petrosal.

Pneumo-gastric nerve.
This nerve leaves the cranium with the nervus accessorius, through a canal in the dura mater behind that for the glosso-pharyngeal. At its entrance into the canal it is composed of a number of separate filaments; but in the foramen jugulare, these soon become imbedded in a small ganglion—the *ganglion of the root of the pneumogastric*. This ganglion, first described by Arnold,[*] is about $\frac{1}{12}$th of an inch in diameter. It is connected by filaments to the sympathetic, to the petrous ganglion of the glosso-pharyngeal, to the spinal accessory and the facial nerves. But its most singular branch is one named by Arnold ' the *auricular*,' because it is distributed to the pinna of the ear. This branch enters a minute foramen in the jugular fossa, near the styloid process, and then proceeds through the substance of the bone to the aqueductus Fallopii, where it divides into two branches; one joins the facial nerve, the other passes to the outside of the head through a canal between the front of the mastoid process and the meatus auditorius, and is distributed to the cartilage of the ear, and the meatus auditorius.

Immediately below this its first ganglion the pneumogastric nerve is joined by two branches from the nervus accessorius, and consequently becomes after this junction a compound nerve. The *ganglion of the trunk*, or inferior ganglion of this nerve below the base of the skull, has been already examined (p. 97).

Portio dura through the temporal bone.
The portio dura or facial nerve, having arrived at the bottom of the meatus auditorius internus, enters the '*aqueductus Fallopii*.[†] This is a tortuous canal excavated through the substance of the temporal bone, and terminating at the stylo-mastoid foramen. When exposed throughout its whole course, we observe that the nerve proceeds

[*] Der Kopftheil des vogel. Nerven System. Heidelberg. 1831.
[†] Fallopius was a distinguished Italian anatomist and professor at Paris, 1561.

from the meatus internus for a short distance outwardly, then makes a sudden bend backwards along the inner wall of the tympanum above the fenestra ovalis, and, lastly, curving downwards at the back of the tympanum, it leaves the skull at the stylo-mastoid foramen. Its branches in the temporal bone are:—

a. A communication between the facial and the auditory nerve at the bottom of the meatus auditorius internus.

b. The *great petrosal* nerve (vidian), which runs to the spheno-palatine ganglion (p. 102).

c. The *lesser petrosal* nerve, which runs to the otic ganglion.

d. Chorda tympani.—This nerve arises from the facial about ½th of an inch before its exit from the stylo-mastoid foramen, ascends for a short distance in a bony canal at the back of the tympanum, and enters that cavity below the pyramid and close to the membrana tympani. It then runs forwards along the tympanum, across the handle of the malleus, to the fissura Glaseri, through which it emerges at the base of the skull, and joining the gustatory nerve, finally proceeds to the submaxillary ganglion, and ends in the tongue. In its passage through the aqueductus Fallopii branches are distributed to the stapedius and laxator tympani muscles.

DISSECTION OF THE NOSE.

Presuming that the dissector is familiar with the bones composing the skeleton of the nose, we shall now describe, 1. The nasal cartilages; 2. The general figure and arrangement of the nasal cavities; 3. The membrane which lines them; and, lastly, the distribution of the olfactory nerves.

Cartilages of the nose.
Two pieces of fibro-cartilage on either side assist in forming the framework of the external nose; and one in the centre completes the septum between the nasal fossæ.

There are two *lateral cartilages*, an upper and a lower. The *upper*, triangular in shape, is connected, superiorly, to the margin of the nasal and superior maxillary bones, anteriorly, to the cartilage of the septum, and inferiorly, to the lower cartilage by means

of a tough fibrous membrane.   The *lower* is sometimes called the
cartilage of the pinna.   It is elongated, and curved upon itself in
such a way as to form the boundary of the external opening of
the nose.   Superiorly, it is connected by fibrous membrane to the
upper lateral cartilage; internally it is in contact with its fellow
of the opposite side, forming the upper part of the 'columna
nasi;' posteriorly, it is attached by fibrous tissue to the superior
maxillary bone: in this tissue, at the base of the ala, are usually
found two or three nodules of cartilage, called '*cartilagines sesa-
moideæ.*'   By their elasticity they keep the nostrils continually
open, and restore them to their ordinary size whenever they have
been expanded by muscular action.

The *cartilage of the septum* is placed perpendicularly in the
middle line: it may lean a little, however, to one side or the
other, and in some instances it is perforated, so that the two nasal
cavities communicate with each other.   The cartilage is smooth
and flat, and its outline is nearly triangular.   The posterior border
is received into a groove in the perpendicular plate of the ethmoid ; the anterior border is much thicker than the rest of the
septum, and is connected, superiorly, with the nasal bones, and on
either side with the lateral cartilages.   The inferior border is
attached to the vomer and the median ridge at the junction of the
palatine processes of the superior maxillæ.

The muscles moving the nasal cartilages have been described
with the dissection of the face (p. 72).

Interior of
the nose.   A vertical section should be made through the right
nasal cavity, a little on the same side of the middle
line, to expose the partly bony and partly cartilaginous
partition of the nasal cavities (*septum narium*).   Each nasal
fossa is narrower above than below.   The greatest perpendicular
depth of each fossa is about the centre, and from this point the
depth gradually lessens, both towards the anterior and the posterior openings of the nose.   Laterally, each fossa is very narrow
in consequence of the projection of the spongy bones towards the
septum: this narrowness in the transverse direction explains the
rapidity with which swelling of the lining membrane from a simple
cold obstructs the passage of air.

The nasal fossæ are bounded by the following bones:—*superiorly*, by the nasal, the nasal spine of the frontal, the cribriform plate of the ethmoid, and the body of the sphenoid; *inferiorly*, by the horizontal plates of the superior maxillary and palate bones; *internally*, is the smooth and flat septum formed by the perpendicular plate of the ethmoid, the vomer, and the cartilage, also by the nasal spine of the frontal, the rostrum of the sphenoid, and the median ridge of the superior maxillary and palate bones; *externally*, by the maxillary, the lachrymal, the ethmoid, the palate, the inferior turbinated bone, and the internal pterygoid plate of the sphenoid.

Meatus of the nose. The outer wall of each nasal cavity is divided by the turbinated bones into three compartments (*meatus*) of unequal size; and in these, are orifices leading to air-cells (*sinuses*) in the sphenoid, ethmoid, frontal, and superior maxillary bones. Each of these compartments should be separately examined.

The *superior meatus* is the smallest of the three, and does not extend beyond the posterior half of the wall of the nose. The posterior ethmoidal and sphenoidal cells open into its anterior part by one wide communication.

The *middle meatus* is larger than the superior. At its anterior part is a long narrow passage (*infundibulum*), which leads upwards to the frontal and the anterior ethmoidal cells. About the middle is a small opening which leads into the antrum of the superior maxilla: this opening in the dry bone is large and irregular, but in the recent state it is reduced nearly to the size of a crow-quill by mucous membrane, so that a very little swelling of the membrane is sufficient to close the orifice entirely.

Notice that the orifices of the frontal and ethmoid cells are so disposed that their secretion will pass, by its own gravity, into the nose. But this is not the case with the sphenoid and maxillary cells; to empty which the head must be inclined on one side. To see all these openings you must raise the respective turbinated bones.

The *inferior meatus* extends nearly along the whole length of the outer wall of the nose. By raising the lower turbinated bone, we observe, towards the front of the meatus, the termination of the nasal duct, through which the tears pass down from the lachrymal sac into the nose. This sac and duct we can now conveniently examine.

Lachrymal sac and nasal duct. This is the passage through which the tears are conveyed from the lachrymal ducts into the nose (p. 70). The lachrymal sac occupies the groove on the nasal side of the orbit, formed by the lachrymal and superior maxillary bones. The upper end is round and closed; the lower gradually contracts into the nasal duct, and opens into the inferior meatus. The sac is composed of a strong fibrous membrane, which adheres very closely to the bone, and is lined by mucous membrane. Its front surface is covered by the tendo oculi and the fascia proceeding from it.

The nasal duct is from half to three quarters of an inch in length, and is directed downwards and backwards. Its termination is guarded by a valvular fold of mucous membrane; consequently, when air is blown into the nasal passages while the nostrils are closed, the lachrymal sac does not become distended. The lachrymal sac and the nasal duct are lined with ciliated epithelium and the canaliculi with the squamous variety.

Behind the inferior turbinated bone is the opening of the Eustachian tube (p. 159). Into this, as well as into the nasal duct, we ought to practice the introduction of a probe. The chief difficulty is to prevent the probe from slipping into the cul-de-sac between the tube and the back of the pharynx.

Mucous or Schneiderian membrane.[*] This membrane lines the cavities of the nose and the air-cells communicating with it, and adheres very firmly to the periosteum. Its continuity may be traced into the pharynx, the various sinuses, the orbits through the nasal ducts, and into the tympana and mastoid cells through the Eustachian tubes. Observe that at the lower border of the turbinated bones it is disposed in thick and loose folds. The membrane varies in thickness and vascularity in different parts of the

* Schneider, De catarrhis. Wittenberg, 1660.

nasal cavities. Upon the lower half of the septum, and the lower turbinated bones it is much thicker than elsewhere, in consequence of a minute plexus of arteries and veins in the submucous tissue. In the sinuses, the mucous membrane is thinner, less vascular, and closely applied upon the periosteum.

The great vascularity of the Schneiderian membrane is obviously intended to elevate the temperature of the inspired air, and to pour out a copious secretion which prevents the membrane from becoming too dry.

Near the nostrils the mucous membrane is furnished with papillæ, a squamous epithelium, like the skin, and a few small hairs (vibrissæ). In the sinuses and all the lower regions of the nose, the epithelium is columnar, and provided with cilia; but in the upper part of the nose, where the sense of smell resides, we no longer find ciliated epithelium, but columnar; beneath which is a stratum of nucleated cells.*

Blood-vessels of the interior nasal branches of the ophthalmic, and the nasal branch of the nose. The arteries of the nose are, the ethmoidal and of the internal maxillary, which enters the nose through the spheno-palatine foramen. The external nose is supplied by the arteria lateralis nasi.

The veins of the nose correspond to the arteries. They communicate with the veins within the cranium through foramina in the cribriform plate of the ethmoid bone, also through the ophthalmic vein and the cavernous sinus. These communications explain the relief afforded by hæmorrhage from the nose in cases of cerebral congestion.

Olfactory nerves. The olfactory nerves, proceeding from each olfactory bulb, in number about twenty on either side, pass through the foramina in the cribriform plate of the ethmoid bone. In its passage each nerve is invested with a coat derived from the dura mater. They are divided into an *inner*, a *middle*, and an *outer* set. The *inner* traverse the grooves on the upper third of the septum. The *middle* supply the roof of the nose. The *outer* pass through grooves in the upper and

* Bowman and Todd's Physiolog. Anatom., cap. xvi.

middle turbinated bones, and are lost in the mucous membrane on the convex surfaces of these bones.*

The olfactory nerves descend between the mucous membrane and the periosteum, and break up into filaments which communicate freely with one another and form minute plexuses. Owing to the difficulty of tracing the ultimate filaments, the exact mode of termination is at present undetermined. Microscopically, the olfactory filaments differ from the other cerebral nerves, in containing no white substance of Schwann, and in being finely granular and nucleated.

The olfactory are nerves of special sense. The common sensibility of the mucous membrane of the nose is supplied by branches from the fifth pair of nerves; namely, the nasal branch of the ophthalmic (p. 178), the nasal branch of the spheno-palatine ganglion (p. 190), and the Vidian nerve. That the sense of smell is independent of the common sensibility of the nose is proved by experiment and by pathology. For instance, any disease affecting the olfactory nerve, even the inflammation of a common cold, impairs the sense of smell, whereas the common sensation of the part continues equally acute, and becomes even more so, as one may readily ascertain by introducing a foreign body into the nostril.

DISSECTION OF THE MUSCLES OF THE BACK.

Those muscles of the back, namely, the trapezius, latissimus dorsi, levator anguli scapulæ, and rhomboidei, which are concerned in the movements of the upper extremity, will be examined in the dissection of the arm. These, therefore, having been removed, we proceed to examine two muscles, named, from their appearance, 'serrati,' which extend from the spine to the ribs.

Serratus posticus superior.

This muscle is situated beneath the rhomboidei. It arises from the ligamentum nuchæ,† the spines of the last cervical, and two or three upper dorsal vertebræ, by

---

* See the plates of Scarpa and Sœmmerring.

† The ligamentum nuchæ is a rudiment of the great elastic ligament of quadrupeds (termed the *park-wax*) which supports the weight of the head. It proceeds from the spine of the occiput to the spines of all the cervical vertebræ except the atlas; otherwise it would interfere with the free rotation of the head.

a sheet-like aponeurosis which makes up nearly half the muscle: the fibres run obliquely downwards and outwards, and are *inserted* by fleshy slips into the second, third, fourth, and sometimes the fifth ribs beyond their angles.   Its *action* is to raise these ribs, and therefore to assist in inspiration.

Serratus posticus inferior.   This muscle is situated beneath the latissimus dorsi. It *arises* from the strong aponeurosis called '*vertebral aponeurosis*,' opposite the two last dorsal and two upper lumbar vertebræ.   It ascends obliquely outwards, and is *inserted* by fleshy slips into the four lower ribs, external to their angles.   The tendency of its *action* is to pull down these ribs, and therefore to assist in expiration.

Vertebral aponeurosis.   The dense and shining aponeurosis which covers the erector spinæ is called 'vertebral aponeurosis.'   It is attached to the crest of the ilium, to the spines of the lower dorsal, all the lumbar, and sacral vertebræ.   Its use is, not only to form a sheath for the erector spinæ, but to give origin to the latissimus dorsi, the serratus posticus inferior, the internal oblique and transverse muscles of the abdomen.   If you make a vertical incision through it and reflect it, you will see that on the outer side of the erector spinæ it is inseparably connected with the tendinous attachments of the internal oblique and transversalis to the transverse processes of the lumbar vertebræ.

The serratus posticus superior must now be reflected from its origin, and turned outwards to expose the following muscle.

Splenius.   This *arises* from the spines of the five or six upper dorsal and the last cervical vertebræ, and from the lower half of the ligamentum nuchæ.   The fibres ascend and divide into two portions, named, according to their respective insertions, *splenius capitis* and *splenius colli*.

a. The *splenius capitis* is inserted into the mastoid process, and the superior curved ridge of the occipital bone beneath the sterno-mastoid.

b. The *splenius colli* is inserted by tendinous slips into the posterior tubercles of the transverse processes of the three upper cervical vertebræ.

The *action* of the splenius, taken as a whole, is to draw the head and the upper cervical vertebræ towards its own side: so far, it co-operates with the opposite sterno-mastoid muscle. When the splenii of opposite sides contract, they extend the cervical portion of the spine, and keep the head erect. The permanent contraction of a single splenius may occasion 'wry neck.' It is necessary to be aware of this, otherwise one might suppose the opposite sterno-mastoid to be affected, considering that the appearance of the distortion is alike in either case.

The splenius and serratus posticus inferior are to be detached from their origins; after reflecting the vertebral aponeurosis from its internal attachment the erector spinæ is exposed.

Erector spinæ. The mass of muscle which occupies the vertebral groove on either side of the spine, is, collectively, called 'erector spinæ,' since it counteracts the tendency of the trunk to fall forwards. Observe that it is thickest and strongest at that part of the spine where it has the greatest weight to support, namely, in the lumbar region; and that its thickness gradually decreases towards the top of the spine.

It *arises* by tendinous fibres from the posterior fifth of the crest of the ilium, the sacrum, and the spines of the lumbar vertebræ. From this extensive origin the muscular fibres ascend, at first as a single mass. Near the last rib, this mass divides into two; an outer, called the '*sacro-lumbalis*;' an inner, the '*longissimus dorsi*.' These two portions should be followed up the back: and there is no difficulty in doing so, because the division is indicated by a longitudinal groove, in which we observe the cutaneous branches of the intercostal vessels and nerves.

Sacro-lumbalis. Tracing the *sacro-lumbalis* upwards, we find that it terminates in a series of tendons which are *inserted* into the angles of the six lower ribs.

Musculus accessorius. By turning outwards the sacro-lumbalis, we observe that it is continued upwards under the name of '*musculus accessorius ad sacro-lumbalem*.' This *arises* by a series of tendons from the angles of the seven or eight lower ribs, and is *inserted* into the angles of the five or six upper ribs.

This is the cervical continuation of the musculus
Cervicalis ascendens. accessorius. It *arises* by tendinous slips from the four
or five upper ribs, and is inserted into the transverse
processes of the three or four cervical vertebræ.

The longissimus dorsi (the inner portion of the erector
Longissi- mus dorsi. spinæ) terminates in tendons which are *inserted* into the
tubercles * at the root of the transverse processes of the
lumbar vertebræ, also into the transverse processes of all the
dorsal vertebræ, and into the greater number of the ribs (varying
from eight to eleven) close to their junction with the transverse
processes.

This is the cervical continuation of the longissimus
Transver- salis colli. dorsi. It *arises* by tendinous slips from the transverse
processes of the second, third, fourth, fifth, and sixth
dorsal vertebræ, and is inserted into the posterior tubercles of the
transverse processes of the four or five lower cervical vertebræ.

This muscle, situated on the inner side of the pre-
Trachelo- mastoid. ceding, is the continuation of the transversalis colli to
the cranium. It arises from the transverse processes
of the fourth, fifth, and sixth dorsal, and the articular processes of
the three or four lower cervical vertebræ, and is inserted by a flat
tendon into the back part of the mastoid process beneath the
splenius.†

* Called 'anapophyses' by Professor Owen.

† Those who are familiar with the transcendental nomenclature of the vertebrate
skeleton, will understand, from the following quotation, the plan upon which the
muscles of the back are arranged :—

'The muscles of the back are either longitudinal or oblique; that is, they either
pass vertically downwards from spinous process to spinous process, from diapophysis
to diapophysis, from rib to rib (pleurapophyses), &c., or they extend obliquely from
diapophysis to spine, or from diapophysis to pleurapophysis, &c.

'The erector spinæ is composed of two planes of longitudinal fibres aggregated
together, below, to form one mass at their point of origin, from the spines and posterior surface of the sacrum, from the sacro-iliac ligament, and from the posterior
third of the iliac crest. It divides into two portions, the sacro-lumbalis and the
longissimus dorsi.

'The former, arising from the iliac crest, or from the pleurapophysis (rib) of the
first sacral vertebra, is inserted by short flat tendons into (1.) the apices of the stunted
lumbar ribs, close to the tendinous origins of the transversalis abdominis; (2.) the

This is a long narrow muscle, situated close to the
Spinalis dorsi. spines of the dorsal vertebræ, and apparently a part of
the longissimus dorsi. It *arises* by tendinous slips
from the spines of the two lower dorsal and two upper lumbar
vertebræ, and is inserted by little tendons into the spines of the
six or eight upper dorsal vertebræ.

The muscles of the spine hitherto examined are all longitudinal
in their direction. We now come to a series which run obliquely
from the transverse to the spinous processes of the vertebræ. And
first of the complexus.

This powerful muscle *arises* from the transverse pro-
Complexus. cesses of the three or four upper dorsal and the last
cervical vertebræ, also from the articular processes of the fourth,
fifth, and sixth cervical vertebræ. It is *inserted* between the two
curved lines of the occiput, near the vertical crest. In the centre
of the muscle there is generally tendinous tissue.[*] The muscle is
perforated by the posterior branches of the second (the great occipital), third, and fourth cervical nerves. Its *action* is to maintain
the head erect.

Cut transversely through the middle of the complexus, and

angles of the eight or nine inferior dorsal ribs; (3.) it is inserted, through the medium
of the musculus accessorius, into the angles of the remaining superior ribs, and into
the long and occasionally distinct pleurapophysial element of the seventh cervical
vertebra; and (4.) through the medium of the cervicalis ascendens, into the pleurapophysial elements of the third, fourth, fifth, and sixth cervical vertebræ. In other
words, the muscular fibres extend from rib to rib, from the sacrum to the third cervical
vertebra.

'The longissimus dorsi, situated nearer the spine than the sacro-lumbalis, is inserted (1.) into the metapophysial spine of the lumbar diapophyses; (2.) into the
diapophyses of all the dorsal vertebræ, near the origin of the levatores costarum;
(3.) through the medium of the transversalis colli into the diapophyses of the second,
third, fourth, fifth, and sixth cervical vertebræ; and (4.) through the medium of the
trachelo-mastoid into the mastoid process, or the only element of a transverse process
possessed by the parietal vertebra. In other words, its fibres extend from diapophysis
to diapophysis, from the sacrum, upwards, to the parietal vertebra.'—*Homologies of
the Human Skeleton*, by H. Coote, p. 75.

[*] The inner border of the complexus is described by some anatomists as a separate
muscle, under the name of 'biventer cervicis,' simply because it consists of two
muscular portions united by an intermediate tendon.

reflect it to see the 'arteria cervicalis profunda' (p. 60), and the posterior branches of the cervical nerves.

Transverso-spinalis This is the mass of muscle which lies in the vertebral groove after the reflection of the complexus and the erector spinæ. It consists of a series of fibres which extend from the transverse and articular processes to the spinous processes of the dorsal and cervical vertebræ, and is usually divided into the '*semispinalis dorsi*' and '*semispinalis colli*.'

a. The *semispinalis dorsi arises* from the transverse processes of the dorsal vertebræ, from the sixth to the tenth, and is *inserted* into the spines of the four upper dorsal and the two or three lower cervical vertebræ.

b. The semispinalis colli arises from the transverse processes of the five or six upper dorsal vertebræ, and the articular processes of the four lower cervical, and is *inserted* into the spines of the axis and the three or four succeeding vertebræ.

Now reflect part of the semispinalis dorsi in order to expose the '*multifidus spinæ*.' This may be considered a part of the preceding muscle, since its fixed points and the direction of its fibres are the same. It consists of a series of little muscles which extend between the spines and transverse processes of the vertebræ from the sacrum to the second cervical vertebra. Those in the lumbar region are the largest. They *arise* by tendinous slips from the transverse processes in the sacral and dorsal region, and from the articular processes in the lumbar and cervical region. They all ascend obliquely, and are *inserted* into the spines and laminæ of all the vertebræ excepting the atlas. It should be observed that their fibres are not of uniform length; some extend only from vertebra to vertebra, while others extend between one, two, or even three vertebræ.[*]

The action of these oblique muscles is not only to assist in

* Beneath the multifidus spinæ we find, in the dorsal region of the spine only, eleven little flat muscles, called by Theile (Müller's Archives f. Anat. &c., 1839), who first described them, '*rotatores spinæ*.' They arise from the upper part of the transverse process, and are inserted into the lower border of the lamina of the vertebra above. These muscles form but a part of the multifidus spinæ.

maintaining the trunk erect, but to bend the spine to one or the
other side.

Levatores costarum. These little muscles *arise* from the apices of the
transverse processes of the dorsal vertebræ, and are
inserted into the rib below. The direction of their
fibres corresponds with that of the outer layer of the intercostal
muscles. They are muscles of inspiration.

Interspinales. The muscles extend between the spines of contiguous
vertebræ. They are arranged in pairs, and only exist
in those parts of the vertebral column which are the most movable. In the cervical region they pass between the spines of the
six lower cervical vertebræ. In the dorsal they are found between
the spines of the first and second, and between those of the
eleventh and twelfth dorsal vertebræ. In the lumbar, between
the spines of the lumbar vertebræ.

Intertransversales. These muscles extend between the transverse processes in the cervical and lumbar regions. In the neck
they are arranged in pairs, like the interspinales, and
the corresponding cervical nerve separates one from the other.
In the loins they are four in number, and are arranged singly.
We have next to examine the muscles concerned in the movements
of the head upon the first and second cervical vertebræ

Rectus capitis posticus major. This is a largely developed interspinal muscle. It
arises by a small tendon from the well-marked spine
of the second cervical vertebra, and, expanding considerably, is *inserted* below the superior curved ridge
of the occipital bone; in other words, into the spine of the occipital vertebra. These two recti muscles, as they ascend to their
insertions, diverge and leave an interval between them in which
are found the recti capitis postici minores.

Rectus capitis posticus minor. This is also an interspinal muscle, but smaller than
the preceding. *Arising* from the feebly developed
spine of the first vertebra, it expands as it ascends, and
is *inserted* into the occipital bone between the inferior curved
ridge and the foramen magnum. The *action* of the two preceding
muscles is to raise the head.

Obliquus inferior. This *arises* from the spine of the second vertebra, and is *inserted* into the transverse process of the first. Its *action* is to rotate the first upon the second vertebra; in other words, to turn the head round.

Obliquus superior. This muscle *arises* from the transverse process of the first vertebra, and ascending obliquely inwards is inserted in the interval between the curved ridges of the occiput. Its *action* is to draw the occiput towards the spine.

Observe that the obliqui and recti muscles of one side form the sides of a triangle, in which we find the branches of the suboccipital or first cervical nerve, the vertebral artery, and the arch of the atlas.

Rectus capitis lateralis. This small muscle extends between the transverse process of the first vertebra and the *eminentia jugularis* of the occiput; but since this eminence is the transverse process of the occipital vertebra, the muscle must be considered as an intertransverse one.

Nerves of the back. The posterior branches of the spinal nerves supply the muscles and skin of the back. They pass backwards between the transverse processes of the vertebræ, and divide into *external* and *internal* branches. The general plan upon which these nerves are arranged is the same throughout the whole length of the spine; but since there are certain peculiarities deserving of notice in particular situations, we must examine each region separately.

Cervical region. The posterior division of the first cervical nerve (the suboccipital) passes between the arch of the atlas and the vertebral artery, and divides into branches which supply the recti and obliqui muscles concerned in the movement of the head upon the first two vertebræ. It sometimes gives off a cutaneous branch which accompanies the occipital artery, and is distributed to the skin of the back of the scalp.

The posterior branch (the great occipital) of the second cervical nerve is the largest of the series, and emerges between the arches of the atlas and axis. It turns upwards beneath the inferior oblique muscles, passes through the complexus, and runs with the occipital artery to the back of the scalp.

The posterior divisions of the six lower cervical nerves divide into *external* and *internal* branches. The *external* are small, and terminate in the splenius, and the continuation of the erector spinæ, viz., the trachelo-mastoid, the transversalis colli, and the cervicalis ascendens. The *internal*, by far the larger, proceed towards the spines of the vertebræ; those of the third, fourth, and fifth lie between the complexus and the semispinalis,* and after supplying the muscles terminate in the integument; those of the sixth, seventh, and eighth lie between the semispinalis and the multifidus spinæ, to which they are distributed.

The posterior divisions of the spinal nerves in this **Dorsal region.** region come out between the transverse processes and the tendons attached to them. They soon divide into *external* and *internal* branches. The *external* pass obliquely over the levatores costarum, between the sacro-lumbalis and the longissimus dorsi; and successively increase in size from above downwards. The upper six terminate in the erector spinæ and the levatores costarum; the rest, after supplying these muscles, pass through the latissimus dorsi, and become the cutaneous nerves of the back. The *internal* successively decrease in size from above downwards. They run towards the spine between the semispinalis dorsi and the multifidus spinæ. The upper six, after giving branches to the muscles, perforate the trapezius and become cutaneous nerves. The lower ones terminate in the muscles of the vertebral groove.

The general arrangement of the nerves in this region **Lumbar region.** resembles that of the dorsal. Their *external* branches, after supplying the erector spinæ, become cutaneous and terminate in the skin over the buttock. The *internal* branches supply the multifidus spinæ.

The posterior divisions of the spinal nerves in this **Sacral region.** region are small. With the exception of the last, they come out of the spinal canal through the foramina in

* The posterior branches of the second, third, and fourth nerves are generally connected, beneath the complexus, by branches in the form of loops. This constitutes the posterior cervical plexus of some anatomists.

the back of the sacrum. The upper two or three divide into *external* and *internal* branches. The *internal* terminate in the multifidus spinæ; the *external* become cutaneous and supply the skin of the gluteal region. The last two sacral nerves proceed, without dividing, to the integument.

The *coccygeal* nerve is exceedingly small, and, after joining a small branch from the last sacral, terminates in the skin.[*]

Vessels of the back. The vessels which supply the back are:—1. Small branches from the occipital; 2. Small branches from the vertebral; 3. The deep cervical; 4. The posterior branches of the intercostal and lumbar arteries.

The *occipital* artery furnishes several small branches to the muscles at the back of the neck; one, larger than the rest (called *arteria princeps cervicis*), descends beneath the complexus, and in some subjects inosculates with the deep cervical artery, and with small branches from the vertebral.

The *deep cervical* artery is the posterior branch of the first intercostal artery. It passes backwards between the transverse process of the last cervical vertebra and the first rib; it then ascends between the complexus and the semispinalis colli.

The *posterior* branches of the intercostal and lumbar arteries accompany the corresponding nerves, and are in all respects similar to them in distribution. Each sends a small branch into the spinal canal.

The *veins* correspond to the arteries.

Præ-vertebral muscles. We have, lastly, to examine three muscles situated in front of the spine; namely, the longus colli, the rectus capitis anticus major, and the rectus capitis anticus minor. In order to have a complete view of the two latter, a special dissection should be made, before the head is removed from the first vertebra.

Longus colli. This muscle is situated in front of the spine, and extends from the third dorsal to the first cervical vertebra. For convenience of description it is divided into three

[*] The branching of the posterior divisions of the several spinal nerves has been accurately described by Mr. Ellis, Med. Gazette, Feb. 10, 1843.

P

sets of fibres, of which one extends *longitudinally* from the body of one vertebra to that of another; the two others extend obliquely between the transverse processes and the bodies of the vertebræ.

The *longitudinal* portion of the muscle arises from the bodies of the two or three upper dorsal and the two lower cervical vertebræ, and is inserted into the bodies of the second, third, and fourth cervical vertebræ.

The *superior oblique* portion, arising from the anterior tubercles of the transverse processes of the third, fourth, and fifth cervical vertebræ, ascends inwards, and is inserted into the front part or body of the first cervical vertebra. The *inferior oblique* portion proceeds from the bodies of the three upper dorsal vertebræ, and is inserted into the transverse processes of the fifth and sixth cervical vertebræ. The *action* of this muscle, taken as a whole, must be to bend the cervical region of the spine. Its nerves come from the deep cervical and brachial plexuses.

This muscle arises from the anterior tubercles of the transverse processes of the third, fourth, fifth, and sixth cervical vertebræ, and is inserted into the basilar process of the occipital bone, in front of the foramen magnum.

Rectus capitis anticus major.

This muscle arises from the root of the transverse process of the first cervical vertebra, and is inserted into the basilar process of the occipital bone, nearer to the foramen magnum than the preceding muscle. The *action* of the recti muscles is to bend the head forwards. They are supplied with nerves from the deep cervical plexus.

Rectus capitis anticus minor.

LIGAMENTS OF THE SPINE.

The vertebræ are connected by their intervertebral fibro-cartilages, by ligaments in front of and behind their bodies, and by ligaments which extend between their arches and their spines. Their articular processes have capsular ligaments, and synovial membranes.

Anterior common ligament. This is a strong band of longitudinal fibres which extends along the front of the bodies of the vertebræ from the axis to the sacrum. The fibres are not all of equal length. The more superficial extend from one vertebra to the fourth or fifth below it; those a little deeper pass from one vertebra to the second or third below it; while the deepest of all proceed from vertebra to vertebra. The ligament becomes broader and stronger in proportion to the size of the vertebræ. By making transverse incisions through it in different situations, we observe that its fibres are more firmly adherent to the intervertebral cartilages, and to the borders of the vertebræ, than to the middle of the bones.

Inter-spinous ligaments. These bands of ligamentous fibres fill up the intervals between the spines of the dorsal and lumbar vertebræ. They are the most marked in the lumbar region. Those fibres which connect the apices of the spines, being stronger than the rest, are described as separate ligaments under the name of *supra-spinous*. Their use is to limit the flexion of the spine.

Ligaments between the arches of the ver-tebræ. These are called, on account of their colour, *ligamenta subflava*.—To obtain a good view of them, the arches of the vertebræ should be removed with a saw. They pass between the arches of the contiguous vertebræ, from the axis to the sacrum; none existing between the occiput and the atlas, or between the atlas and axis. They are composed of yellow elastic tissue, and their strength increases with the size of the vertebræ. This elasticity answers a double purpose: it not only permits the spine to bend forwards, but materially assists in restoring it to its *curve of rest*. They economise muscular force, like the ligamentum nuchæ in animals.

Posterior common ligament. This extends longitudinally, in a similar manner to the anterior common ligament, along the posterior surface of the bodies of the vertebræ, from the occiput to the sacrum.

Intervertebral fibro-cartilage. This substance, placed between the bodies of the vertebræ, is by far the strongest bond of connection between them, and fulfils most important purposes in

the mechanism of the spine. Its peculiar structure is adapted to
break shocks, and to render the spine flexible and resilient. To
see the structure of an intervertebral fibre-cartilage, a horizontal
section must be made through one of them. It is firm and resisting near the circumference, but soft and pulpy towards the centre.
The circumferential portion is composed of concentric layers of
fibro-cartilage, placed vertically. These layers are attached by
their edges to the vertebræ; they gradually decrease in number
from the circumference towards the centre, and the interstices
between them are filled by the soft pulpy tissue. The central
portion is composed almost entirely of this pulpy tissue; and it
bulges when no longer under pressure. Thus the bodies of the
vertebræ, in their motions upon each other, revolve upon a ball of
fluid tightly girt all round by bands of fibrous tissue. These
motions are regulated by the articular processes.

Dissect an intervertebral substance layer after layer in front,
and you will find that the circumferential fibres extend *obliquely*
between the vertebræ, crossing each other like the branches of the
letter X.

The thickness of the intervertebral cartilages is not the same in
front and behind. It is this difference in their thickness, more
than that in the bodies of the vertebræ, which produces the several
curves of the spine. In the lumbar and cervical regions they are
thicker in front; in the dorsal region behind.*

* The structure of the intervertebral cartilages explains the well-known fact, that a
man becomes shorter after standing for some hours; and that he regains his usual
height after rest. The difference between the morning and evening stature amounts
to more than half an inch.

It also explains the fact that a permanent lateral curvature of the spine may be
produced (especially in the young) by the habitual practice of leaning to this or that
side. Experience proves that the cause of lateral curvature depends more frequently
upon some alteration in the structure of the fibro-cartilages than upon the bones.
From an examination of the bodies of one hundred and thirty-four individuals with
crooked spines, it was concluded that in two-thirds the bones were perfectly healthy;
that the most frequent cause of curvature resided in the intervertebral substances; these
being, on the concave side of the curve, almost absorbed, and on the convex side preternaturally developed. As might be expected in these cases, the muscles on the
convex side become lengthened, and degenerate in structure.—On this subject see
Hildebrandt's Anatomie, B. ii. s. 155.

Capsular ligaments.   Each joint between the articular processes has a capsular ligament and a synovial membrane.   The surfaces of the bones are crusted with cartilage.

Inter-transverse ligaments.   These are thin bands of fibres which pass between the transverse processes of the vertebræ.   They are rudimentary in the cervical region, and are sometimes absent.

Motions of the spine.   Though but little movement is permitted between any two vertebræ (the atlas and axis excepted), yet the collective motion between them all is considerable.   The spine can be bent forwards, backwards, or on either side; it also admits of slight rotation.   In consequence of the elasticity of the intervertebral cartilages and the ligamenta subflava, it returns spontaneously to its natural curve of rest like an elastic bow.   Its mobility is greatest in the cervical region, on account of the thickness of the fibro-cartilages, the small size of the vertebræ, the oblique direction of their articulations, and, above all, the horizontal position and the shortness of their spines.   In the dorsal region there is very little mobility, on account of the vertical direction of the articular processes, and the manner in which the arches and the spines overlap each other.   In the lumbar region, the spine again becomes more movable, on account of the thickness of the intervertebral cartilages, and the horizontal direction of the spinous processes.

Ligaments between the occipital bone and the first vertebra.   The occiput is connected to the atlas by an *anterior* (occipito-atlantoid) membrane which passes from the foramen magnum to the front part of the atlas.   The thickest part of this is in the middle.   A *posterior* (occipito-atlantoid) membrane extends in a similar manner from the posterior border of the foramen magnum to the arch of the atlas.   It is perforated by the vertebral artery and the suboccipital nerve.   The movements which take place between these bones are flexion and extension, as in nodding forwards and backwards; and lateral movement, as in inclining the head sideways.

Ligaments between the occipital bone and the axis.

These are the most important; and to see them, the spinal canal must be exposed by removing the arches of the upper cervical vertebræ, and the posterior common ligament, which is here very thick and strong. It descends from the basilar process of the occipital bone over the odontoid and transverse ligaments.

Odontoid or check ligaments.

The odontoid or check ligaments (fig. 44) are two very strong ligaments which proceed from the sides of the odontoid process to the tubercles on the inner sides of the condyles of the occiput. Their use is to limit the rotation of the head. A third or middle odontoid ligament passes from

Fig. 44.

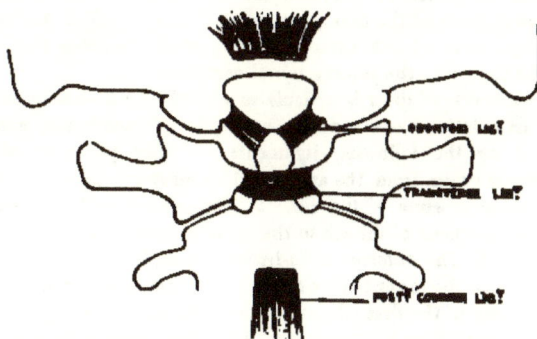

DIAGRAM OF THE ODONTOID AND TRANSVERSE LIGAMENTS.

the apex of the odontoid process to the margin of the foramen magnum. It is sometimes called the *ligamentum suspensorium*.

Articulation between the atlas and the axis.

The odontoid process of the axis forms a pivot upon which the head and atlas rotate. The most important ligament is the *transverse* (fig. 44). It passes behind the odontoid process, and is attached to the tubercles on the inner side of the articular processes of the atlas. From the centre of this ligament a few fibres pass upwards, and others downwards, giving it a cruciform appearance.* Thus it forms with the atlas a ring, into which the odontoid process is received. If this transverse ligament be divided, we observe that the odontoid process is covered with cartilage in front and behind, and is provided with two synovial membranes.

Articulation of the ribs. All the ribs, with the exception of the first and the two last, are articulated with the bodies of two vertebræ, and with the transverse processes.

The head of each rib presents two articular surfaces, corresponding to the bodies of two vertebræ. There are two distinct articulations, each provided with a separate synovial membrane The ligaments are:—1. An *anterior*, which connects the head of the rib with the vertebræ, and with the intervening fibro-cartilage: this, on account of the divergence of its fibres, is called the 'stellate' ligament. 2. An *inter-articular*, which proceeds from the head of the rib to the intervertebral cartilage.

The tubercle of the rib articulates with the transverse process. This articulation has a capsular and synovial membrane, and is secured by the following ligaments:—1. The *posterior costo-transverse* passes from the apex of the transverse process to the apex of the tubercle of the rib. 2. The *middle costo-transverse* connects the neck of the rib to the front surface of the transverse process. 3. The *anterior costo-transverse* ascends from the neck of the rib to the lower border of the transverse process above it.

The head of the first rib articulates with a single vertebra.

The eleventh and twelfth ribs articulate each with a single vertebra, and are not connected to the transverse processes.

Connection between the cartilages of the ribs and the sternum. The cartilages of all the true ribs are received into slight concavities on the side of the sternum. In young subjects we find that the cartilages of the six lower true ribs have distinct articulations provided with synovial membranes. They are secured in front and behind by strong ligamentous fibres, which proceed from the cartilages and radiate upon the sternum, crossing those of the opposite side.

* This is not shown in the diagram.

The *costal cartilages from the sixth to the tenth* are connected by ligamentous fibres.

Articulation of the lower jaw.   The condyle of the lower jaw articulates with the glenoid cavity of the temporal bone. The joint is provided with an inter-articular fibro-cartilage, and with external and internal lateral ligaments (fig. 45).

Fig. 45.

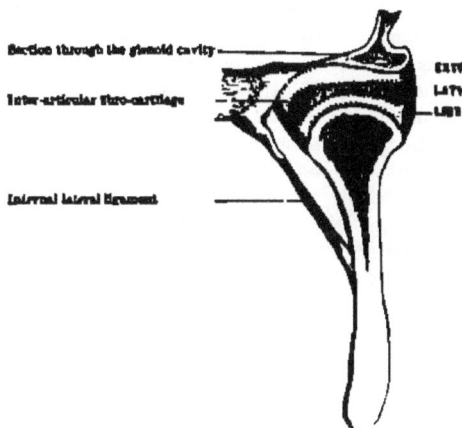

Section through the glenoid cavity

Inter-articular fibro-cartilage

Internal lateral ligament

EXT¹
LAT'V
LIG'T

TRANSVERSE SECTION TO SHOW THE LIGAMENTS AND THE FIBRO-CARTILAGE OF THE JOINT OF THE LOWER JAW.   THE DOTTED LINES REPRESENT THE TWO SYNOVIAL MEMBRANES.

The *external lateral ligament* extends from the tubercle of the zygoma downwards and backwards to the tubercle of the condyle of the jaw.

The *internal lateral ligament* extends from the spinous process of the sphenoid bone to the border of the dental foramen. This 'so-called' ligament cannot in any way contribute to the strength of the joint: the articulation of one side performs the office of internal lateral ligament to the other.

The *inter-articular fibro-cartilage* is of an oval form, and thicker at the margin than at the centre. It is connected on the outer side to the external lateral ligament, and on the inner side some of the fibres of the external pterygoid are inserted into it.

There are *two synovial membranes* for the joint. The larger and looser of the two is situated between the glenoid cavity and the fibro-cartilage. The other is interposed between the fibro-cartilage and the condyle of the jaw. They sometimes communicate through a small aperture in the centre of the fibro-cartilage.

The form of the articulation of the lower jaw admits of motion —upwards and downwards, forwards and backwards, and from side to side. A combination of these motions takes place in mastication: during this act the condyles of the jaw describe an oblique rotatory movement upon the glenoid cavity. The purposes served by this fibro-cartilage in this joint are, that it follows the condyle, and adapts a convenient socket for all its movements; and that, being elastic, it breaks shocks; for shocks here would be almost fatal, considering what a thin plate the glenoid cavity is, and that just above it is the brain.

THE DISSECTION OF THE ARM.

The arm being placed at right angles with the body, make three incisions through the skin: the first, along the middle of the sternum; the second, along the clavicle and down the front of the arm for about four inches; the third, from the ensiform cartilage vertically downwards, to the posterior border of the axilla.

The skin should be carefully separated from the subjacent layer of adipose tissue (called the *superficial fascia*). In doing so, unless the subject be very muscular, you will scarcely notice the thin pale fibres of the broad cutaneous muscle of the neck ('platysma myoides,' p. 13), which arises in this tissue.

Cutaneous nerves.   The numerous nerves which run through the subcutaneous tissue to the skin and mammary gland must be carefully dissected. They are derived from various sources: some, branches of the superficial cervical plexus, descend over the clavicle; others, branches of the intercostal nerves, come through the intercostal spaces close to the sternum, with a small artery; a third series, also branches of the intercostal nerves, come out on the side of the chest, and run forwards over the outer border of the pectoralis major.

The *supra-clavicular* nerves, which descend over the clavicle, are subdivided, according to their direction, into *sternal, clavicular,* and *acromial* branches (diagram, p. 15). The *sternal* cross the inner end of the clavicle to supply the skin over the upper part of the sternum. The *clavicular* pass over the middle of the clavicle, and supply the integument over the front of the chest and the mammary gland. The *acromial* branches cross over the outer end of the clavicle, and distribute their filaments to the skin of the shoulder.

Near the sternum you find the *anterior cutaneous branches of the intercostal nerves.* After traversing the pectoralis major, each nerve sends a filament to the skin over the sternum, and a larger one, which supplies the skin, over the pectoral muscle.

Branches of the internal mammary artery, for the supply of the mammary gland, accompany these nerves. During lactation they increase in size, ramifying tortuously over the surface of the gland. I have seen them nearly as large as the radial at the wrist. They would require a ligature in removal of the breast.

The *lateral cutaneous branches of the intercostal nerves* come out between the digitations of the serratus magnus on the side of the chest. They will be more fully described presently.

Remove the superficial fascia with the mammary gland from the pectoralis major, by dissecting parallel to the course of the fibres. When the muscle has been fully exposed, observe its shape, the course of its fibres, their origin and insertion.

Pectoralis major.   The pectoralis major is the great triangular muscle on the front of the chest. It *arises* from the sternal half of the clavicle, from the front of the sternum, from the cartilages of all the true ribs except the last, and from the aponeurosis of the external oblique muscle of the abdomen. The fibres converge towards the arm, and terminate in a flat tendon, about two inches in breadth, which is *inserted* into the anterior margin of the bicipital groove of the humerus. Their arrangement, as well as the structure of their tendon, is peculiar. The lower fibres which form the boundary of the axilla are folded beneath the rest, and terminate upon the upper part of the tendon, i.e. nearer to the shoulder joint; whereas the upper fibres, which arise from the clavicle, and are frequently separated from the main body of the muscle by a slight interval, descend in front of the lower, and terminate upon the lower part of the tendon. Consequently the upper and lower fibres of the muscle cross each other previously to their insertion.

The object of this arrangement is to enable all the fibres to act simultaneously when the arm is extended.

The upper part of the tendon sends off an 'aponeurosis,' which straps down the long head of the biceps, and is attached to the great tuberosity of the humerus. A second expansion is prolonged backwards to the tendon of the deltoid muscle, and a third is intimately connected with the fascia of the upper arm.

The chief *action* of the pectoralis major is to draw the humerus towards the chest: as in placing the hand on the opposite shoulder, or in pulling an object towards the body. When the arm is raised and made the fixed point, the muscle assists in raising the trunk, as in climbing.

Between the pectoralis major and the deltoid, the great muscle of the shoulder, is an interval varying in extent in different subjects, but always more marked towards the clavicle. It contains a small artery—the *thoracica humeraria*—and the *cephalic vein*, which ascends on the outer side of the arm, and empties itself into the axillary. This interval is the proper place to feel for the coracoid process. In doubtful injuries about the shoulder, this point of bone is a good landmark in helping the surgeon to arrive at a correct diagnosis.

The pectoralis major is supplied with nerves by the anterior

thoracic branches of the brachial plexus; with blood, by the long
and short thoracic branches of the axillary artery.

Anatomy of the infraclavicular region. Reflect from the clavicle, the clavicular portion of
the pectoralis major, and in doing so, a small nerve,
the anterior thoracic, must be noticed entering the
under surface of the muscle. Beneath the portion so
reflected, part of the pectoralis minor will be exposed. Between
the upper border of this muscle and the clavicle, is an important
space, in which you must dissect and examine the relative position
of the following objects—

Costocoracoid fascia. a. A strong ligamentous expansion, called the costo-
coracoid fascia, which extends from the cartilage of
the first rib to the coracoid process. Between these
points it is attached to the clavicle, and forms a complete investment for the subclavius muscle. It presents a crescent-shaped
edge, which arches over, and protects the axillary vessels and
nerves: from this edge is prolonged a fascia, which passes in front
of the axillary vessels forming the anterior portion of their sheath;
the posterior being formed by a prolongation of the deep cervical
fascia. The front portion of this sheath is perforated by the
cephalic vein, thoracica acromialis artery, and anterior thoracic
nerve. This fascia must be removed.

b. The subclavius muscle enclosed in its fibrous sheath.

c. The axillary vein, artery, and brachial plexus of nerves.

d. A short arterial trunk (the thoracic axis), which divides into
several radiating branches.

e. The termination of the cephalic vein in the axillary.

f. Two nerves (the anterior thoracic), which descend from the
brachial plexus below the clavicle, cross in front of the axillary
vessels to supply the pectoral muscles.

Subclavius. This muscle lies between the clavicle and the first
rib. It *arises* from the cartilage of the first rib by a
round tendon, and is *inserted* into a groove on the under surface
of the clavicle between its two tubercles. Its nerve comes from
the brachial plexus. Its *action* is to depress the clavicle, and
prevent its too great elevation.

In the space now before us are the great vessels and nerves of the axilla in the first part of their course. They lie at a great depth from the surface. They are surrounded by a sheath of fascia, which descends with them beneath the clavicle, and are situated with regard to each other in the following manner. The axillary vein lies in front of the artery, and rather to its thoracic side. The axillary (brachial) plexus of nerves is situated above the artery, and on a posterior plane. The plexus consists of two, or sometimes three large cords, which result from the union of the anterior branches of the last four cervical and the first dorsal.

Relative position of the axillary vessels and nerves.

Thoracic axis. This is the first branch of the axillary artery. It comes off above the pectoralis minor, and soon divides into three branches—the *superior or short thoracic*, the *thoracica humeraria*, and the *thoracica acromialis*. The *superior or short thoracic* runs between the pectoralis major and minor, supplying ramifications to both, and anastomosing with the intercostal and internal mammary arteries. The *thoracica humeraria* descends with the cephalic vein, in the interval between the pectoralis major and deltoid, and ramifies in both. The *thoracica acromialis* passes over the coracoid process to the under surface of the deltoid, which it supplies, and communicates with the circumflex branches of the axillary. All these arteries are accompanied by veins, which most frequently empty themselves into the cephalic, but occasionally into the axillary vein itself.

Cephalic vein. The cephalic vein is one of the principal cutaneous veins of the arm. Commencing on the back of the thumb and forefinger, it runs up the radial side of the forearm, over the front of the elbow-joint; thence ascending along the outer edge of the biceps, it runs up the interval between the pectoralis major and deltoid, pierces the costo-coracoid fascia, and finally empties itself into the axillary vein.[*]

---

[*] The cephalic vein, in some cases, runs over the clavicle to join the external jugular; or there may be a communication (termed jugulo-cephalic) between these veins.

Anterior
thoracic
nerves.
These nerves come from the brachial plexus, to supply the pectoral muscles. There are generally two—an external and an internal—one for each pectoral muscle (p. 62). The external arises from the outer cord of the brachial plexus, passes over the axillary artery, and supplies the pectoralis major; the internal comes from the internal cord, and emerges between the axillary artery and vein, to enter the under surface of the pectoralis minor.

Difficulty of tying the first part of the axillary artery.
From this view of the relations of the axillary artery in the first part of its course, some idea may be formed of the difficulty of passing a ligature round it in this situation. In addition to its great depth from the surface, varieties sometimes occur in the position of the nerves and veins, which would render the operation still more embarrassing. For instance, the anterior thoracic nerves may be more numerous than usual, and form by their mutual communication a plexus around the artery. A large nerve is often seen crossing obliquely over the artery, immediately below the clavicle, to form one of the roots of the median nerve. The cephalic vein may ascend higher than usual, and open into the subclavian; and, as it receives large veins corresponding to the thoracic axis, a concourse of veins would be met with in front of the artery. Again, it is by no means uncommon to find a deep-seated vein (e.g. the supra-scapular) crossing over the artery to join the axillary vein.

DISSECTION OF THE AXILLA.

The skin having already been reflected, it is necessary to notice the axillary sebaceous glands, and afterwards to make out the axillary fascia.

Sebaceous glands.
In close contact with the skin, near the roots of the hairs in the axilla, are numerous sebaceous glands. They are of a reddish brown colour, and rather larger than a pin's head.

Axillary fascia.
This tough membrane, which lies immediately beneath the skin of the axilla, is a continuation of the general investment of the muscles. It closes in and forms the floor of the cavity of the axilla. Externally it is strengthened by fibres from the tendons of the pectoralis major and latissimus dorsi, and is continuous with the fascia of the arm; internally, it is prolonged on the side of the chest, over the serratus magnus muscle; in front and behind, it divides so as to inclose between its layers the muscles which form the boundaries of the axilla. Thus the anterior layer incloses the two pectoral muscles, and is connected with the coracoid process, the costo-coracoid ligament, and the clavicle; the posterior layer incloses the latissimus dorsi, and passes backwards to the spine.

A subcutaneous artery, sometimes of considerable size, often runs in the substance of the axillary fascia. It generally arises from the brachial, or from the lower part of the axillary, and runs across the floor of the axilla towards the lower edge of the pectoralis major. So far as I know, it has not hitherto been named; but it is worth remembering, because it would occasion much hæmorrhage if wounded in opening an abscess.

Contents of axilla.
Remove the axillary fascia, and display the boundaries and the contents of the axilla. The dissection of this cavity is difficult, and you must proceed cautiously. Bear in mind that the trunk blood-vessels and nerves run through the *upper* part of the axilla; that the long thoracic artery runs along the anterior border, and the subscapular artery along the posterior. Commence working, therefore, in the middle; break down with the handle of the scalpel the loose connective tissue, fat, and absorbent glands, which occupy the cavity. You will soon discover some cutaneous nerves coming out between the ribs, and then crossing the axillary space. These nerves are the *lateral cutaneous branches of the intercostal nerves*; they perforate the intercostal spaces between the digitations of the serratus magnus, midway between the sternum and the spine, and divide into anterior and posterior branches. The *anterior* turn over the pectoralis major, to supply the skin on the front of the chest and

the mammary gland. The *posterior* pass backwards over the
latissimus dorsi, and are distributed to the skin covering this
muscle and the scapula.

Intercosto-
humeral
nerves.
The perforating branch of the second intercostal
nerve requires a special description; it is larger than
the others, and is called the '*intercosto-humeral*,' because it supplies the integuments of the arm. It comes through
the second intercostal space, traverses the upper part of the axilla,
where it receives a branch of the lesser internal cutaneous nerve
(nerve of Wrisberg), and terminates in filaments, which are distributed to the skin on the inner side of the arm, as low as the
internal condyle. The perforating branch of the third intercostal
is also an '*intercosto-humeral*' nerve. It receives a branch from
the second, and runs a similar course. The distribution of these
nerves may account for the pain down the arm which is sometimes
experienced in pleurisy.

Boundaries
of the axilla.
The axilla may be described as a conical space, of
which the summit is beneath the clavicle, and the base
between the pectoralis major and the latissimus dorsi. Now,
what are its boundaries? On the *inner* side, it is bounded by the
ribs, covered by the serratus magnus; on the *outer* side by the
humerus, covered by the coraco-brachialis and biceps; in *front*
by the pectoralis major and minor; *behind* by the latissimus
dorsi, teres major, and subscapularis. Its anterior and posterior
boundaries converge from the chest, so that the axilla becomes
narrower towards the arm. With a full view of the axilla before
you, think what serious consequences may follow suppuration
here; the matter may burrow under the pectoral muscles, or under
the scapula, or it may run up beneath the clavicle and point in
the neck.

Axillary
absorbent
glands.
The axillary glands form a continuous chain beneath
the clavicle, with the cervical glands. They are from
twelve to fifteen in number, of a reddish brown colour,
and variable size. Most of them lie near some large blood-vessel;
others are imbedded in the loose tissue of the axilla; sometimes
one or two small ones are observed along the lower border of the

pectoralis major. They are supplied with blood by a branch (*thoracica alaris*) of the axillary artery, and by branches from the thoracic and infra-scapular arteries.

These glands receive the absorbents from the arm, from the front and side of the chest, and from the outer half of the mammary gland.

Now reflect the pectoralis major from its origin, to expose the pectoralis minor, and the ramifications of the short and long thoracic arteries. Preserve the arteries as much as possible in connection with the main trunks.

Pectoralis minor. This muscle *arises* from the third, fourth, and fifth ribs, near the costal cartilages. The fibres run upwards and outwards, and converge to a strong tendon, which is *inserted* into the anterior surface of the coracoid process. The tendon is connected to that of the coraco-brachialis by a strong fascia, which forms a protection for the subjacent axillary vessels and nerves. The action of this muscle is to draw the scapula downwards and forwards.

Latissimus dorsi. This muscle forms the posterior margin of the axilla. It *arises* from the crest of the ilium, from the spines of the two or three upper sacral, all the lumbar, and six lower dorsal vertebræ, and by digitations from the three lower ribs, corresponding with those of the external oblique. It is *inserted* by a broad flat tendon (which runs behind the axillary vessels and nerves), into the bottom of the bicipital groove of the humerus.

Teres major. This muscle lies behind the latissimus dorsi, is closely connected with it, and assists in forming the posterior boundary of the axilla. It *arises* from the lower angle of the back of the scapula, and is *inserted* by a broad flat tendon into the posterior margin of the bicipital groove of the humerus. A bursa or sac, containing serum, to prevent friction, intervenes between this tendon and that of the latissimus dorsi. The action of this and the preceding muscle is to draw the humerus inwards and backwards.

Subscapularis. This muscle occupies the internal surface of the scapula. It *arises* from the internal surface of the

Q

scapula, with the exception of the angles and neck, and terminates in a strong tendon, which passes under the axillary vessels and nerves, over the inner side of the shoulder-joint, and is *inserted* into the lesser tuberosity of the humerus. The tendon of the muscle is intimately connected with the capsular ligament of the shoulder-joint, and between the coracoid process and the tendon is a bursa, which frequently communicates with the joint. Its action is to rotate the humerus inwards.

Serratus magnus.

This muscle covers the side of the chest like a girth. It *arises* from the eight upper ribs by nine slips or digitations, the second rib having two. Its fibres converge and are *inserted* into the posterior border of the scapula. Its action is to draw the scapula forwards; but of this more hereafter. It is supplied by the following nerve, which you see on its outer surface.

External respiratory nerve of Bell.

This nerve supplies the serratus magnus only. It comes from the fifth and sixth cervical nerves; and after passing through the scalenus medius, runs behind the axillary vessels, to the outer surface of the serratus magnus; each digitation receiving a separate filament.*

Having surveyed the muscles which bound the axilla, study next the axillary artery, and its branches: to this end, reflect the subclavius from its insertion, and the pectoralis minor from its origin.

Course and relations of the axillary artery.

This artery, a continuation of the subclavian, takes the name of 'axillary' at the outer border of the first rib. It runs downwards and outwards, through the upper part of the axilla, beneath the two pectoral muscles, and along the inner edge of the coraco-brachialis, as far as the lower border of the tendon of the teres major, where it takes the name of 'brachial.' Its course may be divided into three portions: one above the pectoralis minor; one behind it; and the third below it. The artery in the

---

* It may be asked why this nerve is called the 'external respiratory.' It was so named by Sir C. Bell, who considered the serratus magnus as the external respiratory muscle.

first part of its course is covered by the pectoralis major and the costo-coracoid sheath; and is crossed by the cephalic vein. On the inner side is the axillary vein; on the outer, the brachial plexus of nerves; and behind it, is the first intercostal space and the second digitation of the serratus magnus. In the *second* part, it lies behind the pectoralis minor; on its inner side is the axillary vein, separated however from the artery by the brachial plexus, which here surrounds the artery. The artery rests upon loose cellular tissue. In the *third* part, i.e. below the pectoralis minor, the artery lies upon the subscapularis, and then upon the tendons of the latissimus dorsi and teres major. On the outer side is the coraco-brachialis; on its inner side, the axillary vein. The brachial plexus here breaks up into its various divisions, which are generally arranged in the following manner: in *front* of the artery are the two roots of the median nerve, which converge like the letter V; on the *outer* side are the musculo-cutaneous and external root of the median; on the *inner*, the ulnar, the two internal cutaneous, and the internal root of the median; *behind* it, the musculo-spiral and circumflex nerves.

Branches of the axillary artery.
The number and origin of these branches often vary, but their general course is in most cases similar, and they usually arise in the order in which they are here described.

The *thoracic axis* arises above the pectoralis minor, and divides into branches, which have been already described (p. 221).

The *alar thoracic* is variable in its origin, supplies the glands and cellular tissue of the axilla

The *inferior or long thoracic artery*, sometimes called the external mammary, runs along the lower border of the pectoralis minor. It supplies the mammary gland, the serratus magnus and pectoral muscles, and maintains a free anastomosis with the short thoracic, internal mammary, and intercostal arteries.

The *subscapular* is the largest branch of the axillary; it arises opposite the lower border of the subscapularis, and soon divides into an anterior and posterior branch.

a. The *anterior branch* is the continued trunk; it runs along

q 2

the anterior edge of the subscapularis towards the lower angle of
the scapula. Its numerous branches supply the subscapularis,
latissimus dorsi, and serratus magnus, and anastomose with the
intercostal and thoracic arteries, as well as the posterior scapular
(a branch of the subclavian).

b. The *posterior branch* (dorsalis scapulæ) runs to the back of
the scapula, through a triangular space, bounded in front by the

Fig. 40.

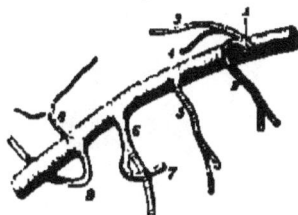

PLAN OF THE BRANCHES OF THE AXILLARY ARTERY.

1. Thoracic axis, giving off	6. Subscapular.
2. Short thoracic.	7. Dorsalis scapulæ.
3. Thoracica acromialis.	8. Anterior circumflex.
4. Thoracica humeraria.	9. Posterior circumflex.
5. Long thoracic.	

long head of the triceps; below, by the teres major; and above,
by the subscapular and teres minor (diagram, p. 229). On the
back of the scapula, it divides into branches, which ramify close
to the bone, supplying the infra-spinatus and teres minor, and
anastomose with the supra-scapular and posterior scapular arteries
(diagram, p. 60). The subscapular vein empties itself into the
axillary vein.

Anterior and
posterior
circumflex
arteries.
There are two circumflex arteries—an *anterior* and
a *posterior*, so called from the manner in which they
encircle the neck of the humerus. The *posterior circumflex artery* is as large as the subscapular, close to
which it is given off; or both may arise from a common trunk
from the axillary. It passes backwards through a quadrilateral

space, bounded above by the subscapularis and teres minor, below
by the teres major, externally by the neck of the humerus, and
internally by the long head of the triceps (fig. 47). It then winds
round the back of the neck of the humerus, and is distributed to
the under surface of the deltoid.

Fig. 47.

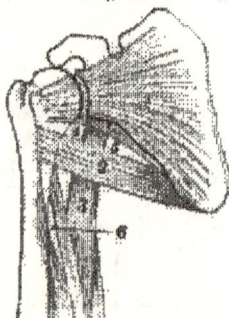

DIAGRAM OF THE ORIGINS OF THE TRICEPS.

1. Subscapularis.
2. Teres major.
3. Long head of triceps.
4. Square space for circumflex a. and n.
5. Triangular space for dorsalis scapulæ a.
6. Space for musculo-spiral a., and superior
profunda a.

Besides the deltoid, the posterior circumflex artery supplies the
long head of the triceps, the head of the humerus, and the shoulder-
joint. It inosculates above with the acromio-thoracic and supra-
scapular arteries, below with the ascending branch of the superior
profunda (a branch of the brachial), and in front with the anterior
circumflex artery. If you cannot find the posterior circumflex
artery in its normal position, look for it (as a branch of the
brachial) below the tendon of the teres major.

The *anterior circumflex artery*, much smaller than the posterior, runs in front of the neck of the humerus, above the tendon
of the latissimus dorsi. It passes directly outwards beneath the
coraco-brachialis and short head of the biceps, close to the bone,

and terminates in the under surface of the delloid, where it inosculates with the posterior circumflex artery.

The most remarkable branch of the anterior circumflex artery is one which runs with the long tendon of the biceps up the groove of the humerus, and is called, on that account, the bicipital artery. It supplies the shoulder-joint and the neck of the humerus.

Axillary vein. The *axillary vein* is formed by the junction of the venæ comites of the brachial artery, near the lower border of the subscapularis. It receives the subscapular and the other veins corresponding to the branches of the axillary artery, with the exception of the circumflex, which usually join either the subscapular or one of the venæ comites. The axillary also receives the cephalic, and sometimes the basilic vein.

The axillary vein in the first part of its course lies in front of the artery, and close to its sternal side; in the lower two thirds of its course the vein lies still to the sternal side of the artery, but is separated from it by some of the nerves of the brachial plexus.

Axillary or brachial plexus of nerves. This plexus is formed by the anterior branches of the four lower cervical and first dorsal nerves, and receives also a small communicating branch from the fourth cervical nerve. The plexus is broad at the lower part of the neck, where it emerges between the anterior and middle scalene muscles; but it gradually contracts as it descends beneath the clavicle into the axilla.

The arrangement of the nerves in the formation of the plexus is usually thus:—The fifth and sixth cervical unite to form a single cord; the eighth cervical and the first dorsal form another cord; the seventh cervical runs for a short distance alone, and then splits into two branches, one of which joins the cord formed by the fifth and sixth cervical, the other, that formed by the eighth cervical and first dorsal. The branch joining the trunk formed by the eighth cervical and first dorsal usually receives a large reinforcement from the conjoined fifth and sixth cervical. Thus two great trunks are formed, which lie for some distance above and to the outer side of the subclavian artery. Beneath the clavicle, a third cord is formed by the junction of a fasciculus from each of the two primary trunks, so that in the axilla there are three large cords,

Fig. 48.

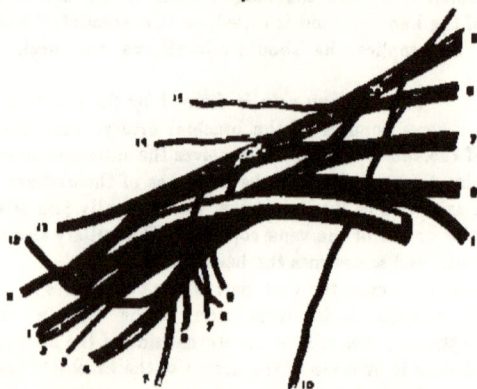

DIAGRAM OF THE BRACHIAL PLEXUS OF NERVES, AND THEIR RELATION TO THE AXILLARY ARTERY.

1. Ulnar.	8–9. Anterior thoracic n. to pectoral
2. Internal cutaneous.	muscle.
3. Lesser int. cutaneous (n. of Wris-	10. N. to serratus magnus.
berg).	11. Median.
4. Musculo-spiral.	12. Circumflex.
5. N. to latissimus dorsi.	13. External cutaneous.
6. N. to teres major.	14. Supra-scapular.
7. N. to subscapularis.	15. Posterior scapular.

one external to the axillary artery, one internal to it, the third behind it.*

The axillary plexus gives off some branches above the clavicle; these were dissected with the neck (p. 63). Below the clavicle, it gives off the following:—

From the outer cord, an anterior thoracic branch, the external

---

* This seems, from a number of dissections, to be the most frequent arrangement of the nerves forming the brachial plexus. This arrangement is, however, very variable, often differing on the two sides in the same subject.

cutaneous, and the outer head of the median ; from the inner cord, another anterior thoracic nerve, the inner head of the median, the ulnar, the internal, and the lesser internal cutaneous. From the posterior cord, the three subscapular nerves, the circumflex and the musculo-spiral.

The anterior thoracic nerves have been described (p. 222).

Subscapular nerves.   The three 'subscapular' nerves are found on the surface of the subscapularis. They come from the posterior cord of the brachial plexus, and supply respectively the latissimus dorsi, teres major, and subscapularis. The nerve for the latissimus dorsi (called the long subscapular nerve) runs with the anterior branch of the subscapular artery.

The *nerve for the teres major* is either a branch of the preceding, or comes distinct from the plexus. It lies nearer to the humerus than the long subscapular, and after supplying a branch to the latissimus dorsi, terminates in the teres major.

The proper *nerve of the subscapularis* arises from the plexus higher than the others.

Circumflex nerve.   The posterior circumflex artery is accompanied by the circumflex nerve which supplies the deltoid. This large nerve comes from the posterior part of the brachial plexus, in common with the musculo-spiral and subscapular nerves, and, after sending a branch to the teres minor, terminates in the under surface of the deltoid. The nerve supplies the skin covering the deltoid by branches which turn round the posterior border of the muscle ; other branches are distributed to the skin over the long head of the triceps.

DISSECTION OF THE UPPER ARM.

Let the incision be continued down the inner side of the arm as far as two inches below the elbow. Reflect the skin, and trace the following cutaneous nerves.

Cutaneous nerves.   The filaments of the *intercosto-humeral nerves* run down the inner and posterior part of the arm, to the olecranon; on the inner side of the arm, one joins a branch from the nerve of Wrisberg.

The branches of the *internal cutaneous nerve* perforate the fascia about the middle of the inner side of the arm, and subdivide into filaments which supply the anterior and posterior surface of the forearm, as low as the wrist.

The *lesser internal cutaneous (nerve of Wrisberg)* perforates the fascia about the lower third of the arm, and supplies the skin over the internal condyle and olecranon.

The *internal cutaneous branch of the musculo-spiral nerve*, sometimes wanting, and always small, comes through the fascia near the middle of the inner side of the arm.

The nerves which perforate the fascia near the middle of the outer part of the arm, are the *external cutaneous branches of the musculo-spiral.* They are accompanied by a small branch from the superior profunda artery. They divide into filaments, one of which is to be traced down the outer and back part of the forearm, nearly as low as the wrist.

On the outer side of the tendon of the biceps the *external cutaneous* nerve perforates the fascia, and divides into many branches, which supply the skin of the outer part of the forearm.

Disposition of veins in front of the elbow.　　The next object of attention should be the disposition of the veins in front of the elbow. In cleaning these veins, take care not to divide the branches of the internal and external cutaneous nerves which pass both above and below them.

The following is the ordinary arrangement of the superficial veins at the bend of the elbow: On the outer side is the radial; on the inner side is the ulnar vein; in the centre is the median, which divides into two branches; the external of which, uniting with the radial to form the cephalic vein, is called the *median cephalic*; the internal, uniting with the ulnar to form the basilic, is named the *median basilic.* Near its bifurcation, the median vein communicates by a branch (mediana profunda) with the deep veins which accompany the arteries of the forearm.

Trace the *cephalic vein* up the arm. It runs along the outer border of the biceps to the groove between the pectoralis major and the deltoid, where it terminates in the axillary.

Fig. 49.

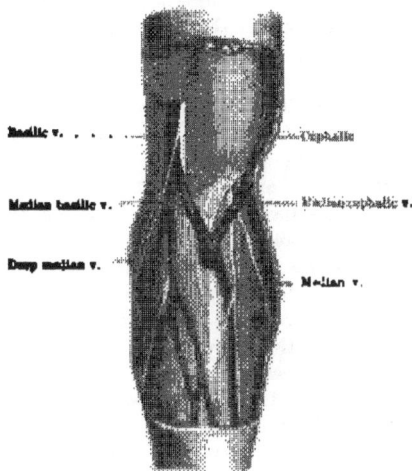

Basilic v. ....Cephalic

Median basilic v. ....Median cephalic v.

Deep median v. ...

Median v.

SUPERFICIAL VEINS AND NERVES AT THE BEND OF THE LEFT ELBOW.

The *basilic vein* ascends along the inner side of the arm with the internal cutaneous nerve. Near the upper third of the arm, it perforates the fascia, and empties itself either into the internal vena comes of the brachial artery, or into the axillary vein.

Relation of nerves and veins at elbow. The principal branches of the nerves pass beneath the veins; but many small filaments cross in front which are exposed to injury in venesection.

Relation of median basilic vein to brachial artery. Since the median basilic vein is larger than the median cephalic, and, on account of the strong fascia beneath, more easily compressible, it is usually chosen for venesection; its position therefore, in reference to the brachial artery, becomes very important. The vein is only separated from the artery by the fascia, derived from the tendon of the biceps. This fascia is in some subjects remarkably thin, or even absent. It sometimes happens that the artery lies above the fascia, in absolute contact with the vein. In choosing, therefore, this vein for venesection, there is a risk of wounding the artery; hence the practical rule, to bleed either from the median cephalic, or from the median basilic above the situation where it crosses the brachial artery.

Immediately above the internal condyle, in the neighbourhood of the basilic vein, we find one or two small *absorbent glands*. Others may be higher up along the inner side of the arm. I have seen a gland at the bend of the elbow; but never below this joint. These little glands are the first which become tender and enlarged after an injury to the hand.

Muscular fascia. The fascia which invests the muscles of the upper arm is a continuation of the fascia from the trunk and the axilla. This membrane varies in density; thus it is thin over the biceps, stronger on the inner side of the arm, to protect the brachial vessels and nerves, and strongest over the triceps. What are its connections? At the upper part of the arm it is connected with the coracoid process and the clavicle; it is strengthened at the axilla by an expansion from the tendons of the pectoralis major and latissimus dorsi; posteriorly, it is attached to the spine of the scapula. The fascia surrounds the brachial vessels with a sheath, and furnishes partitions which separate the muscles from each other. Of these partitions the most marked are the *external* and *internal intermuscular septa*, which divide the muscles on the anterior from that on the posterior surface of the upper arm. These septa are attached to the condyloid ridges of the humerus and to the condyles. The *internal* septum, the stronger of the two, begins at the insertion of the coraco-brachialis, and separates the triceps extensor from the brachialis anticus. The *external septum* commences from the insertion of the deltoid, and separates the brachialis anticus, the supinator longus, and the extensor carpi radialis longior in front, from the triceps behind.

At the lower part of the upper arm, the fascia is remarkably strong, especially where it covers the brachialis anticus, and the

brachial vessels, and is continued over the muscles on the inner
side of the forearm. At the back of the elbow, the fascia is
attached to the tendon of the triceps, and the olecranon.

Now remove the fascia in order to study the muscles on the
front of the arm; namely, the biceps, the coraco-brachialis, and
the brachialis anticus.

Biceps.   The biceps, as its name implies, arises by two heads
—a long and a short. The *short* or internal *head*
arises from the point of the coracoid process of the scapula, by a
thick flat tendon which is common to a slender muscle on its
inner side, called the coraco-brachialis. The *long head* of the
biceps *arises* from the upper border of the glenoid cavity of the
scapula by a long round tendon, which traverses the shoulder-
joint and passes over the head of the humerus, and down the
groove between the two tuberosities. The tendon is retained in
the groove by a fibrous bridge derived from the capsule of the
joint, and connected with the tendon of the pectoralis major.
Divide this bridge and see that the synovial membrane of the
joint is reflected round the tendon, and accompanies it for about
two inches down the groove, thus forming a sort of synovial fold.
The object of this is to facilitate the play of the tendon, and to
carry little arteries (from the anterior circumflex) for its supply.
The two heads unite about the middle of the arm, and form a
single muscle, which terminates in a strong flat tendon of considerable length; this sinks deep into the triangular space at the
bend of the elbow, and, after a slight twist upon itself, is *inserted*
into the posterior part of the tubercle of the radius. The anterior
part of the tubercle, over which the tendon plays, is crusted with
cartilage, and a *bursa mucosa* intervenes to prevent friction. The
most internal fibres of the muscle are inserted into a *strong broad
aponeurosis,* which is prolonged from the inner border of the
tendon to the fascia on the inner side of the forearm. This
aponeurosis, called the *semi-lunar fascia of the biceps,* protects
the brachial vessels and the median nerve at the bend of the
elbow.

The *action* of the biceps is twofold. 1. It is a flexor of the forearm: 2. It is a supinator of the forearm, in consequence of its insertion into the *posterior* part of the tubercle of the radius. Its power of supination is greatest when the arm is bent, because its tendon is then inserted at a right angle. Why does the long tendon pass through the shoulder-joint? It acts like a strap, and confines the head of the humerus in its proper centre of motion. But for this tendon, the head of the bone, when the deltoid acts, would be pulled directly upwards and strike against the under surface of the acromion. When the tendon is ruptured or dislocated from its groove a man can move his arm backwards and forwards, but he cannot raise the smallest weight. The biceps is supplied with blood by an artery (from the brachial), which runs into the middle of it, and then divides into ascending and descending branches. Its nerve comes from the external cutaneous (musculo cutaneous).

Coraco-brachialis.   This thin muscle is situated at the upper part of the arm, and runs parallel to the inner border of the short head of the biceps. It *arises* by fleshy fibres from the point of the coracoid process, in common with the short head of the biceps, and from a fibrous septum which lies between them. The muscle terminates in a flat tendon, which is *inserted* into the inner side of the middle of the humerus, between the brachialis anticus and the inner head of the triceps. Its action is to draw the humerus forwards and inwards, e.g. in bringing the gun up to the shoulder.

Concerning the coraco-brachialis remember, 1. That the external cutaneous nerve runs through it; 2. That its inner fleshy border is the guide to the axillary artery in the last part of its course; 3. That the brachial artery lies upon its flat tendon of insertion, and can here be effectually compressed by the finger or the tourniquet.

The coraco-brachialis and biceps are covered at their upper part by the deltoid and pectoralis major. The head of the humerus rolls beneath the coraco-brachialis and short origin of the biceps; and a large *bursa* is interposed between these muscles and the tendon of the subscapularis, which covers the head of the bone.

Brachialis anticus.   This muscle is situated close to the lower half of the humerus, and is partially concealed by the biceps. Between the two muscles you find the external cutaneous nerve, which supplies them both.

It arises from the humerus by a fleshy digitation on either side of the tendon of the deltoid; from the front surface of the bone below this point, and from the intermuscular septa. The muscle, becoming thicker and broader as it descends, covers the front of the capsule of the elbow-joint, and terminates in a tendon, which is inserted in a pointed manner into the coronoid process of the ulna. Its action is to bend the forearm.

Now examine the course and relations of the brachial vessels and nerves.

Course and relations of the brachial artery.   The brachial artery, a continuation of the axillary, takes its name at the lower border of the teres major. It runs down the inner side of the arm, along the *inner border of the coraco-brachialis and biceps*, to the front of the elbow, where it divides, near the coronoid process of the ulna, into the radial and ulnar arteries.

Thus its direction corresponds with a line drawn from the anterior part of the axilla to the central point between the condyles of the humerus.

In the upper part of its course it lies on the long and inner heads of the triceps (from the long head it is separated by the musculo-spiral nerve and superior profunda artery); in the middle, it lies on the tendon of the coraco-brachialis; in the lower part, on the brachialis anticus.

The artery is accompanied by two veins (*venæ comites*), and the median nerve, all of which are invested in a common sheath of fascia. The median nerve crosses obliquely in front of the artery, lying, near the axilla, on its outer side, near the elbow on its inner.

The *ulnar* nerve at first runs along the inner side of the artery, but below is separated from it by the internal intermuscular septum, where it passes behind the internal condyle. Superficial to the artery, we find the internal cutaneous nerve and the basilic vein.

Observe particularly that the artery is more or less overlapped, in the first part of its course, by the coraco-brachialis, lower down by the fleshy belly of the biceps; these muscles in their respective situations are the best guides to the artery.

About the middle of the humerus, the artery lies for nearly two inches on the tendon of the coraco-brachialis, and is so close to the bone that it can be effectually compressed; here, too, it is crossed by the median nerve.

At the bend of the elbow the artery is protected by the semi-lunar fascia from the tendon of the biceps. It enters a triangular space, bounded by the pronator radii teres internally, and by the supinator radii longus externally. It sinks into this space, with the tendon of the biceps to its outer side, and the median nerve to its inner; all three rest upon the brachialis anticus. Opposite the coronoid process of the ulna it divides into the radial and ulnar arteries.

Two veins, of which the internal is the larger, lie in close contact with the brachial artery, and communicate at frequent intervals by transverse branches.

Branches of brachial artery. The brachial artery gives off three branches, which arise from its inner side; namely, the superior profunda, the inferior profunda, and the anastomotica magna. It also gives off muscular branches to the coraco-brachialis and biceps.

The *profunda superior* arises from the brachial artery, immediately below the tendon of the teres major.[*] It winds round the posterior part of the humerus, between the outer and inner heads of the triceps, with the musculo-spiral nerve (p. 229), and a little above the middle of the arm divides into two branches, which run for some distance on either side of the nerve. One of these runs in the substance of the triceps muscle to the olecranon, and anastomoses with the ulnar recurrent, the interosseous recurrent, and anastomotica magna arteries; the other branch accompanies the

[*] If you cannot find the profunda in its usual place, look for it above the tendon of the latissimus dorsi, when you will probably find that it is given off from a common trunk with the posterior circumflex.

musculo-spiral nerve to the outer side of the arm, descends deep
in the fissure between the brachialis anticus and supinator radii
longus, and terminates in numerous ramifications, some of which
pass in front of the external condyle, and others behind it, to
inosculate with the radial and interosseous recurrent arteries.

Fig. 50.

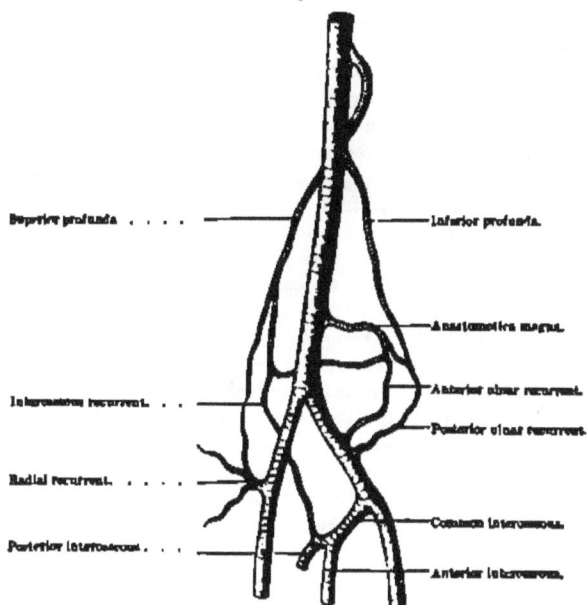

Superior profunda . . . .   Inferior profunda.

                                   Anastomotica magna.

                                   Anterior ulnar recurrent.

Interosseous recurrent. . .   Posterior ulnar recurrent.

Radial recurrent. . . . .

                                   Common interosseous.

Posterior interosseous . . .   Anterior interosseous.

PLAN OF THE BRANCHES OF THE BRACHIAL ARTERY AND THE ARTERIAL
INOSCULATIONS ABOUT THE RIGHT ELBOW-JOINT.

Before its division, the superior profunda sends several branches
to the triceps, some of which inosculate minutely with the circumflex arteries. These would assist in establishing a collateral

circulation if the brachial artery were tied above the origin of the profunda.

The *profunda inferior* arises from the brachial, opposite to the insertion of the coraco-brachialis, or sometimes by a common trunk with the superior profunda. It runs with the ulnar nerve on the inner head of the triceps (which it supplies), to the interval between the internal condyle and the olecranon, where it inosculates with the posterior ulnar recurrent and anastomotica magna arteries.

The *medullary artery* of the humerus arises sometimes from the brachial, sometimes from the inferior profunda. It pierces the tendon of the coraco-brachialis, runs obliquely downwards through the bone, and in the medullary canal divides into ascending and descending branches, which anastomose with the nutrient vessels of the bone derived from the periosteum.

The *anastomotica magna* arises from the inner side of the brachial, about two inches above the elbow, runs tortuously inwards across the brachialis anticus, and divides into branches, some of which pass in front of, others behind the internal condyle, anastomosing with the superior profunda, the inferior profunda, and the anterior ulnar recurrent arteries.

Numerous unnamed *muscular branches* arise from the outer side of the brachial artery; one of these, more constant than the rest, supplies the biceps; another runs transversely beneath the coraco-brachialis and biceps, over the insertion of the deltoid, supplying this muscle and the brachialis anticus.

Venæ comites. The two veins which accompany the brachial artery are continuations of the deep radial and ulnar veins. The internal is usually the larger, since it generally receives the veins corresponding to the principal branches of the artery. In their course they are connected at intervals by transverse branches either in front of, or behind the artery. Near the subscapularis, the *vena comes externa* crosses obliquely in front of the axillary artery to join the vena comites interna, which then takes the name of 'axillary.'

Now trace the great nerves of the upper arm, which proceed

R

from the brachial plexus near the tendon of the subscarplaris;
namely, the median, the external cutaneous, ulnar, and musculo-
spiral or radial.

Median nerve. The median nerve arises by two roots, which converge in front of the axillary artery (p. 231). The
external root is derived from a trunk in common with the external
cutaneous; the internal from a trunk in common with the ulnar
and internal cutaneous. In its course down the arm, the nerve is
situated at first on the outer side of the brachial artery, between
it and the coraco-brachialis; about the middle of the arm the
nerve crosses obliquely over the vessel, or perhaps beneath it, so
that at the bend of the elbow it is found on the inner side of the
artery, lying upon the brachialis anticus, and covered by the
semilunar fascia from the biceps.*

The eventual distribution of the median nerve is to the two

---

* I have observed the following *varieties* relating to the median nerve, and its course
in regard to the artery:—

a. The roots may be increased in number by one on either side of the artery; or the
internal root may be deficient.

b. They may vary in their position with regard to the artery; both may be situated
behind the vessel, or one behind, and the other in front of it.

c. The nerve, formed in the usual manner, may be joined lower down by a large
branch from the external cutaneous; such a case presents a junction of two large
nerves in front of the brachial artery, in the middle of the arm.

d. The nerve in many cases crosses under, instead of over the artery.

e. The nerve sometimes runs parallel and external to the artery; or it may run
parallel to, and in front of the artery.

In one hundred arms the relative position of the nerve to the artery in its course
down the arm was as follows:—

        In 72, the nerve took the ordinary course.

        „ 20, the nerve crossed obliquely under the artery.

        „ 5, the nerve ran parallel and superficial to the artery.

        „ 3, the nerve ran parallel and external to the artery.

These varieties of the median nerve are of practical importance, for this reason:
whenever, in the operation of tying the brachial artery, we do not find the nerve in
its normal position, we may expect to find some irregular distribution of the arteries,
e.g. a high division of the brachial, or even, which I have often seen, a 'vas aberrans'
coming from the upper part of the brachial, and joining either the radial or ulnar
arteries.

pronators and all the flexors of the forearm (except the flexor carpi ulnaris and the ulnar half of the flexor profundus digitorum), to the muscles of the ball of the thumb, to both sides of the thumb, fore and middle fingers, and the radial side of the ring finger.

External cutaneous nerve. This nerve (often called the musculo-cutaneous or 'perforans Casserii') arises in common with the external root of the median, from the external cord of the brachial plexus, and is situated on the outer side of the axillary artery. It perforates the coraco-brachialis, and then runs down between the biceps and the brachialis anticus. A little above the elbow-joint, between the tendon of the biceps and the supinator radii longus, the nerve becomes subcutaneous, and, passing under the median cephalic vein, divides into branches, for the supply of the integuments of the forearm.

The external cutaneous nerve, in the upper part of its course, sends branches to the coraco-brachialis and the short head of the biceps, and, as it descends between the biceps and the brachialis anticus, it supplies both. Consequently, if the nerve were divided in the axilla, the result would be inability to bend the arm.* This nerve also sends some small branches to supply the elbow-joint.

Ulnar nerve. This nerve arises from the inner cord of the brachial plexus, in common with the internal cutaneous and the inner head of the median. It descends along the inner side of the brachial artery, as far as the insertion of the coraco-brachialis. The nerve then diverges from the artery, perforates the internal intermuscular septum, and runs with the inferior profunda artery, behind the internal condyle.

---

* In some instances the external cutaneous nerve descends on the inner side of the coraco-brachialis without perforating the muscle; in these cases it often sends a larger branch than usual to the median nerve.

The trunk of the external cutaneous nerve may come from the median at any point between the axilla and the middle of the arm. In some subjects the nerve is absent; all its branches are then supplied by the median, which is larger than usual. Such anomalies are easily explained by the fact of the two nerves having always a common origin.

The eventual distribution of the nerve is to the flexor carpi ulnaris, half the flexor profundus digitorum, all the interosseous muscles of the hand, both sides of the little finger, and the ulnar side of the ring finger; also to the muscles of the ball of the little finger.

Previous to the examination of the musculo-spiral nerve, we should have some knowledge of the great muscle which occupies the whole of the posterior part of the humerus—viz., the triceps.

Tric-ps extensor cubiti.   This muscle has three distinct origins, named from their position, *external, internal,* and *middle* or *long* head (p. 229). The *middle* or *long* head *arises* by a flat tendon from the inferior border of the scapula, close to the glenoid cavity. The *external* head *arises* from the humerus immediately below the insertion of the teres minor. The *internal* head *arises* from the humerus below the insertion of the teres major. The three heads unite near the middle of the arm to form a single fleshy mass, which covers the posterior part of the elbow-joint, and is *inserted* by a thick tendon into the summit and sides of the olecranon.

Musculo-spiral or radial nerve.   This, the largest of the brachial nerves, arises, in common with the circumflex, from the posterior cord of the axillary plexus (p. 231). It descends at first behind the axillary artery, and then winds obliquely round the posterior part of the humerus, between the external and internal heads of the triceps, in company with the superior profunda artery. About the lower third of the outer side of the arm, the nerve runs deeply imbedded between the brachialis anticus and the supinator radii longus. A little above the elbow-joint it divides into its two principal branches—the *radial,* which accompanies the radial artery along the forearm—and the *posterior interosseous,* which perforates the supinator brevis, and supplies all the muscles on the back of the forearm.

What is the distribution of this great nerve? In a word, it supplies *all* the extensors of the forearm, wrist, thumb, and fingers; and all the supinators except one, namely, the biceps (supplied by the external cutaneous nerve).

DISSECTION OF THE FRONT OF THE FOREARM.

Prolong the incision down to the wrist, and at its termination make another transversely. Reflect the skin, and carefully dissect the subcutaneous veins and nerves.

Cutaneous veins.   On the inner side is found the *anterior ulnar vein*, which commences on the front of the little finger and wrist, and is then continued upwards on the inner side of the forearm as far as the elbow, where it is joined by the posterior ulnar vein to form the basilic (p. 234).

The veins on the back of the hand commence at the extremities of the fingers, run up *between* the knuckles, and unite on the back of the hand in the shape of an arch, with its concavity upwards. The *posterior ulnar vein* arises from this arch by a branch (vena salvatella) situated over the fourth interosseous space, and runs up on the back of the forearm towards the inner condyle, to join the anterior ulnar vein.

The *radial vein*, situated on the outer side of the forearm, commences on the back of the hand from the venous arch, runs up the outer side of the front of the forearm to the elbow, where it becomes the cephalic.

Running up in front of the middle of the forearm is the *median vein*: near the bend of the elbow it is joined by a deep branch—*mediana profunda*—after which it divides into two branches, an outer or *median cephalic*, which joins the cephalic, and an inner or *median basilic*, which joins the basilic.

Cutaneous nerves.   On the radial side of the forearm, as low down as the wrist, are found the terminal branches of the musculo-cutaneous nerve. At the lower part of the forearm, these filaments are situated over the radial artery. On the ulnar side is the anterior division of the internal cutaneous nerve, while its posterior branch passes to the back of the forearm, supplying it as far as the middle. On the outer and back part of the forearm near the elbow, the external cutaneous branch of the musculo-spiral is seen running down as far as the wrist. At the lower third of the radial side of the forearm, the radial nerve

becomes superficial, and turns over the radius to supply the back of
the hand and fingers. Near the styloid process of the ulna, the
dorsal branch of the ulnar nerve perforates the fascia to reach the
back of the hand.

Deep fascia
of the fore-
arm.

The muscles of the forearm are enveloped by a dense
shining aponeurosis, which is continuous with that of
the upper arm. Its thickness increases as it approaches
the wrist, in order that the tendons in this situation
may be effectually maintained in their position. It is composed
of fibres which cross each other obliquely, and is attached above
to the condyles of the humerus and olecranon ; internally, to the
ridge on the posterior part of the ulna. At the back of the
wrist it forms the posterior annular ligament, and in front is
continuous with the anterior annular ligament. Above, the fascia
is strengthened by fibres from the tendons of the biceps and
brachialis anticus. The aponeurotic expansion from the inner
edge of the tendon of the biceps is exceedingly strong. It braces
the muscles on the inner side of the forearm, and interlaces at
right angles with the fibres of the fascia attached to the internal
condyle. The under surface of the fascia gives origin to the
muscular fibres in the upper part of the forearm, and furnishes
septa which separate the muscles, and form so many distinct
sheaths for them. The fascia is perforated at various parts for the
passage of the cutaneous vessels and nerves of the forearm.

Remove the fascia from the muscles by incisions corresponding
to those for reflecting the skin ; taking care of the cutaneous
branches of the median and ulnar nerves close to the wrist.

At the bend of the elbow, a triangular space is found, with its
base towards the humerus ; on the inner side it is bounded by
the pronator teres ; on the outer, by the supinator radii longus.
In it are found the following objects, which must be carefully
dissected :—1. The brachial artery (with its companion veins)
dividing into the radial and ulnar ; 2, on the outer side of the
artery is the tendon of the biceps ; 3, on the inner, the median
nerve ; 4, the musculo-spiral nerve, partly concealed by the
supinator longus ; 5, the radial recurrent artery ; 6, the anterior

ulnar recurrent; 7, the common interosseous branch of the ulnar artery.

Muscles of forearm.

The muscles of the forearm are arranged in two groups; one, consisting of supinators and extensors, is attached to the outer condyloid ridge and condyle; the other, consisting of pronators and flexors, is attached to the inner condyle. The inner group should be examined first: they arise by a common tendon, and are arranged in the following order: pronator teres; flexor carpi radialis; palmaris longus; flexor carpi ulnaris, and flexor sublimis digitorum.

Pronator radii teres.

This muscle forms the inner boundary of the triangular space at the elbow. It *arises* from the anterior surface of the internal condyle, from the common tendon, and from the septum between it and the flexor carpi radialis. It has also a small tendinous origin from the coronoid process of the ulna. From these two origins, between which the median nerve passes, the muscle proceeds obliquely downwards, and is inserted by a flat tendon into a rough surface on the outer and back part of the middle third of the radius. In amputating the forearm, it is very desirable to save the insertion of this muscle, that the stump may have a pronator.

Flexor carpi radialis.

This muscle *arises* by the common tendon from the internal condyle, from the intermuscular septa, and from the fascia of the forearm. The fleshy fibres terminate near the middle of the forearm, in a flat tendon, which runs in a separate sheath outside the anterior annular ligament of the wrist, passes through a groove in the os trapezium, lined by a synovial membrane, and is *inserted* into the bases of the second and third metacarpal bones. Note that the outer border of its tendon is the guide to the radial artery in the lower half of the forearm.

Palmaris longus.

This slender muscle arises from the common tendon at the internal condyle, from the intermuscular septa, and from the fascia of the forearm. About the middle of the forearm it terminates in a flat tendon, which descends vertically down the middle of the forearm to the wrist, lying upon

the flexor sublimis digitorum; it then passes over the anterior
annular ligament, and is continued into the palmar fascia. This
muscle is a tensor of the palmar fascia.*

Flexor carpi ulnaris.   This muscle *arises* by two heads; one from the
internal condyle, the common tendon, and the inter-
muscular septum; the other from the inner edge of
the olecranon: these two origins form an arch under which the
ulnar nerve passes. It also arises from the upper two-thirds of
the posterior edge of the ulna, through the medium of the aponeurosis, which is common to this muscle and the flexor profundus
digitorum. The tendon appears on the radial side of the muscle,
about the lower third of the forearm, and receives fleshy fibres on
its ulnar side as low as the wrist. It is inserted into the os pisi-
forme, and thence by a strong tendon into the os unciforme and
the base of the fifth metacarpal bone.

The tendon of the flexor carpi ulnaris is the guide to the ulnar
artery, which lies close to its radial side, and is *overlapped* by it.
As it passes over the annular ligament, the tendon furnishes a
fibrous expansion to protect the ulnar artery and nerve.

Flexor sublimis digi-torum.   This muscle is situated beneath those previously mentioned, and has two distinct origins. The longer origin
takes place from the internal condyle, from the internal
lateral ligament, the common tendon, the intermuscular septa,
and the coronoid process of the ulna; the shorter origin takes place
by tendinous and fleshy fibres from an oblique ridge on the front
of the radius, extending to about an inch below the insertion of
the pronator teres. This, called its *radial origin*, is partly concealed by the pronator teres. The muscle thus formed passes down
the middle of the forearm, and divides into four distinct muscular
slips: from these, four tendons arise, which pass beneath the annular ligament into the palm, and on to the fingers, where they split
to allow the passage of the deep flexor tendons, and are *inserted*

* The palmaris longus is sometimes absent. The situation of its muscular portion is
subject to variety; sometimes occupying the middle, sometimes the lower third of the
forearm. The tendon is in some instances wholly inserted into the anterior annular
ligament.

into the sides of the second phalanges. Its *action* is, therefore, to bend the second joint of the fingers.

Having finished the superficial muscles on the inner side of the forearm, notice one of those on the outer side, named supinator radii longus, before you trace the vessels and nerves of the forearm.

Supinator radii longus.

This muscle forms the external boundary of the triangular space at the bend of the elbow. It *arises* from the upper two-thirds of the external condyloid ridge of the humerus, commencing a little below the insertion of the deltoid. The muscular fibres terminate about the middle of the forearm in a flat tendon, which is *inserted* into the base of the styloid process of the radius. The inner border of the muscle is the guide to the radial artery. It supinates the hand, but acts much more powerfully as a flexor of the forearm.

Radial artery.

The radial artery, one of the divisions of the brachial, runs down the radial side of the forearm to the wrist, where it turns over the external lateral ligament of the carpus, beneath the extensor tendons of the thumb, and sinks into the space between the first and second metacarpal bones to form the deep palmar arch. Thus, a line drawn from the middle of the bend of the elbow to the front of the styloid process of the radius indicates its course. In the upper third of the forearm, the artery lies between the pronator teres on the inner, and the supinator longus on the outer side; the fleshy border of the latter overlaps it in muscular subjects. In the lower two-thirds of the forearm the artery is more superficial, and is placed between the tendons of the supinator longus on the outer, and the flexor carpi radialis on the inner side. In its course, it lies successively on the following: first upon the tendon of the biceps; secondly, upon the supinator radii brevis; thirdly, upon the tendon of the pronator teres; fourthly, upon the radial origin of the flexor sublimis; fifthly, upon the flexor longus pollicis; sixthly, upon the pronator quadratus; and, lastly, upon the radius. It is accompanied by two veins, which communicate at frequent intervals, and join the venæ comites of the brachial artery at the bend of the elbow.

In the middle third of its course the artery is accompanied by the radial nerve (a branch of the musculo-spiral) which lies to its outer side. Below this point, the nerve leaves the artery, and passes under the tendon of the supinator longus to the back of the hand.

Thus, in the situation where the pulse is felt, the radial nerve no longer accompanies the artery; nevertheless, the vessel is not without a nerve, for it is accompanied by a branch of the musculo-cutaneous (or external cutaneous), which runs superficial to it.

The radial artery sends off in the forearm the following branches, besides offsets, which supply the muscles on the outer side of the forearm.

The *radial recurrent* is given off just below the elbow; it passes outwards to supply the long and short supinators and the two radial extensors. One of its ramifications runs up with the musculo-spiral nerve between the supinator longus and brachialis anticus, and forms a delicate inosculation with the superior profunda (p. 240).

The *arteria superficialis volæ* arises from the radial, about half an inch, or more, above the lower end of the radius; it runs superficially over the anterior annular ligament, above or perhaps through the origin of the muscles of the ball of the thumb, into the palm of the hand, where it inosculates with the superficial branch of the ulnar, and completes the superficial palmar arch.[*]

The *anterior* and *posterior carpal* arteries are small branches of the radial, which run beneath the tendons, and supply the synovial membrane and bones of the carpus, anastomosing with the anterior interosseous, the carpal branches of the ulnar, and the recurrent carpal branch of the deep palmar arch.

Radial nerve.   The radial nerve, a branch of the musculo-spiral, is given off above the bend of the elbow, deep between the supinator radii longus and brachialis anticus; it descends on

---

[*] There is great variety in the size and origin of the superficialis volæ; sometimes it is very large, arises higher than usual, and runs to the wrist parallel with the radial; sometimes it is very small, terminating in the muscles of the thumb; or it may be absent.

the outer side of the radial artery, covered by the supinator radii longus. In the upper third of the forearm the nerve is at some distance from the artery; in the middle third it approaches nearer to it; but in the lower third, the nerve leaves the artery, passes underneath the tendon of the supinator longus, perforates the fascia on the outer side of the forearm, and divides into two branches, which supply the back of the thumb, fore, and half the middle finger.

Ulnar artery. This artery, the larger of the two divisions of the brachial, comes off at the middle of the elbow, runs obliquely inwards along the ulnar side of the forearm to the wrist, passes over the annular ligament near the pisiform bone, and entering the palm, forms the superficial palmar arch, by inosculating with the superficialis volæ.

In the upper half of its course the artery describes a gentle curve with the concavity towards the radius, and lies deep beneath the superficial layer of muscles, the pronator teres, flexor carpi radialis, palmaris longus, and flexor sublimis digitorum. It is also crossed in its upper part by the median nerve. In the lower part of its course it descends between the flexor sublimis and flexor carpi ulnaris, of which the tendon partially overlaps it at the wrist. The artery lies for a short distance on the brachialis anticus; in the remainder of its course it lies on the flexor profundus digitorum.

The ulnar nerve is at first separated from the artery by a considerable interval: but about the middle of the forearm it joins the artery, and accompanies it in the rest of its course, lying close to its inner side. Both pass over the anterior annular ligament of the carpus, lying close to the pisiform bone,—the nerve being nearer to the bone. A strong expansion from the tendon of the flexor carpi ulnaris protects them in this exposed situation.

Observe particularly the depth of the ulnar artery under the many muscles which cover it in the upper third of its course. In the middle third it is partially overlapped by the flexor carpi ulnaris. In the lower third it lies under the radial border of the flexor carpi ulnaris, which is the *proper guide* to the vessel. The artery is accompanied by two veins which join the venæ comites of the brachial.

The ulnar artery furnishes the following branches in the forearm :—

The *anterior* and *posterior ulnar recurrent* arise immediately below the elbow-joint,—sometimes by a common trunk. The *anterior* passes upward between the brachialis anticus and the pronator teres, and inosculates with the inferior profunda and anastomotica magna. The *posterior* ascends between the flexor sublimis and the flexor profundus digitorum, to the space between the internal condyle and the olecranon : it then passes up between the two heads of the flexor carpi ulnaris, where it inosculates with the same arteries as the anterior (p. 240).

The *common interosseous* artery arises from the ulnar, about an inch and a half below the division of the brachial ; and soon divides into the anterior and posterior interosseous, which we shall examine presently.

The *anterior* and *posterior carpal* branches communicate with corresponding branches from the radial, and supply the synovial membrane and bones of the carpus.

Ulnar nerve.   This nerve runs behind the internal condyle, between the two origins of the flexor carpi ulnaris. In its course down the upper part of the forearm, the nerve is still covered by this muscle, and lies upon the flexor profundus digitorum. About the middle third of the forearm, the nerve joins the ulnar artery, and runs along its inner side over the annular ligament into the palm.

The ulnar nerve gives off some filaments which are distributed to the elbow-joint, and supplies two muscles in the forearm ; namely, the flexor carpi ulnaris and the inner half of the flexor profundus digitorum.

About one inch and a half above the styloid process of the ulna, the nerve gives off a large cutaneous branch to the back of the hand. It crosses under the tendon of the flexor carpi ulnaris, and, immediately below the styloid process of the ulna, appears on the back of the hand, where it divides into branches, which supply the back of the little finger, the ring, and half the middle finger; here also it sends a branch which communicates with the radial nerve.

Median nerve.   This nerve, at the bend of the elbow, lies on the inner side of the brachial artery. It then passes between the two origins of the pronator teres, and descends along the middle of the forearm, between the flexor sublimis and the flexor profundus digitorum. At the lower part of the forearm it becomes more superficial, lying about the middle of the wrist, between the outer tendon of the flexor sublimis, and the inner border of the tendon of the flexor carpi radialis: it then enters the palm beneath the anterior annular ligament, and divides into five branches for the supply of the thumb, both sides of the fore and middle fingers, and the outer side of the ring finger.*

Immediately below the elbow, the median nerve sends branches to the pronator teres and all the flexor muscles of the forearm, except the flexor carpi ulnaris and the inner half of the flexor profundus, which are supplied by the ulnar. The *interosseous* branch of the median runs with the anterior interosseous artery, upon the interosseous membrane between the flexor longus pollicis and flexor profundus digitorum: it supplies both these muscles and the pronator quadratus.

Before the median nerve passes beneath the annular ligament, it sends off its *superficial palmar* branch, which passes over the ligament, and divides into small filaments to supply the skin of the palm and ball of the thumb.

Now reflect the superficial layer of muscles, to see those more deeply seated. Preserve the principal vessels and nerves.

The deep-seated muscles are the flexor digitorum profundus, and the flexor longus pollicis; beneath both, near the wrist, lies the pronator quadratus. Close to the interosseous membrane run the anterior interosseous artery and nerve.

Flexor profundus digitorum.   This is the thickest muscle of the forearm. It *arises* from the upper two-thirds of the anterior surface of the ulna, from the same extent of its internal surface, from

---

* If the tendon of the palmaris longus happen to be broader than usual, it may partially cover the median nerve near the wrist; but most frequently the nerve is immediately beneath the fascia, the tendon lying to its ulnar side.

the aponeurosis attached to the posterior edge of the ulna, and from the inner two-thirds of the interosseous ligament. About the middle of the forearm it divides into four muscular slips, which terminate in flat tendons. These tendons lie upon the same plane, and pass beneath the annular ligament under those of the superficial flexor, into the palm. On the first phalanx of the fingers, the tendons of the deep flexor perforate those of the superficial, and are *inserted* into the base of the third or ungual phalanx.

Flexor longus pollicis.   This muscle is situated on the front surface of the radius, outside the preceding. It arises from the front surface of the radius, between the tubercle and the pronator quadratus, and from the interosseous membrane.* Its tendon proceeds beneath the annular ligament to the last phalanx of the thumb.

Pronator quadratus.   This square muscle *arises* from the lower fourth of the ulna; its fibres pass transversely outwards, and are *inserted* into the lower fourth of the radius. It rotates the radius on the ulna.

Interosseous artery.   Nearly on a level with the insertion of the biceps, the ulnar artery gives off from its outer side the *common interosseous*, which runs backwards for about half an inch, and divides into the *anterior* and *posterior interosseous*.

The *anterior interosseous* artery runs down close to the interosseous membrane, lying between the flexor profundus digitorum and flexor longus pollicis. At the upper edge of the pronator quadratus it divides into two branches; one of which, the smaller, passes behind the muscle, supplies it and the front of the carpal bones, communicating with the anterior carpal arteries from the radial and ulnar; the other, the most important, perforates the interosseous membrane, and helps to supply the muscles on the back of the forearm.

A branch, the *arteria comes nervi mediani*, which almost always accompanies the median nerve, is an offset from the anterior interosseous. It lies in close contact with the nerve, sometimes in its

---

* Sometimes by a slip from the coronoid process.

very centre; though usually of small size, it may be as large as the ulnar artery itself, and in such cases passes under the annular ligament with the nerve to join the palmar arch.   This is interesting, because it helps to explain the recurrence of hæmorrhage from a wound in the palm, even after the radial and ulnar arteries have been tied.

The anterior interosseous artery also gives off branches to the muscles on either side, and the nutrient arteries, which enter the radius and ulna from below upwards, near the centre of the forearm, to supply the medullary membrane.

Anterior interosseous nerve.   This nerve is a branch of the median ; it is close to the artery, supplies the flexor longus pollicis, half the flexor profundus digitorum, and the pronator quadratus.

DISSECTION OF THE PALM OF THE HAND.

Make a vertical incision along the centre of the palm, and a transverse one along the bases of the fingers; from this transverse cut continue vertical incisions along the front of the fingers, and reflect the skin; taking care not to remove a small cutaneous muscle—the palmaris brevis—situated near the ball of the little finger, and also two small cutaneous branches of the median and ulnar nerves, which are found in the fat of the palm.

Observe how closely, in the centre of the palm, the skin adheres to the palmar fascia beneath it.   On the ball of the little finger and the distal ends of the metacarpal bones, the subcutaneous structure is composed of a dense filamentous tissue, which contains numerous pellets of fat, forming a kind of elastic pad.   A similar padding protects the palmar surfaces of the fingers.   These cushions on the ends of the fingers defend them in the powerful actions of the hand ; they are also useful in subservience to the nerves of touch.

The palm is supplied with nerves by two small branches—one, the palmar branch of the median, passes in front of the anterior annular ligament to the centre of the palm ; the other, a branch of the ulnar, supplies the inner aspect of the hand.

This small cutaneous muscle is situated on the inner
Palmaris brevis. side of the palm. It arises from the inner edge of the
central palmar fascia, and terminates in the skin on the
inner side of the palm. Its use is to support the pad on the inner
edge of the palm: it acts powerfully as we grasp; it raises the
edge of the palm and hollows it, forming the ' cup of Diogenes.'
It is supplied by the ulnar nerve.

This fascia has a silvery lustre, and, in the centre of
Palmar fascia. the palm, is remarkably dense and strong. It is divided
into three portions, a central—by far the strongest; an
external, covering the muscles of the thumb; and an internal,
covering the muscles of the little finger. From the deep surface
of the fascia two septa dip down, so as to divide the palm into
three separate compartments; one for the ball of the thumb, a
second for that of the little finger, and a third for the centre of the
palm.

The fascia is formed by a prolongation from the anterior annular
ligament. It is also strengthened by the expanded tendon of the
palmaris longus.

The central portion of the fascia is triangular, with the apex at
the wrist. About the middle of the palm it splits into four portions,
which are connected by transverse tendinous fibres, extending completely across the palm, and corresponding pretty nearly to the
transverse furrow of the skin in this situation.

Examine any one of these four portions of the fascia, and you
will find that it splits into two strips which embrace the corresponding flexor tendons, and are intimately connected with the
transverse metacarpal ligament. The effect of this is that the
flexor tendons of each finger are kept in place in the palm, by a
fibrous ring. Between the four divisions of the palmar fascia the
digital vessels and nerves emerge, and descend in a line with the
clefts between the fingers.

In the hands of mechanics, in whom the palmar fascia is usually
very strong, we find that slips of it are lost in the skin at the
lower part of the palm, and also for a short distance along the
sides of the fingers.

The chief use of the palmar fascia is to protect the vessels and nerves from pressure when anything is grasped in the hand. It also confines the flexor tendons in their proper place.

Between the interdigital folds of the skin, we find aponeurotic fibres to strengthen them, constituting what are called the *transverse ligaments* of the fingers. They form a continuous ligament across the lower part of the palm, in front of the digital vessels and nerves.

Cut through the palmar fascia at its attachment to the anterior annular ligament, and reflect it towards the fingers, to expose the vessels, nerves, and tendons in the palm. The vessels lie above the nerves, and the tendons still deeper. There is an abundance of loose cellular tissue to allow the free play of the tendons. When suppuration takes place in the palm, it is seated in this tissue. Reflect for a moment, what mischief is likely to ensue. The matter cannot get to the surface through the dense palmar fascia, or on the back of the hand; it will therefore run up under the annular ligament, and make its way deep amongst the tendons of the forearm.

Superficial palmar arch.

The ulnar artery, having passed over the annular ligament near the pisiform bone, describes a curve across the upper part of the palm beneath the palmar fascia towards the thumb, and, gradually diminishing in size, inosculates with the superficialis volæ, and very commonly with a branch from the arteria radialis indicis, to form the superficial palmar arch. The curve of the arch is directed towards the ball of the thumb. How are we to ascertain its exact position in the hand? Most commonly its greatest convexity descends as low as a horizontal line drawn across the junction of the upper with the middle third of the palm.

In its passage over the annular ligament, the artery is protected in a furrow, between the pisiform and unciform bones, and by an expansion from the tendon of the flexor carpi ulnaris to the palmaris longus. The ulnar nerve lies close to its inner side. In the palm, the artery rests for a short distance upon the muscles of the little finger, then it lies upon the superficial flexor tendons

s

and the divisions of the ulnar and median nerves; and is covered
by the palmaris longus and the palmar fascia.

Fig. 51.

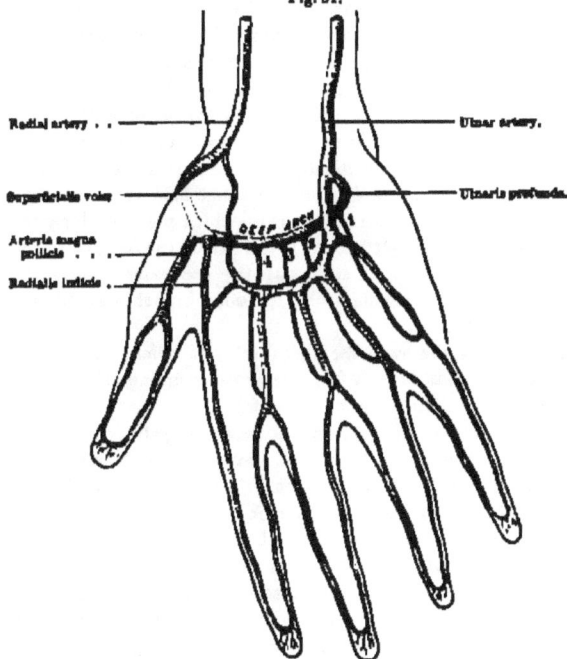

DIAGRAM OF THE SUPERFICIAL AND DEEP PALMAR ARCHES.

1, 2, 3, 4. Interosseous branches.

Immediately below the pisiform bone, the ulnar
artery gives off the *ulnaris profunda*, which sinks
deeply into the palm between the abductor and flexor
brevis minimi digiti, to assist in forming the deep palmar arch. It is accompanied by the deep branch of the ulnar nerve.

Branches of the ulnar artery in the palm.

From the concavity of the arch small branches ascend to the carpus, and inosculate with the other carpal branches of the radial and ulnar arteries.

From the convexity of the arch arise *four digital arteries*, which supply all the fingers, excepting the radial side of the index finger. Observe carefully the course of these arteries, because you may have to open abscesses in the palm. The first descends over the muscles on the inner side of the palm, to the ulnar side of the little finger, along which it runs to the apex. The second, third, and fourth descend nearly vertically between the tendons, *in a line with the clefts* between the fingers, and about half an inch above the clefts each divides into two branches, which proceed along the opposite sides of the fingers nearly to the end of the last phalanges, where they unite to form an arch with the convexity towards the end of the finger; from this arch numerous branches supply the papillæ of the skin.

In the palm of the hand the digital arteries before they divide are joined by a small branch from the corresponding interosseous artery (a branch of the deep palmar arch).

The digital arteries freely communicate, on the palmar and dorsal aspect of the fingers, by transverse branches, which supply the joints and the sheaths of the tendons. Near the ungual phalanx, a considerable branch passes to the back of the finger, and forms a network of vessels round the root of the nail.

The *ulnar nerve* passes over the annular ligament
Ulnar nerve in the palm. into the palm, on the inner side of the ulnar artery, and a little behind it. It lies in a groove between the pisiform and unciform bones, so that it is perfectly secure from pressure in this apparently exposed situation. Immediately below the pisiform bone, the nerve divides into a superficial and a deep palmar branch. The *deep* branch supplies the muscles of the little finger, and accompanies the ulnaris profunda artery into the palm, to supply *all* the interosseous muscles, and the two inner lumbricales. The *superficial* branch sends filaments to the palmaris brevis, to the integument on the inner side of the palm, and then divides into two digital nerves, one for the supply of the

s 2

ulnar side of the little finger, and the other for the contiguous sides of the little and ring fingers.

The digital branches run along the sides of the fingers to their extremities superficial to their corresponding arteries. The more external of the two branches communicates with the median nerve behind the superficial palmar arch.

Anterior annular ligament of the carpus. This exceedingly strong and thick ligament confines the flexor tendons of the fingers and thumb, and fastens together the bones of the carpus. It is attached externally to the scaphoid and trapezium; internally to the pisiform and unciform. Its upper border is continuous with the aponeurosis in front of the wrist; its lower terminates in the palmar fascia; its anterior surface receives the expanded tendon of the palmaris longus, and gives origin to most of the muscles constituting the ball of the thumb and little finger.

Cut vertically through the ligament, and observe, that, with the carpal bones, it forms an elliptical canal, with the broad diameter transversely. This canal is lined by a synovial membrane which is reflected loosely over the tendons. Superficial to the ligament, pass the palmaris longus, the ulnar artery and nerve, and the palmar branch of the median nerve; beneath it, pass the superficial and deep flexor tendons of the fingers, the long flexor tendon of the thumb, and the median nerve. The tendon of the flexor carpi radialis does not run with the other tendons, but is contained in a distinct sheath, lined by a separate synovial membrane, formed partly by the annular ligament and partly by the groove in the trapezium.

Median nerve in the palm. In its passage under the annular ligament, the median nerve is enveloped in a fold of synovial membrane. It lies between the tendons of the flexor sublimis and those of the flexor profundus, and is rather nearer to the radial than the ulnar side of the wrist. As soon as it appears in the palm, the nerve lies superficial to all the tendons, and then divides into two branches; the external gives off branches to the muscles of the ball of the thumb, namely, to the abductor pollicis, the opponens pollicis, and the outer head of the flexor brevis pollicis, and then terminates in three digital nerves, two of which are distributed to the thumb, and the third to the outer side of the index finger; the internal gives off two digital branches which supply the rest of the forefinger, the middle finger, and the radial side of the ring finger.

The two nerves to the thumb proceed, one on each side of the long flexor tendon, to the last phalanx.

The third digital nerve runs along the radial side of the index finger. The fourth descends towards the cleft between the index and middle fingers, and subdivides into two branches, which supply their opposite sides. The fifth is joined by a filament from one of the ulnar digital nerves, and then subdivides above the cleft between the middle and ring fingers, to supply their opposite sides.

Two small branches are given off from the third and fourth digital nerves, to supply the two outer lumbricales; the two inner being supplied by the ulnar.

About an inch and a quarter above the clefts between the fingers, each digital nerve subdivides into two branches, between which the digital artery passes and bifurcates lower down; therefore a vertical incision down the cleft would divide the artery before the nerve.

In their course along the fingers and thumb, the nerves lie superficial to the arteries, and nearer to the flexor tendons. About the middle of the first phalanx each nerve sends a branch, which runs along the back of the finger nearly to the extremity, communicating with the dorsal branches, derived from the radial and ulnar nerves.[*] Near the ungual phalanx another branch is dis-

---

[*] We find upon the cutaneous nerves of the hand and feet, little bodies termed, after their discoverer, corpuscles of 'Pacini.' Some of them will be found, by carefully examining the trunk of a nerve, or one of its smaller branches, in the subcutaneous tissue at the root of a finger. Each corpuscle is about $\frac{1}{20}$th of an inch long, and is attached by a slender fibro-cellular pedicle to the nerve upon which it is situated; through the pedicle, a single primitive nerve fibril passes into the corpuscle. The corpuscle itself is composed of a series of concentric capsules, varying from twenty to fifty in number, and separated by intervals containing fluid: and the nerve fibril terminates by a dilated extremity in a central cavity, which exists in the axis of the corpuscle. Their function is unknown.

tributed to the skin around and beneath the root of the nail. Each
nerve terminates near the end of the finger in a brush of filaments,
with their points directed to the papillæ of the skin.

Flexor ten-
dons and
their sheaths. Immediately below the annular ligament the tendons
separate from each other; near the metacarpal joints
they pass in pairs, through strong fibrous rings (p. 256)
formed by the divisions of the palmar fascia. Below the metacarpal joint the two tendons for each finger enter the sheath
(theca), which confines them in their course along the phalanges.
It is formed by a strong fibrous membrane, which is attached to
the ridges on the phalanges, and converts the groove in front of
these bones into a complete canal, exactly large enough to contain
the tendons. The density of the sheath varies in particular
situations, otherwise there would be an obstacle to the easy
flexion of the fingers. To ascertain this, cut open one of the
sheaths along its entire length ; you will then see that it is much
stronger between the joints than over the joints themselves.
Through these sheaths, inflammation commencing in the integuments of the finger may readily extend to the synovial membrane
of the tendon.

In cases of whitlow, when matter forms in the theca, the incision
should be made deep enough to lay open this fibro-osseous canal,
without which the incision will be of no use. It is obvious that
the incision should be made down the *centre* of the finger, to avoid
the digital nerves and arteries. If this opening be not timely
made, the flexor tendons are likely to slough, and the finger
becomes stiff.*

But what protects the joints of the fingers where the flexor

---

* On closer inspection it will be observed that the sheath is composed of bands of
fibres, which take different directions, and have received distinct names. The
strongest are called the '*ligamenta vaginalia.*' They constitute the sheath over the
body of the phalanx, and extend transversely from one side of the bone to the other.
The '*ligamenta cruciata*' are two slips, which cross obliquely over the tendons. The
'*ligamenta annularia*' are situated immediately in front of the joints, and may be
considered as thin continuations of the ligamenta vaginalia. They consist of delicate
fibres, which are attached on either side of the joints to the glenoid ligaments, and
pass transversely over the tendons.

tendons play over them? Look into an open sheath, and you
will see that in front of the joints the tendons glide over a smooth
fibro-cartilaginous structure, called the 'glenoid' ligament.

To facilitate the play of the tendons, the interior of the sheath,
as well as the tendons, is lined by a synovial membrane, of the
extent of which it is important to have a correct knowledge. With
a probe you may easily ascertain that the synovial membrane is
reflected from the sheath upon the tendons, a little above the
metacarpal joints of the fingers; that is, nearly in a line with the
transverse fold in the skin in the lower third of the palm. Towards
the distal end of the finger, the synovial sheath stops short of the last
joint, so that it is not injured in amputation of the ungual phalanx.

And now notice how beautifully the tendons are adapted to each
other in their course along the finger. The superficial flexor, near
the root of the finger, becomes slightly grooved to receive the deep
flexor; about the middle of the first phalanx it splits into two
portions, through which the deep flexor passes. The two portions
reunite below the deep tendon so as completely to embrace it, and
then divide a second time into two slips, which interlace with
each other and are inserted into the sides of the second phalanx.
The *deep* flexor, having passed through the opening of the superficial one, is inserted into the base of the last phalanx.*

In what way are the tendons supplied with blood? Raise and
separate the tendons, and you will see that slender folds of synovial
membrane (vincula tendinum) run up from the phalanges to the
tendons; when minutely injected, these folds are full of blood-
vessels.

The *tendon of the flexor longus pollicis* lies on the radial side of
the other tendons beneath the annular ligament. It passes between
the two portions of the flexor brevis pollicis and the two sesamoid
bones of the thumb, enters its proper sheath, and is *inserted* into

---

* In the museum of the College of Surgeons, a preparation is put up which shows
a beautiful piece of animal mechanics about the flexor tendons; namely, that in its
passage along the phalanges the deep flexor forms at the first phalanx a kind of little
patella for the superficial one; but at the second phalanx the superficial flexor lies
deeper than the other, and forms a little patella for it. This is a very pretty mechanical ingenuity to increase the leverage in each case.

the base of the last phalanx. Its synovial sheath is prolonged
from the large bursa of the flexor tendons beneath the annular
ligament, and accompanies it down to the last joint of the
thumb; consequently the sheath is injured in amputation of the
last phalanx.

Bursal sac of the carpus. A large and loose synovial sac, called the bursa of the
carpus, facilitates the play of the tendons beneath the
anterior annular ligament. It lines the under surface of
the ligament and the groove of the carpus, and is reflected in loose
folds over the tendons. It is prolonged up the tendons for an inch
and a half, or two inches, and forms a 'cul-de-sac' above the
ligament. Below the ligament the bursa extends into the palm,
and sends off prolongations for each of the flexor tendons, which
accompany them down to the middle of the hand. You will easily
understand that, when the bursa is inflamed and distended by fluid,
there will be a bulging above the annular ligament, and another in
the palm, with perceptible fluctuation between them; the unyielding ligament causing a constriction in the centre.*

Lumbricales. These four slender muscles, one for each finger, are
attached to the deep flexor tendons in the palm. All
of them *arise* from the radial side of the deep tendon of their
corresponding finger: the third and fourth often arise from the
adjacent sides of two tendons. Each terminates in a broad thin
tendon which passes over the radial side of the first joint of the
finger, and is *inserted* into the extensor tendon on the back of the
finger. Their *action* is to bend the first joint of the fingers. Being
inserted near the centre of motion, they can move the fingers with
great rapidity. As they produce the quick motions of the musician's
fingers, they are called by anatomists 'fidicinales.'

The two inner lumbricales are supplied by the deep branch of

* I have met with only one instance in which this bursa communicated with the
wrist joint. It communicates always with the synovial sheath of the long flexor of
the thumb, in most cases with that of the flexor of the little finger, and but rarely
with that of the index, middle, and ring fingers. On this account inflammation of the
sheath of the thumb or little finger is more liable to be attended with serious consequences than either of the others.

the ulnar nerve; the two outer by the third and fourth digital branches of the median.

Let us now proceed to the muscles composing the ball of the thumb and the little finger. The dissection of them requires considerable care.

Muscles of the ball of the thumb. The great strength of the muscles of the ball of the thumb (unde nomen pollicis), is one of the distinguishing features of the human hand. This strength is necessary in order to oppose that of all the fingers. In addition to its strength, the thumb enjoys perfect mobility. It has no less than eight muscles to work it :—namely, an abductor, an opponens, two flexors, three extensors, and an adductor. Take first the muscles of the ball.

Abductor pollicis. This is the most superficial. It is a thin, flat muscle, and *arises* from the os scaphoides and the annular ligament; and is *inserted* by a flat tendon into the base of the first phalanx of the thumb. Its *action* is to draw the thumb away from the fingers. Reflect it from its insertion to expose the following—

Flexor ossis metacarpi pollicis or opponens. This muscle *arises* from the os trapezium and the annular ligament, and is inserted into the whole length of the metacarpal bone of the thumb. The *action* of this powerful muscle is to oppose the thumb to all the fingers. Reflect it from its insertion, to expose the following—

Flexor brevis pollicis. This muscle has two origins; one from the annular ligament and os magnum, the other from the os trapezoides, os magnum, and the base of the third metacarpal bone. It is *inserted* by two strong tendons into the base of the first phalanx of the thumb; the superficial tendon being connected with the abductor pollicis, and the deep one with the adductor pollicis. A sesamoid bone is found in each of the tendons. The tendons of insertion of this muscle are separated by the long flexor tendon of the thumb and the arteria magna pollicis. Its *action* is to bend the first phalanx of the thumb.

Adductor pollicis. This muscle *arises* from the palmar aspect of the shaft of the metacarpal bone of the middle finger; its fibres converge and are *inserted*, along with the inner portion of the flexor brevis pollicis, into the base of the first phalanx of the thumb. Its *action* is to draw the thumb towards the palm, as when we bring the tips of the thumb and little finger into contact. It is supplied by the deep branch of the ulnar nerve, which also supplies the inner head of the flexor brevis pollicis. The other muscles of the ball of the thumb are supplied by the median nerve.

Muscles of the ball of the little finger.
The muscles of the little finger correspond in some measure with those of the thumb. Thus we have an abductor, a flexor brevis, and an opponens minimi digiti.

Abductor minimi digiti.
This, the most superficial of the muscles of the little finger, *arises* from the pisiform bone, and from the tendinous expansion of the flexor carpi ulnaris : it is *inserted* by a flat tendon into the base of the first phalanx of the little finger. Its *action* is to draw this finger from the rest.

Flexor brevis minimi digiti.
This slender muscle may fairly be considered as a portion of the preceding. It *arises* from the unciform . bone and annular ligament, and is *inserted* with the tendon of the abductor into the base of the first phalanx of the little finger. Its *action* is similar to that of the abductor. Between the origins of the abductor and flexor brevis minimi digiti, the deep branch of the ulnar artery and nerve sinks down to form the deep palmar arch.

Opponens digiti minimi.
The last two muscles must be reflected from their insertion, to expose the *opponens digiti minimi*. It *arises* from the unciform bone and the annular ligament, and is inserted along the shaft of the metacarpal bone of the little finger. Its *action* is to draw this bone, the most movable of all the metacarpal bones of the fingers, towards the thumb. Thus it greatly strengthens the grasp of the palm.

Now cut through all the flexor tendons, and remove the deep fascia of the palm, to see the deep arch of arteries and its branches.

Branches of the radial artery in the palm.
The radial artery enters the palm at the angle between the first and second metacarpal bones (between the inner head of the flexor brevis and the

adductor pollicis), and gives off three branches — the arteria magna pollicis, the radialis indicis, and the palmaris profunda, which unites with the ulnar to form the deep arch.

The *arteria magna pollicis* runs in front of the abductor indicis (first dorsal interosseous), close along the metacarpal bone of the thumb: in the interval between the lower portions of the flexor brevis pollicis, the artery divides into two branches, which proceed one on either side of the thumb, and inosculate at the apex of the last phalanx. Their distribution and mode of termination are similar to those of the other digital arteries.

The *arteria radialis indicis* runs between the abductor indicis and adductor pollicis, along the radial side of the index finger to the extremity, where it forms an arch with the other digital artery, a branch of the ulnar. Near the lower margin of the adductor pollicis, the radialis indicis generally receives a branch from the superficial palmar arch.

The *palmaris profunda* is considered as the continuation of the radial artery. It enters the palm between the inner head of the flexor brevis and the adductor pollicis, resting upon the bases of the metacarpal bones and the interosseous muscles, and inosculates with the deep branch of the ulnar artery, thus completing the deep palmar arch. From the curve of the arch small recurrent branches ascend to supply the bones and joints of the carpus, inosculating with the other carpal arteries. From the convexity of the arch four small branches, called *palmar interosseous* (fig. 51, p. 258), descend to supply the interosseous muscles, and near the clefts of the fingers communicate with the digital arteries. These palmar interosseous branches are sometimes of considerable size, and take the place of one or more of the digital arteries, ordinarily derived from the superficial palmar arch. Other branches, called ' *perforating*,' pass between the upper ends of the metacarpal bones to the back of the hand, and communicate with the carpal branches of the radial and ulnar.

Deep branch of the ulnar nerve.   This nerve sinks into the palm with the ulnaris profunda artery, between the abductor and flexor brevis minimi digiti. It then runs with the deep palmar arch towards the radial side of the palm, and terminates in the adductor pollicis, and inner head of the flexor brevis pollicis. Between the pisiform and unciform bones, the nerve gives a branch to each of the muscles of the little finger. Subsequently it sends branches to each interosseous muscle and to the two inner lumbricales.

The tendon of the flexor carpi radialis in the palm must now be followed to its insertion into the bases of the second and third metacarpal bones.

The dissection of the remaining muscles of the palm, called, from their position, '*interossei*,' must be for the present postponed.

MUSCLES OF THE BACK CONNECTED WITH THE ARM.

Make an incision down the spine from the occiput to the sacrum; another from the last dorsal vertebra upwards and outward to the acromion; and a third from the sacrum along the crest of the ilium; then reflect the skin outwards from the dense subcutaneous tissue, in which will be found the following cutaneous nerves.

Cutaneous nerves of the back. These are derived from the posterior branches of the spinal nerves, and correspond generally to the number of the vertebræ. The posterior primary branches, much smaller than the anterior, divide between the transverse processes into external and internal branches. From the internal, which become superficial near the spines of the vertebræ, are derived those branches which supply the skin in the cervical and upper dorsal regions; from the external, which appear near the angles of the ribs, those which supply the skin of the lower dorsal and lumbar regions. In the cervical and upper dorsal region, the cutaneous nerves perforate the complexus, splenius, and trapezius; in the lower dorsal and lumbar region they perforate the serratus posticus inferior and latissimus dorsi. As might be expected, the external branches are the larger, especially in the loins, where some of them descend over the crest of the ilium, and terminate in the skin of the buttock.

Of these cutaneous nerves notice particularly the following:—

The *posterior branch of the second cervical nerve* is called the *great occipital.* It perforates the complexus, and ramifies upon the scalp, with the branches of the occipital artery.

The *cutaneous branch of the third cervical nerve* also sends a branch to the back of the scalp.

The *cutaneous branch of the second dorsal nerve* is the largest of all the dorsal cutaneous nerves. It may be traced outwards towards the spine of the scapula.

The *posterior branch of the second lumbar nerve* perforates the fascia lumborum near the posterior superior spine of the ilium, and runs over the crest of the ilium, to supply the skin of the buttock.

The trapezius and latissimus dorsi, which form the first layer of muscles, must now be cleaned by dissecting in the course of their fibres.

Trapezius.   Alone, this muscle is triangular; with its fellow, it presents a trapezoid form. It *arises* from the inner fourth, more or less, of the superior curved line of the occiput; from the ligamentum nuchæ,* from the spines of the seventh cervical, and all the dorsal vertebræ, and from their supraspinous ligaments. The fibres converge towards the shoulder. The upper are *inserted* fleshy into the external third of the clavicle; the middle, into the inner border of the acromion and spine of the scapula; the lower terminate in a thin tendon, which plays over the triangular surface at the back of the scapula, and is inserted into the beginning of the spine. The insertion of the trapezius exactly corresponds to the origin of the deltoid, and the two

---

* The 'ligamentum nuchæ' is, in man, only a rudiment of the great elastic ligament which supports the weight of the head in quadrupeds. It extends from the spine of the occiput to the spines of all the cervical vertebræ except the atlas; otherwise it would impede the free rotation of the head. In the giraffe this ligament is six feet long, and as thick as a man's forearm. I am told by Professor Quekett, that when divided it shrinks at least two feet.

muscles are connected by a thin aponeurosis over the spine and acromion. If both the trapezius muscles be exposed, you will see that, between the sixth cervical and the third dorsal vertebra, their origin presents an aponeurotic space of an elliptical form.

The fixed point of the muscle being at the spine, all its fibres tend to raise the shoulder. The deltoid cannot raise the humerus beyond an angle of sixty degrees: beyond this the elevation of the arm is principally effected by the action of the trapezius rotating the scapula. It is in strong action when a weight is borne upon the shoulders; again, its middle and inferior fibres act powerfully in drawing the scapula backwards, as in preparing to strike a blow. If both muscles act, they draw the head backwards; if one, it draws the head to the same side. It is supplied by the nervus accessorius and the cervical plexus, and by the superficialis colli artery.

Latissimus dorsi.
This broad flat muscle occupies the lumbar and lower dorsal region, and thence extends to the arm, where it forms part of the posterior boundary of the axilla. It arises from the posterior third of the external lip of the crest of the ilium, from the spinous processes of the two upper sacral, all the lumbar and the six lower dorsal vertebræ by a strong aponeurosis; and, lastly, from the three or four lower ribs by digitations, which correspond with those of the external oblique muscle of the abdomen. All the fibres converge towards the axilla, where they form a thick muscle, which curves round the inferior angle of the scapula, and is *inserted* by a broad, flat tendon, into the bottom of the bicipital groove of the humerus. The tendon is about two inches broad, and lies in front of that of the teres major, from which it is separated by a large *bursa*.*

The latissimus dorsi draws the humerus inwards and backwards; rotating it also inwards. It also co-operates with the pectoralis major in pulling any object towards the body: if the humerus be the fixed point, it raises the body, as in climbing. The object of

* The latissimus dorsi sometimes receives a distinct accessory slip from the inferior angle of the scapula. It is supplied by the long subscapular nerve.

the muscle arising so high up the back is, that the transverse fibres of the muscle may strap down the inferior angle of the scapula. It sometimes happens that the scapula slips above the muscle: this displacement is readily recognised by the unnatural projection of the lower angle of the bone, and the impaired movements of the arm.[*]

Between the base of the scapula, the trapezius, and the upper border of the latissimus dorsi, a triangular space is observed when the arm is raised, in which the lower fibres of the rhomboideus major and part of the sixth intercostal space, are exposed. Immediately above the crest of the ilium, between the free margins of the latissimus dorsi and external oblique, there is, also, an interval in which a little of the internal oblique can be seen.

Vertebral aponeurosis.

This dense shining aponeurosis of the back is situated between the serrati postici and the erector spinæ, of which muscle it forms the posterior part of the sheath. It is pointed above, where it is continuous with the deep cervical fascia, broader and stronger below. It consists of tendinous fibres, which are attached internally to the spines of the six or seven lower dorsal, all the lumbar and sacral vertebræ; externally, to the angles of the ribs; and inferiorly it is blended with the tendons of the serratus posticus inferior and latissimus dorsi. When suppuration takes place in the loins, constituting 'lumbar abscess' in connection with spinal disease, the matter is seated beneath this aponeurosis, and is therefore a long time in coming to the surface.

Reflect the trapezius from its insertion. On its under surface see the ramifications of its nutrient artery, the *superficialis colli* (a branch of the posterior scapular). A large nerve, the *spinal accessory*, enters its under surface near the clavicle, and divides into filaments, some of which ascend, others descend in its substance.

---

[*] We have seen an instance of this displacement. There was great projection of the inferior angle of the scapula, especially when the man attempted to raise the arm. He could not raise the arm beyond a right angle, unless firm pressure was made on the lower angle of the scapula, so as to supply the place of the muscular strap. Whether the scapula can be replaced or not, apply a firm bandage round the chest.

Spinal accessory nerve. This nerve is one of the three divisions of the eighth pair of cerebral nerves. It arises from the lateral part of the cervical portion of the spinal cord by several roots, some of which are as low as the sixth cervical vertebra. Formed by the union of these roots, the nerve enters the skull through the foramen magnum, and leaves it again through the foramen jugulare. It then runs behind the internal jugular vein, traverses obliquely the upper third of the sterno-mastoid, and crosses the posterior triangle of the neck to the trapezius, which it supplies (p. 15).

Beneath the trapezius we have to examine the second layer, consisting of three muscles connected with the scapula; namely, the levator anguli scapulæ, the rhomboideus major and minor. The scapula must be adjusted so as to stretch their fibres.

Levator anguli scapulæ. This muscle is situated at the side of the neck. It arises by four tendons from the posterior tubercles of the transverse processes of the four upper cervical vertebræ. The muscular slips to which the tendons give rise, form a single muscle, which descends down the side of the neck, and is *inserted* into the posterior border of the scapula between its spine and superior angle. Its *action* is to raise the posterior angle of the scapula; as, for instance, in shrugging the shoulders. Its nerve comes from the fifth and sixth cervical.

Rhomboideus major and minor. These flat muscles extend from the spinous processes of the vertebræ to the base of the scapula. They often appear like a single muscle. The rhomboideus minor, the higher of the two, *arises* by a thin aponeurosis from the spinous processes of the last cervical and the first dorsal vertebra, and is *inserted* into the base of the scapula opposite its spine. The rhomboideus major *arises* by tendinous fibres from the spinous processes of the four or five upper dorsal vertebræ, and is *inserted* by fleshy fibres into the base of the scapula between its spine and inferior angle. The *action* of these muscles is to draw the scapula upwards and backwards. They are the antagonists of the serratus magnus.

The *nerve of the rhomboid muscles* (posterior scapular) is a branch of the fifth and sixth cervical. It passes outwards beneath the lower part of the levator anguli scapulæ, to which it sends a branch, and is lost in the under surface of the rhomboidei.

Omo-
hyoideus.
This muscle extends from the scapula to the os hyoides, and consists of two long narrow muscular portions, connected by an intermediate tendon beneath the sterno-mastoid. The posterior portion only can be seen in the present dissection. It *arises* from the scapula, close behind the notch, and from the ligament above the notch. From thence the slender muscle passes forwards across the lower part of the neck, beneath the sterno-mastoid, where it changes its direction and ascends nearly vertically, to be attached to the os hyoides at the junction of the body with the greater cornu (p. 22). Thus the two portions of the muscle form beneath the sterno-mastoid an obtuse angle, of which the apex is tendinous, and of which the angular direction is maintained by a layer of fascia, proceeding from the tendon to the first rib and the clavicle. Its *action* is to depress the os hyoides. Its nerve comes from the descendens noni.

Supra-scapu-
lar artery.
This artery (transversalis humeri), a branch of the thyroid axis, runs beneath and parallel with the clavicle, over the lower end of the scalenus anticus to the upper border of the scapula, where it usually passes above the ligament, bridging over the notch. It ramifies in the supra spinous fossa, supplying the supra-spinatus, and then passes under the acromion to the infra-spinous fossa, where it inosculates freely with the dorsalis scapula, a branch of the subscapular. It sends off the *supra-acromial* branch, which ramifies upon the acromion, anastomosing with the other acromial arteries derived from branches of the axillary. The supra-scapular vein terminates either in the subclavian or in the external jugular.

The *supra-scapular* nerve, a branch of the fifth and sixth cervical, runs with the corresponding artery, and after passing through the supra-scapular notch, is distributed to the supra-spinatus and infra-spinatus. In the supra-spinous fossa, this nerve sends a small branch to the shoulder-joint.

T

Posterior scapular artery.   This artery, sometimes called the 'transversalis colli,' is usually described as arising from the thyroid axis, but it comes very frequently from the subclavian in the third part of its course. It runs across the lower part of the neck, above, or between the nerves of the brachial plexus, towards the posterior superior angle of the scapula. Here it pursues its course along the posterior border of the scapula beneath the levator anguli scapulæ and the rhomboidei, anastomosing with branches of the supra-scapular and sub-scapular arteries. The corresponding vein joins the external jugular or the subclavian.

Divide the rhomboid muscles near their insertion, and trace the artery to the inferior angle of the scapula, where it terminates in the rhomboidei, serratus magnus, and latissimus dorsi.

Numerous muscular branches arise from the posterior scapular. One, the *superficialis colli*, is given off near the upper angle of the scapula for the supply of the trapezius.

Divide and reflect the latissimus dorsi below the inferior angle of the scapula, and draw the scapula forcibly outwards, to have a more perfect view of the extent of the serratus magnus than was seen in the axilla. The abundance of cellular tissue in this situation is necessary for the play of the scapula on the chest.

Serratus magnus.   This broad flat muscle intervenes between the scapula and the ribs. It *arises* by nine fleshy digitations from the eight upper ribs, each rib giving origin to one, and the second to two. The four lower digitations correspond with those of the external oblique muscle of the abdomen. All the fibres pass backwards, and converge to be *inserted* along the posterior border of the scapula, chiefly near the upper and lower angles.

This is the most important of the muscles which regulate the movements of the scapula; it draws the scapula forwards—and thus gives additional reach to the arm; it counteracts all forces which tend to push the scapula backwards; for instance, when a man falls forwards upon his hands, the serratus magnus sustains the shock, and prevents the scapula from being driven back to the spine. Supposing the fixed point to be at the scapula, some anatomists ascribe to it the power of raising the ribs; hence Sir Charles Bell called it the external respiratory muscle, as opposed to the internal respiratory muscle, the diaphragm.

The nerve which supplies it is a branch of the fifth and sixth cervical nerve: it descends along its outer surface (p. 226).

Divide the serratus magnus near the scapula, and remove the arm by sawing through the middle of the clavicle, cutting through the axillary vessels and nerves. These should be tied to the coracoid process. After the removal of the arm, examine the precise insertion of the preceding muscles.

DISSECTION OF THE MUSCLES OF THE SHOULDER.

Dissect first the cutaneous nerves of the shoulder; Cutaneous nerves of the shoulder. these are derived, partly from the branches of the cervical plexus which descend over the acromion (p. 17), partly from the circumflex nerve, of which one or two branches turn round the posterior border of the deltoid; others perforate the muscle, each accompanied by a small artery.

Notice the strong layer of fascia upon the surface of the deltoid, which extends from the aponeurosis covering the muscles on the back of the scapula, and is continuous with the fascia of the arm. It dips down between the fibres of the muscle, dividing it into large bundles. This fascia must be removed.

Deltoid. The great muscle which covers the shoulder-joint is named deltoid, from its resemblance to the Greek Δ reversed. It arises from the external third of the clavicle, from the acromion, and from the spine of the scapula down to the triangular surface at its root. This origin, which corresponds to the insertion of the trapezius, is tendinous and fleshy everywhere, except at the commencement of the spine of the scapula, where it is simply tendinous, and connected with the infra-spinous aponeurosis. The muscular fibres descend, the anterior backwards, the posterior forwards, the middle perpendicularly; all converge to a tendon which is *inserted* into a rough surface on the outer side of

the humerus, a little above the middle of the shaft. The insertion
of the tendon extends one inch and a half along the humerus, and
terminates in a smaller V-shaped form, the origin of the brachialis
anticus being on either side.

The muscular bundles composing the deltoid have a peculiar
arrangement: a peculiarity arising from its broad origin and its
narrow insertion. It consists in the interposition of tendons
between the bundles for the attachment of the muscular fibres.
The annexed woodcut shows this beautiful arrangement better
than any description. The action of the muscle is not only concentrated upon one point, but its power is also greatly increased,
by this arrangement.

Action of the deltoid. It raises the arm; but it cannot do so beyond an
angle of sixty degrees. The elevation of the arm
beyond this angle is effected through the elevation of
the shoulder by the trapezius and serratus magnus. Its anterior
fibres draw the arm forwards; its
posterior, backwards.

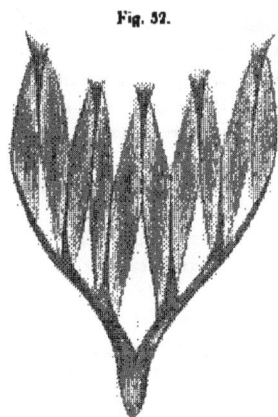

Fig. 52.

ANALYSIS OF THE DELTOID.

This powerful muscle is well supplied with blood, by the anterior
and posterior circumflex, the thoracica humeraria, the thoracica
acromialis, all from the axillary
artery; also by the deltoid branch
of the brachial. Its nerve is the
circumflex.

The deltoid gives the rotundity
to the shoulder. When the head
of the humerus is dislocated into
the axilla, the fibres of the muscle
run vertically to their insertion;
hence the flattening of the deltoid,
and the greater prominence of the
acromion.

Below the deltoid we generally meet with ununited fracture of
the humerus; owing to the muscle raising the upper fragment.

Reflect the deltoid from its origin, and turn it downwards. Observe the ramifications of the circumflex artery and nerve, on its under surface: also the large bursa between it and the tendons inserted into the head of the humerus. See how the muscle protects the shoulder-joint; how it covers the coraco-acromial ligament, the head, neck, and upper part of the humerus, as well as the tendons inserted into the greater tuberosity.

Bursa under the deltoid. — A bursa of large size is situated between the deltoid, and the tendons inserted into the head of the humerus. It extends for some distance beneath the acromion and the coraco-acromial ligament, and covers the great tuberosity of the humerus. I have seen it communicating by a wide opening with the shoulder-joint, but this is a rare exception. Its use is to facilitate the movements of the head of the bone under the acromial arch.

Posterior circumflex artery. — This artery is given off from the axillary: it runs behind the surgical neck of the humerus, through a quadrilateral opening, bounded above by the subscapularis and teres minor, below by the teres major, externally by the neck of the humerus, and internally by the long head of the triceps (p. 229). Its branches terminate on the under surface of the deltoid, anastomosing with the anterior circumflex, acromial thoracic, and supra-scapular arteries.

From the posterior circumflex, a branch descends in the substance of the long head of the triceps, to inosculate with the superior profunda; this is one of the channels through which the circulation would be carried on, if the axillary were tied in the last part of its course.

Circumflex nerve. — This nerve, a branch of the posterior cord of the axillary plexus, runs with the posterior circumflex artery. It sends a branch to the teres minor, one or two to the integuments of the shoulder, and terminates in the substance of the deltoid. The proximity of this nerve to the head of the humerus explains the occasional paralysis of the deltoid, after dislocation or fracture of the humerus. The nerve is apt to be injured, if not actually lacerated by the pressure of the bone,

In the summer of 1840, a man was admitted into the hospital
with a severe injury to the shoulder, and died of delirium tremens.
On examination the humerus was found broken high up, the
capsule of the joint opened, and the circumflex nerve torn completely across.[*]

The muscles of the dorsum of the scapula are covered by a
strong aponeurosis, firmly attached to the spine and borders of the
bone. At the posterior edge of the deltoid, it divides into two
layers, one of which passes over, the other under, the muscle.
Remove the aponeurosis, so far as it can be done without injury
to the muscular fibres which arise from its under surface.

Infra-
spinatus.
This muscle *arises* from the posterior two-thirds of
the infra-spinous fossa, and from the aponeurosis which
covers it. The fibres converge to a tendon, which is at
first contained in the substance of the muscle, and then proceeds
over the capsule of the shoulder-joint to be *inserted* into the
greater tuberosity of the humerus. Its nerve comes from the
supra-scapular.

Teres minor.
This long narrow muscle is situated below the infra-
spinatus, along the inferior border of the scapula. It
arises from the dorsum of the scapula, close to the inferior border.
The fibres ascend parallel with those of the infra-spinatus, and
terminate in a tendon, which passes over the capsule of the
shoulder-joint, and is *inserted* into the lowest depression on the
great tuberosity of the humerus, and by muscular fibres into the
bone below it. It is supplied by a branch of the circumflex
nerve, which has usually a small ganglion upon it.

The *action* of the infra-spinatus and teres minor is to rotate the
humerus outwards.

Teres major.
This muscle is closely connected with the latissimus
dorsi, and extends from the inferior angle of the scapula
to the humerus, contributing to form the posterior boundary of the
axilla. It *arises* from the flat surface at the inferior angle of the
back of the scapula, and from its inferior border, and terminates

[*] See preparation in Museum of St. Bartholomew's Hospital, series 3, no. 42.

upon a flat tendon, two inches in breadth, which is *inserted* into the inner edge of the bicipital groove of the humerus, behind and a little below the tendon of the latissimus dorsi. Its *action* is to draw the humerus backwards. It is supplied by the middle subscapular nerve.

You will find a bursa in front of, and another behind the tendon of the teres major; the former separates it from the latissimus dorsi, the latter from the bone.

Supra-spinatus.   This muscle *arises* from the posterior two-thirds of the supra-spinous fossa, and from its aponeurotic covering. It passes under the acromion, over the shoulder-joint, and is *inserted* by a strong tendon into the greater tuberosity of the humerus. To see its insertion, the acromion should be sawn off near the neck of the scapula. Its *action* is to assist the deltoid in raising the arm. Its nerve is derived from the supra-scapular.

Subscapularis.   This muscle occupies the subscapular fossa. It *arises* from the posterior three-fourths of the fossa, from three or four tendinous septa attached to the oblique ridges on its surface. The fibres converge towards the neck of the scapula, where they terminate upon three or four tendons, which are concealed amongst the muscular fibres, and are *inserted* into the lesser tuberosity of the humerus. Its broad insertion is closely connected with the capsule of the shoulder-joint, which it completely protects upon its inner side. Its *action* is to rotate the humerus inwards. The nerve which supplies it comes from the posterior cord which gives off the circumflex and musculo-spiral.

The coracoid process, with the coraco-brachialis and short head of the biceps, form an arch, under which the tendon of the subscapularis plays. There are several *bursæ* about the tendon. One of considerable size on the upper surface of the tendon, facilitates its motion beneath the coracoid process and the coracobrachialis: this sometimes communicates with the large bursa under the deltoid. Another is situated between the tendon and the capsule of the joint, and almost invariably communicates with it.

Now reflect the muscles from the surfaces of the scapula, to trace the arteries which ramify upon it.

Continuation of supra-scapular artery. This artery, a branch of the thyroid axis, runs under and parallel with the clavicle, and passes above the notch of the scapula, into the supra-spinal fossa: it sends a branch to the supra-spinatus, another to the shoulder-joint, and then descends over the neck of the scapula into the fossa below the spine, where it inosculates directly with the dorsalis scapulæ. Its branches ramify upon the bone, and supply the infra-spinatus and teres minor.

The supra-scapular nerve passes most frequently through the notch of the scapula, accompanies the corresponding artery, and supplies the supra and infra-spinatus.

Dorsalis scapulæ artery. This artery, after passing through the triangular space (p. 229), curves round the inferior border of the scapula, which it sometimes grooves, to the infra-spinous fossa, where it ascends close to the bone, and anastomoses with the supra and posterior scapula arteries.

The frequent communications about the scapula between the branches of the subclavian and axillary arteries, would furnish a free current of blood to the arm, if the subclavian were tied above the clavicle (p. 60).

Triceps extensor cubiti. This muscle, which arises by three heads, and was only partially seen in the dissection of the upper arm (p. 229), should now be fully examined. The long head arises immediately below the glenoid cavity of the scapula, by a strong tendon which is connected with the capsule of the shoulder-joint. The second or external head *arises* from the posterior part of the humerus, below the insertion of the teres minor; the third or internal head *arises* from the posterior part of the humerus, below the teres major. The precise origin of these heads from the humerus may be ascertained by following the superior profunda artery and musculo-spiral nerve, which intervene between them. The three portions of the muscle terminate upon a broad tendon, which covers the back of the elbow-joint, and is *inserted* into the summit and sides of the olecranon; it is also connected with the fascia on the back of the forearm. The reason of this connection is, that the same muscle which extends the forearm may at the same time tighten the fascia which gives origin to the extensors of the wrist and fingers. This is just what we observed in the case of the biceps, and its semi-lunar expansion in the fascia of the forearm.

Between the tendon and olecranon is a *bursa*, commonly of small size, but sometimes so large as to extend upwards behind the capsule of the joint. This bursa must not be mistaken for that which is always found between the skin and the olecranon, and is so often injured by a fall on the elbow.

By dividing the triceps transversely a little above the elbow, and turning down the lower portion, it will be observed that some of the muscular fibres terminate upon the capsule of the joint. They have been described by some anatomists as a distinct muscle, under the name of *subanconeus*;' their use is to draw up the capsule, so that it may not be injured during extension of the arm. The subanconeus is in this respect analogous to the sub-cruraeus muscle of the thigh. Observe the *bursa* under the tendon, and the arterial arch formed upon the back part of the capsule by the superior profunda and the anastomotica magna (fig. 50, p. 240).

Trace the continuation of the superior profunda artery (p. 239), and musculo-spiral nerve round the posterior part of the humerus. They lie in a groove on the bone, between the external and internal heads of the triceps, and are protected by an aponeurotic arch thrown over them by the external head of the triceps. After supplying the muscles, the artery continues along the outer side of the arm between the brachialis anticus and supinator radii longus, and inosculates with the radial recurrent. It gives off a branch which runs down between the triceps and the bone, and inosculates at the back of the elbow with the anastomotica magna and posterior interosseous recurrent. The musculo-spiral nerve which accompanies the artery sends branches to supply the three portions of the triceps, the supinator radii longus, and extensor carpi radialis longior.* It then divides into the posterior inter-

---

* In some (rare) instances, the brachialis anticus receives a branch from the musculo-spiral.

osseous and radial nerves. A small branch of this nerve, which passes through the substance of the triceps to supply the anconeus, must be made out. The cutaneous branches of the musculo-spiral nerve have been already dissected (p. 233).

DISSECTION OF THE BACK OF THE FOREARM.

Remove the skin from the back of the forearm, hand, and fingers. Observe the subcutaneous *bursa* over the olecranon. It is commonly of considerable size, and, if distended, would appear nearly as large as a walnut. Another *bursa* is sometimes found a little lower down upon the ulna. A subcutaneous *bursa* is generally placed over the internal condyle, another over the external. A *bursa* is also situated over the styloid process of the ulna; this sometimes communicates with the sheath of the extensor carpi ulnaris. Small *bursæ* are sometimes developed in the cellular tissue over each of the knuckles.

The cutaneous veins from the back of the hand and forearm join the venous plexus at the bend of the elbow (see p. 234).

Cutaneous nerves of the back of the forearm and hand.

They are the external cutaneous branches of the musculo-spiral, branches of the internal cutaneous, and of the external cutaneous. The greater number of these nerves may be traced down to the back of the wrist.

The skin on the back of the hand is united to the subjacent tendons by an abundance of loose connective tissue, in which we find large veins, and branches of the radial and ulnar nerves. The dorsal branch of the ulnar nerve passes beneath the tendon of the flexor carpi ulnaris, over the internal lateral ligament of the wrist; and divides upon the back of the hand into filaments, which supply the back of the little finger, the ring finger, and the ulnar side of the middle finger. The radial nerve passes obliquely beneath the tendon of the supinator longus, and subdivides into branches, which supply both sides of the back of the thumb and forefinger, and the radial side of the middle finger.*

The radial nerve commonly gives off a branch which joins that division of the ulnar nerve which supplies the radial border of the ring and contiguous side of the middle finger.

The *fascia on the back of the forearm* is composed of fibres interlacing and stronger than that upon the front of the forearm. It is attached to the condyles of the humerus and to the olecranon, and is strengthened by an expansion from the tendon of the triceps. Along the forearm it is attached to the ridge on the posterior part of the ulna. Its upper third gives origin to the fibres of the muscles beneath it, and separates them by septa, to which their fibres are also attached.

Posterior annular ligament. This should be considered as a part of the fascia of the forearm, strengthened by oblique aponeurotic fibres on the back of the wrist to confine the extensor tendons. These fibres are attached to the styloid process of the radius, and thence pass obliquely inwards to the inner side of the wrist, where they are connected with the pisiform and cuneiform bones. Observe that they pass below the styloid process of the ulna, to which they are in no way attached, otherwise the rotation of the radius would be impeded.

From the deep surface of this 'so-called' ligament, processes are attached to the ridges on the back of the radius, so as to form six distinct sheaths for the passage of the extensor tendons. Counting from the radius, the first sheath contains the tendons of the extensor ossis metacarpi and the extensor primi internodii pollicis; the second, the tendons of the extensor carpi radialis longior and brevior; the third, the tendon of the extensor secundi

---

* The relative share which the radial and ulnar nerves take in supplying the fingers varies. Under any arrangement the thumb and each finger has two dorsal nerves, one on either side, of which the terminal branches reach the root of the nail. They supply filaments to the skin on the back of the finger, and have frequent communications with the palmar digital nerves. In some instances one or more of the dorsal nerves do not extend beyond the first phalanx; their place is then supplied by a branch from the palmar nerve.

internodii pollicis; the fourth, the tendons of the indicator and
the extensor communis digitorum; the fifth, the tendon of the
extensor minimi digiti; and the sixth, the tendon of the extensor
carpi ulnaris. All the sheaths are lined by synovial membranes,
which extend nearly to the insertions of their tendons. In a few
instances, one or more of them communicate with the wrist-
joint.

The *fascia of the metacarpus* consists of a thin fibrous layer,
continued from the posterior annular ligament. It separates the
extensor tendons from the subcutaneous veins and nerves, and is
attached to the radial side of the second metacarpal bone, and the
ulnar side of the fifth.

Superficial
muscles on
the back of
the forearm.
The fascia must be removed from the muscles, without injuring the muscular fibres which arise from its
under surface. Preserve the posterior annular ligament. The following muscles are now exposed, and
should be examined in the order in which they are placed, proceeding from the radial to the ulnar side:—1. The supinator radii
longus (already described, p. 249). 2. The extensor carpi radialis longior. 3. The extensor carpi radialis brevior. 4. The
extensor communis digitorum. 5. The extensor minimi digiti.
6. The extensor carpi ulnaris. 7. The anconeus.

A little below the middle of the forearm, the extensors of the
wrist and fingers diverge from each other, leaving an interval, in
which are seen the three extensors of the thumb—the extensor
ossis metacarpi pollicis, the extensor primi internodii pollicis, and
the extensor secundi internodii pollicis. The two former cross the
radial extensors of the wrist, and pass over the lower third of the
radius.

Between the second and third extensors of the thumb, we observe a part of the lower end of the radius, which is not covered
either by muscle or tendon. This subcutaneous portion of the
bone is immediately above the prominent tubercle in the middle
of its lower extremity, and, since it can be easily felt through the
skin, it presents a convenient place for examination in doubtful
cases of fracture.

Extensor carpi radialis longior. This muscle is partly covered by the supinator radii longus. It *arises* from the lower third of the ridge, leading to the external condyle of the humerus, and from the intermuscular septum, descends along the outer side of the forearm, and terminates about the middle, in a flat tendon, which passes beneath the extensor ossis metacarpi, and primi internodii pollicis, traverses a groove on the outer and back part of the radius, lined by a synovial membrane, and is *inserted* into the radial side of the carpal end of the metacarpal bone of the index finger. Previous to its insertion, the tendon is crossed by the extensor secundi internodii pollicis. It is supplied by a branch from the musculo-spiral nerve.

Extensor carpi radialis brevior. This muscle *arises* from the external condyle and from the external lateral ligament of the elbow-joint. The muscular fibres terminate near the middle of the forearm, upon the under surface of a flat tendon, which descends, covered by that of the extensor carpi radialis longior, beneath the first two extensors of the thumb. The tendon traverses a groove on the back of the radius, on the same plane with that of the long radial extensor, but lined by a separate synovial membrane, and is *inserted* into the radial side of the metacarpal bone of the middle finger. A bursa is generally found between the tendon and the bone. Its nerve comes from the posterior interosseous nerve.

Extensor digitorum communis. This muscle *arises* from the common tendon attached to the external condyle, from the septa between it and the contiguous muscles, and from its strong fascial covering. About the middle of the forearm the muscle divides into three or four fleshy slips, terminating in as many flat tendons, which pass beneath the posterior annular ligament, through a groove on the back of the radius lined by synovial membrane. On the back of the hand they become broader and flatter, and diverge from each other towards the metacarpal joints of the fingers, where they become thicker and narrower, and give off on each side a fibrous expansion, which covers the sides of the joint. Over the first phalanx of the finger, each tendon again spreads out, receives the expanded tendons of the lumbricales and interossei muscles, and divides at the second phalanx into three portions, of which the middle is inserted into the upper end of the second phalanx; the two lateral, reuniting over the lower end of the second phalanx, are inserted into the upper end of the third.[*]

Observe the oblique aponeurotic slips which connect the tendons on the back of the hand. They are subject to great variety. The tendon of the index finger is commonly free; it is situated on the radial side of the proper indicator tendon, and becomes united with it at the metacarpal joint.

The tendon of the middle usually receives a slip from that of the ring-finger. The tendon of the ring finger generally sends a slip to the tendons on either side of it, and in some cases entirely furnishes the tendon of the little finger.

It is not only a general extensor of the fingers, but it can extend some of the phalanges independently of the rest: e.g. it can extend the first phalanges while the second and third are flexed; or it can extend the second and third phalanges during flexion of the first.

Extensor digiti minimi or auricularis. This long slender muscle, which is situated on the inner side of the common extensor muscle, arises from the common tendon from the external condyle, and from the septa between it and the contiguous muscles. Its slender tendon runs beneath the annular ligament immediately behind the joint between the radius and ulna, in a special sheath lined by synovial membrane. At the first joint of the little finger, the tendon is joined by that of the common extensor, and both expand upon the first and second phalanges, terminating in the same manner as the extensor tendons of the other fingers. Its nerve comes from the posterior interosseus.

Extensor carpi ulnaris. This muscle *arises* from the common tendon from the external condyle, from the septum between it and the extensor minimi digiti, and from the aponeurosis of the forearm. The fibres terminate upon a strong broad tendon,

---

[*] The extensor tendons are only inserted into the periosteum, whereas the flexor tendons are inserted into the substance of the bone. This accounts for the facility with which the former will tear off the bones in cases of necrosis, while the latter will adhere so tightly as to require cutting before the phalanx can be removed.

which traverses a distinct groove on the back of the ulna, close to the styloid process, and is inserted into the carpal end of the metacarpal bone of the little finger. Below the styloid process of the ulna, the tendon passes beneath the posterior annular ligament, over the back of the wrist, and is here contained in a very strong fibrous canal, which is attached to the back of the cuneiform, pisiform, and unciform bones, and is lined by a continuation from the synovial membrane in the groove of the ulna. The *action* of this muscle is to extend the band, and incline it towards the ulnar side. It is supplied by the posterior interosseous nerve.

In pronation of the forearm, the lower end of the ulna projects between the tendons of the extensor carpi ulnaris and the extensor minimi digiti. A subcutaneous *bursa* is sometimes found above the bone in this situation.

Anconeus.
This small triangular muscle is situated at the outer and back part of the elbow. It is covered by a strong layer of fascia, derived from the tendon of the triceps, and appears like a continuation of that muscle. It *arises* tendinous from the posterior part of the external condyle of the humerus, and is *inserted* into the triangular surface on the upper fourth of the outer part of the ulna. Part of the under surface of the muscle is in contact with the capsule of the elbow-joint. Its *action* is to assist in extending the forearm. Its nerve comes from the musculo-spiral.

Deep-seated muscles on the back of the forearm.
To expose the deep layer of muscles, detach from the external condyle, the extensor carpi radialis brevior, the extensor communis digitorum, the extensor minimi digiti, and the extensor corpi ulnaris; and after noticing the vessels and nerves which enter their under surface, turn them down. The deep-seated muscles, with the posterior interosseous artery and nerve, must be cleaned. The muscles exposed are: 1. The extensor ossis metacarpi pollicis. 2. Extensor primi internodii pollicis. 3. Extensor secundi internodii pollicis. 4. Extensor indicis or indicator. 5. The supinator radii brevis. They are all supplied by branches from the posterior interosseous nerve.

Extensor ossis metacarpi pollicis.

This muscle *arises* from the posterior surface of the ulna below the supinator brevis, from the posterior surface of the radius, and from the interosseous ligament. The muscle crosses the radial extensors of the wrist about three inches above the carpus, and terminates in a tendon, which passes along a groove, lined by synovial membrane, on the outer part of the lower end of the radius, and is *inserted* into the base of the metacarpal bone of the thumb, and frequently also by a tendinous slip into the trapezium.

Extensor primi internodii pollicis.

This muscle *arises* from the posterior surface of the radius and ulna, below the preceding, and from the interosseous ligament. It turns over the radial extensors of the wrist, and terminates upon a tendon which passes beneath the annular ligament, through the groove on the outer part of the radius, and is *inserted* into the radial side of the base of the first phalanx of the thumb.

Extensor secundi internodii pollicis.

Arises from the posterior surface of the ulna, and from the interosseous membrane. The tendon receives fleshy fibres as low as the wrist, passes beneath the annular ligament, in a distinct groove on the back of the radius, crosses the tendons of the radial extensors of the wrist, proceeds over the metacarpal bone and the first phalanx of the thumb, and is *inserted* into the base of the last phalanx.

The tendons of the three extensors of the thumb may be easily distinguished in one's own hand. The extensor ossis metacarpi, and primi internodii pollicis, cross obliquely over the radial artery, where it lies on the external lateral ligament of the carpus; the extensor secundi internodii pollicis crosses the artery just before it sinks into the palm, between the first and second metacarpal bones, and is a good guide to the vessel. The *action* of the three extensors of the thumb is implied by their names.

Extensor indicis, or indicator.

This muscle *arises* from the posterior surface of the ulna, and from the interosseous ligament. The tendon passes beneath the posterior annular ligament, in the same groove on the back of the radius with the tendons of the extensor digitorum communis. It then proceeds over the back of the hand to the first phalanx of the index finger, where it is united to the ulnar border of the common extensor tendon. By the *action* of this muscle, the index finger can be extended independently of the others.

Reflect the extensor carpi radialis longior and the anconeus from their origins, to expose the following muscle.

Supinator
radii brevis.   This muscle embraces the upper third of the radius. It *arises* from the external lateral ligament of the elbow-joint, from the annular ligament surrounding the head of the radius, from an oblique ridge on the outer surface of the ulna below the insertion of the anconeus, and by fleshy fibres from the triangular excavation below the lesser sigmoid notch of the ulna. The muscular fibres turn over the neck and upper part of the shaft of the radius, and are *inserted* into the upper third of this bone, as far forwards as the ridge leading from the tubercle to the insertion of the pronator teres. The muscle is perforated obliquely by the posterior interosseous nerve, one of the terminal divisions of the musculo-spiral nerve, and its upper part is in contact with the capsule of the elbow-joint. It is a powerful supinator of the forearm, some of its fibres acting at nearly a right angle to the axis of the radius.

Posterior
interosseous
artery.   This artery comes from the ulnar by a common trunk with the anterior interosseous (p. 254), and supplies the muscles on the back of the forearm. It passes between the radius and ulna above the interosseous membrane, and appears between the supinator radii brevis and the extensor ossis metacarpi pollicis. After supplying branches to all the muscles in this situation, the artery descends, much diminished in size, between the superficial and deep layer of muscles to the wrist, where it inosculates with the carpal branches of the anterior interosseous, and the posterior carpal branches of the radial and ulnar arteries.

But the largest branch of this artery is the *recurrent*. It ascends beneath the anconeus muscle to the space between the external condyle and the olecranon, where it inosculates with the branch of the superior profunda, which descends in the substance of the triceps.

In the lower part of the back of the forearm, a branch of the anterior interosseous artery is seen passing through the interosseous membrane to reach the back of the wrist (see p. 254).

Posterior interosseous nerve. The nerve which supplies the muscles on the back of the forearm is the *posterior interosseous*, a branch of the musculo-spiral. It passes obliquely through the supinator radii brevis, and descends between the superficial and deep layer of muscles on the back of the forearm, sending to each a filament, generally in company with a branch of the posterior interosseous artery. It sends a branch to the extensor carpi radialis brevior, and supplies the supinator brevis in passing through its substance. The supinator radii longus and the extensor carpi radialis longior are supplied by distinct branches from the musculo-spiral.

The continuation of the posterior interosseous nerve descends beneath the extensor secundi internodii pollicis and the tendons of the extensor digitorum communis to the back of the wrist. Behind the common extensor tendons the nerve forms a kind of gangliform enlargement from which filaments are sent to the carpal and metacarpal joints.

Radial artery on the back of the wrist. Trace the continuation of the radial artery over the external lateral ligament of the carpus, beneath the extensor tendons of the thumb, to the upper part of the interval between the first and second metacarpal bones, where it sinks between the two origins of the abductor indicis, and entering the palm, forms the deep palmar arch. In this part of its course it is crossed by filaments of the radial nerve; observe, also, that the tendon of the extensor secundi internodii pollicis passes over it immediately before it sinks into the palm. It supplies the following small branches to the back of the hand:—

a. *Posterior carpal artery.*—This branch passes across the carpal bones, beneath the extensor tendons. It inosculates with the termination of the anterior interosseous artery, and with a corresponding branch from the ulnar artery. The carpal artery sends off small branches, called the *dorsal interosseous*, which descend along the third and fourth interosseous spaces, beneath the extensor tendons, inosculating near the carpal ends of the metacarpal bones with the perforating branches from the deep palmar arch.

b. The *first dorsal interosseous artery* is generally larger than the others. It descends over the second interosseous muscle to the cleft between the index and middle fingers, communicating here with a perforating branch of the deep palmar arch, and terminates in small branches, some of which proceed along the back of the fingers, others inosculate with the palmar digital arteries.

c. The *dorsal artery of the index-finger*, a branch of variable size, passes over the first interosseous muscle to the radial side of the back of the index finger.

d. The *dorsal arteries of the thumb* are two small branches which arise from the radial opposite the head of the first metacarpal bone, and run along the back of the thumb, one on either side. They are often absent.

These dorsal interosseous arteries supply the extensor tendons and their sheaths, the interosseous muscles, and the skin on the back of the hand, and the first phalanges of the fingers.

Remove the tendons from the back and from the palm of the hand : observe the deep palmar fascia which covers the interosseous muscles. It is attached to the ridges of the metacarpal bones, forms a distinct sheath for each interosseous muscle, and is continuous inferiorly with the transverse metacarpal ligament. On the back of the hand the interosseous muscles are covered by a thin fascia, which is attached to the adjacent borders of the metacarpal bones.

Transverse metacarpal ligament   This consists of strong bands of ligamentous fibres, which pass transversely between the digital extremities of the metacarpal bones. These bands are intimately united to the fibro-cartilaginous ligament of the metacarpal joints, and are of sufficient length to admit of a certain degree of movement between the ends of the metacarpal bones.

Remove the fascia which covers the interosseous muscles, and separate the metacarpal bones by dividing the transverse meta-

c 2

carpal ligament. A *bursa* is frequently developed between their digital extremities.

These muscles, so named from their position, extend from the sides of the metacarpal bones to the bases of the first phalanges and the extensor tendons of the fingers. In each interosseous space (except the first, in which there is only an abductor) there are two, one of which is an abductor, the other an adductor of a finger. According to this arrangement there are *seven* in all; four of which, situated on the back of the hand, are called dorsal; the remainder, seen only in the palm, are called palmar.

Interosseous muscles.

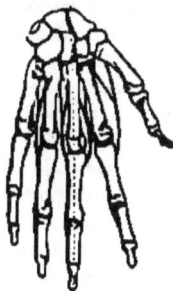

Fig. 53.

DIAGRAM OF THE FOUR DORSAL IN-
TEROSSEI, DRAWING FROM THE
MIDDLE LINE.

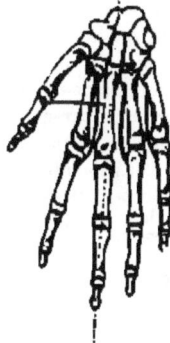

Fig. 54.

DIAGRAM OF THE THREE PALMAR IN-
TEROSSEI, AND ALSO THE ADDUCTOR
POLLICIS, DRAWING TOWARDS THE
MIDDLE LINE.

Each dorsal interosseous muscle *arises* from the opposite sides of two contiguous metacarpal bones (fig. 53). From this double origin the fibres converge to a tendon, which passes between the metacarpal joints of the finger, and is *inserted* into the side of the base of the first phalanx ;

Dorsal interossei.

it is also connected by a broad expansion with the extensor tendon on the back of the finger.

The *first* dorsal interosseous muscle (abductor indicis) is larger than the others, and occupies the interval between the thumb and fore-finger. It arises from the upper half of the ulnar side of the first metacarpal bone, and from the entire length of the radial side of the second : between the two origins, the radial artery passes into the palm. Its fibres converge on either side to a tendon, which is inserted into the *radial* side of the first phalanx of the index finger and its extensor tendon.

The *second* dorsal interosseous muscle occupies the second metacarpal space. It is inserted into the radial side of the first phalanx of the middle finger and its extensor tendon.

The *third* and *fourth*, occupying the corresponding metacarpal spaces, are inserted, the one into the ulnar side of the middle, the other into the ulnar side of the ring finger.

If an imaginary line be drawn longitudinally through the middle finger, as represented by the dotted line in fig. 53, we shall find that all the dorsal interosseous muscles are abductors from that line; consequently, they separate the fingers from each other.

Palmar interosseous. It requires a careful examination to distinguish this set of muscles, because the dorsal muscles protrude with them into the palm. They are smaller than the dorsal, and each arises from the lateral surface of only one metacarpal bone, that, namely, connected with the finger into which the muscle is inserted (fig. 54). They terminate in small tendons, which pass between the metacarpal joints of the fingers, and are inserted, like the dorsal muscles, into the sides of the first phalanges and the extensor tendons on the back of the fingers.

The *first* palmar interosseous muscle arises from the ulnar side of the second metacarpal bone, and is inserted into the ulnar side of the index finger. The *second* and *third* arise, the one from the radial side of the fourth, the other from the radial side of the fifth metacarpal bone, and are inserted into the same sides of the ring and little fingers.

The palmar interosseous muscles are all adductors to an imaginary line drawn through the middle finger (fig. 54). They are, therefore, the opponents of the dorsal interosseous muscles, and move the fingers towards each other.

The palmar and dorsal interossei are supplied by offsets from the deep branch of the ulnar nerve.

DISSECTION OF THE LIGAMENTS.

The inner end of the clavicle articulates with a shallow excavation on the upper and outer part of the sternum. The security of the joint depends upon the strength of its ligaments. There are two synovial membranes, and an intervening fibro-cartilage.

Joint between the clavicle and the sternum.

The *anterior sterno-clavicular ligament* (fig. 55), consists of a

Fig. 55.

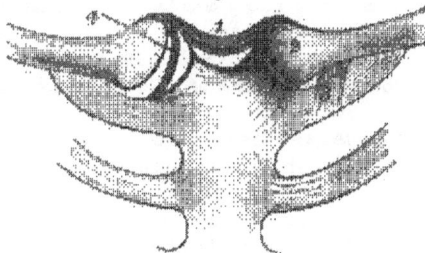

DIAGRAM OF THE STERNO-CLAVICULAR LIGAMENTS.

1. Interclavicular ligament.
2. Anterior sterno-clavicular ligament.
3. Costo-clavicular ligament.
4. Interarticular fibro-cartilage.

broad band of ligamentous fibres, which pass obliquely downwards and inwards over the front of the joint, from the end of the clavicle to the anterior surface of the sternum.

A similar band, the *posterior sterno-clavicular* ligament, extends over the back of the joint, from the back of the clavicle to the back of the sternum.

The clavicles are connected by the *inter-clavicular ligament.* It extends transversely above the notch of the sternum, and has a broad attachment to the upper border of each clavicle. Between the clavicles it is more or less attached to the sternum, so that it forms a curve with the concavity upwards.

The three ligaments just described are so closely connected, that, collectively, they form a complete fibrous capsule of great strength for the joint.

A ligament, called the *costo-clavicular* or *rhomboid*, connects the clavicle to the cartilage of the first rib. It ascends from the cartilage of the rib to a rough surface beneath the sternal end of the clavicle. Its use is to limit the elevation of the clavicle. There is such constant movement between the clavicle and the cartilage of the first rib, that a well-marked *bursa* is commonly found between them.

Interarticular fibro-cartilage.—To see this, cut through the rhomboid, the anterior and posterior ligaments of the joint, and raise the clavicle. It is nearly circular in form, and thicker at the circumference than the centre, in which there is sometimes a perforation. Inferiorly, it is attached to the cartilage of the first rib, close to the sternum; superiorly, to the upper part of the clavicle and the inter-clavicular ligament. Its circumference is inseparably connected with the fibrous capsule of the joint.

The joint is provided with two synovial membranes: one between the articular surface of the sternum and the inner surface of the fibro-cartilage; the other, between the articular surface of the clavicle and the outer surface of the fibro-cartilage.

This interarticular fibro-cartilage is a structure highly elastic, without admitting of any stretching. It equalises pressure, prevents shocks, and also acts as a ligament, preventing the clavicle from being driven inwards towards the mesial line.

Observe the relative form of the cartilaginous surfaces of the bones: that of the sternum is slightly concave in the transverse, and convex in the antero-posterior direction; that of the clavicle is the reverse.

The form of the articular surfaces and the ligaments of a joint being known, it is easy to understand the movements of which it is capable. The clavicle can move upon the sternum in a direction either vertical or horizontal: thus it admits of circumduction. These movements, though limited at the sternum, are considerable at the apex of the shoulder.

CONNEXION OF THE CLAVICLE WITH THE SCAPULA. The outer end of the clavicle articulates with the acromion, and is connected by strong ligaments to the coracoid process of the scapula.

Joint between the acromion and the clavicle.—The clavicle and the acromion articulate with each other by two flat oval cartilaginous surfaces, of which the planes slant inwards, and the greater diameters are in the antero-posterior direction.

The *superior ligament*, a broad band of ligamentous fibres, strengthened by the aponeurosis of the trapezius, extends from the upper surface of the acromion to the upper surface of the clavicle.

The *inferior ligament*, of less strength, extends along the under surface of the joint from bone to bone.

An *interarticular fibro-cartilage* is sometimes found in this joint: but it is incomplete, and seldom extends lower than the upper half. There is only one synovial membrane.

Coraco-clavicular ligament.—The clavicle is connected to the coracoid process of the scapula by two strong ligaments—the *conoid* and *trapezoid*, which, being continuous with each other, might fairly be considered as one. The *trapezoid* ligament is the more anterior and external. It arises from the back part of the coracoid process, and ascends obliquely outwards to the clavicle, near its outer end. The *conoid* ligament is fixed at its apex to the root of the coracoid process, ascends vertically, and is attached by its base to the clavicle, near the posterior border. When the clavicle is fractured in the line of the attachment of the coraco-clavicular ligament, there is no displacement of the fractured ends; these being kept in place by the ligament.

Ligaments proper to the scapula.—There are two: the *coracoid* ligament, attached to the margins of the supra-scapular notch; and the *coraco-acromial* or *triangular* ligament, attached by its apex to the acromion, and by its base to the outer border of the coracoid process. It is separated from the upper part of the capsule of the shoulder-joint by a large *bursa.*

The articular surface of the head of the humerus,
forming rather more than one-third of a sphere, moves
upon the shallow glenoid cavity of the scapula, which
is of an oval form, with the broader end downwards, and the long
diameter nearly vertical. The security of the joint depends, not
upon any mechanical contrivance of the bones, but upon the great
strength and number of the tendons which surround it.

To admit the free motion of the head of the humerus upon the
glenoid cavity, it is requisite that the *capsular ligament* of the
joint be loose and capacious. Accordingly, the head of the bone,
when detached from its muscular connections, may be separated
from the glenoid cavity to the extent of an inch, or more, without
laceration of the capsule. This explains the elongation of the arm
observed in some cases in which effusion takes place into the joint;
also in cases of paralysis of the deltoid.

The *capsular ligament* is attached above, round the circumference of the glenoid cavity; and below, round the anatomical
neck of the humerus. It is strengthened on its upper and posterior part by the tendons of the supra-spinatus, infra-spinatus,
and teres minor; its inner part is strengthened by the broad tendon
of the subscapularis, its lower part by the long head of the triceps.

Thus the circumference of the capsule is surrounded by tendons
on every side, excepting a small space towards the axilla. If the
humerus be raised, it will be found that the head of the bone rests
upon this unprotected portion of the capsule between the tendons
of the subscapularis and the long head of the triceps : through this
part of the capsule the head of the bone usually protrudes in dislocations into the axilla.

At the upper and inner side of the joint, a small opening (*foramen ovale*) is observable in the capsular ligament, through which
the tendon of the subscapularis passes, and comes in contact with
the synovial membrane.

The upper surface of the capsule is strengthened by a strong
band of ligamentous fibres, called the *coraco-humeral* or *accessory
ligament*. It is attached to the root of the coracoid process,
expands over the upper surface of the capsule, with which it is

inseparably united, and is fixed into the greater tuberosity of the humerus.

Open the capsule to see the tendon of the long head of the biceps. It enters the joint through the groove between the two tuberosities, becomes slightly flattened, and passes over the head of the bone to be attached to the upper border of the glenoid cavity. It is loose and movable within the joint; and it acts like a strap, keeping down the head of the bone.

The tendon of the biceps does not perforate the synovial membrane of the joint. It is inclosed in a tubular sheath, which is reflected over it at its attachment to the glenoid cavity, and accompanies it for two inches down the groove of the humerus. During the earlier part of fœtal life it is connected to the capsule by a fold of synovial membrane, which subsequently disappears.

The margin of the glenoid cavity of the scapula is surrounded by a fibro-cartilaginous band of considerable thickness, called the *glenoid ligament*. This not only enlarges but deepens the cavity. Superiorly, it is continuous on either side with the tendon of the biceps; inferiorly, with the tendon of the triceps: in the rest of its circumference it is attached to the edge of the cavity.

The cartilage covering the head of the humerus is thicker at the centre than at the circumference. The reverse is the case in the glenoid cavity.

The *synovial membrane* lining the under surface of the capsule is reflected around the tendon of the biceps, and passes with it in the form of a cul-de-sac, down the bicipital groove. On the inner side of the joint it always communicates with the bursa beneath the tendon of the subscapularis.

The shoulder-joint has a more extensive range of motion than any other joint in the body; it is, in fact, a universal joint. It is capable of motion forwards and backwards; of adduction, abduction, circumduction, and rotation.

Elbow-joint.   The elbow-joint is a perfect hinge. The larger sigmoid cavity of the ulna is adapted to the trochlea upon the lower end of the humerus, admitting of simple flexion and extension; while the shallow excavation upon the head of the radius admits not only of flexion and extension, but of rotation upon the rounded articular eminence (*capitellum*) of the humerus. The joint is secured by two strong lateral ligaments. No ligament is attached to the head of the radius, otherwise its rotatory movement would be impeded. It is simply surrounded by a ligamentous collar, called the annular ligament, within which it freely rolls.

Internal lateral ligament.—This is triangular. Its apex is attached to the internal condyle of the humerus: from this point the fibres radiate, and are inserted into the greater sigmoid cavity of the ulna.

A transverse band of ligamentous fibres extends from the olecranon to the coronoid process across a notch observable on the inner side of the sigmoid cavity: through this notch vessels pass into the joint.

External lateral ligament.—This is attached to the external

Fig. 56.

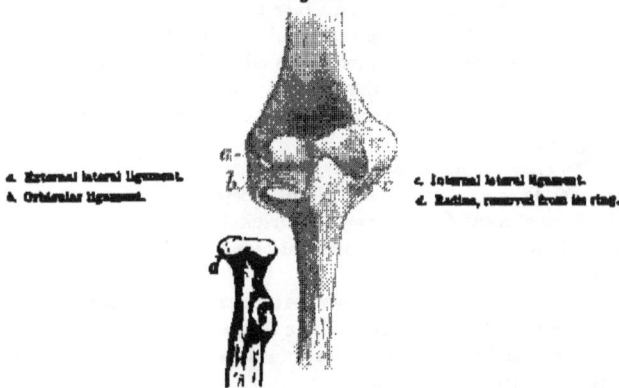

a. External lateral ligament.
b. Orbicular ligament.

c. Internal lateral ligament.
d. Radius, removed from its ring.

LIGAMENTS OF THE ELBOW.

condyle of the humerus; the fibres spread out as they descend, and are interwoven with the annular ligament, surrounding the head of the radius.

The *anterior* and *posterior* ligaments of the elbow-joint consist merely of a few thin ligamentous fibres spread over the capsule of the joint in front and behind. There is no need of ligaments to limit flexion and extension in this joint : for the coronoid process limits the one ; the olecranon the other.

The preceding ligaments, collectively, form a continuous capsule for the joint.

The orbicular or *annular ligament of the radius* (fig. 56) is attached to the anterior and the posterior border of the lesser sigmoid cavity of the ulna. With this cavity, it forms a complete collar, which encircles the head and part of the neck of the radius. The lower part of the collar is narrower than the upper, in order to clasp the neck of the radius, and maintain it more accurately in position.

Synovial membrane of the elbow-joint.—Open the joint by a transverse incision in front, and observe the relative adaptation of the cartilaginous surfaces of the bones. The synovial membrane lines the interior of the capsule, and forms a cul-de-sac between the head of the radius and its orbicular ligament. It is widest and loosest under the tendon of the triceps. Where the membrane is reflected from the bones upon the ligaments, there is more or less adipose tissue, particularly in the fossæ on the front and back part of the lower end of the humerus.

Interosseous ligament or membrane. This is an aponeurotic septum, stretched between the bones of the forearm, of which the chief purpose is to afford an increase of surface for the attachment of muscles. The septum is deficient above, to permit free rotation of the radius. Its fibres extend obliquely downwards from the radius to the ulna. It is perforated in its lower third by the anterior interosseous vessels.

The name of *round* or *oblique ligament* is given to a thin band of ligamentous fibres, which extends obliquely between the bones of the forearm in a direction contrary to those of the interosseous membrane. It is attached, superiorly, to the front surface of the ulna, near the outer side of the coronoid process; inferiorly, to the radius immediately below the tubercle. Between this ligament and the upper border of the interosseous membrane is a triangular interval through which the posterior interosseous artery passes to reach the back of the forearm. A *bursa* intervenes between the oblique ligament and the insertion of the tendon of the biceps. The use of this ligament is to limit supination of the radius.

RADIO-CAR-PAL OR WRIST JOINT. This joint is formed by the lower end of the radius, which articulates with the scaphoid and semilunar bones of the carpus: the lower end of the ulna is excluded from the joint by a triangular fibro-cartilage, which articulates with a small portion of the cuneiform bone. The joint is secured by an anterior, a posterior, and two lateral ligaments, forming, together, an uninterrupted capsule around it.

The *external lateral ligament* extends from the styloid process of the radius, to the scaphoid bone and the anterior annular ligament (p. 302).

The *internal lateral ligament* proceeds from the extremity of the styloid process of the ulna, to the cuneiform bone. Some of its fibres are attached to the pisiform bone, and the anterior annular ligament.

The *anterior ligament* consists of two or more broad bands of ligamentous fibres, which extend from the lower end of the radius, to the first row of carpal bones.

The *posterior ligament*, weaker than the preceding, proceeds from the posterior surface of the lower end of the radius, and is attached to the posterior surfaces of the first row of carpal bones.

The *synovial membrane* lines the under aspect of the triangular fibro-cartilage at the end of the ulna, is reflected over the several ligaments of the joint, and thence upon the first row of the carpal bones.

JOINT BE-TWEEN THE LOWER ENDS OF THE RA-DIUS AND ULNA. The inner surface of the lower end of the radius presents a slight concavity, which rotates upon the convex head of the ulna: this mechanism is essential to the pronation and supination of the hand. These corresponding surfaces are crusted with a thin layer of cartilage, and are provided with a very loose synovial membrane. The joint is strengthened in front and behind by a thin transverse

ligament, which extends from the anterior and posterior borders
of the sigmoid cavity of the radius, to the anterior and posterior
surfaces of the styloid process of the ulna. But the principal
uniting medium between the bones is a strong fibro-cartilage.

Fibro-cartilage between the radius and ulna.—Saw through
the bones of the forearm, and separate them by cutting through
the interosseous membrane, and opening the synovial membrane
of the joint between the lower ends. Thus a good view is ob-

Fig. 57.

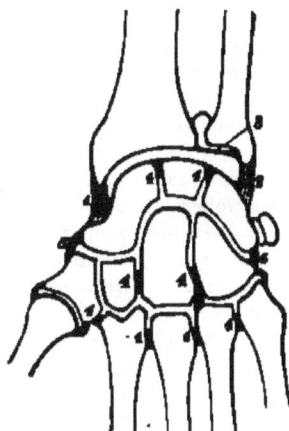

1. External lateral ligament.
7. Internal lateral ligament.
8. Interarticular fibro-car-
    tilage.

4. Interosseous liga-
    ments.

5. Lateral ligaments of
    the intercarpal joint.

DIAGRAM OF THE WRIST-JOINT.

tained of the fibro-cartilage which connects them (fig. 57). It is
triangular, and placed transversely at the lower end of the
ulna, filling up the interval caused by the greater length of the
radius. Its base is attached to the lower end of the radius, and
its apex to the root of the styloid process of the ulna. It is thin
at the base and the centre, thicker at the apex and the sides. Its
upper surface is in contact with the ulna, and covered by the
synovial membrane of the radio-ulnar joint; its lower surface,

forming a part of the wrist-joint, corresponds to the cuneiform bone. Its borders are connected with the anterior and posterior ligaments of the wrist. In some instances there is an aperture in the centre.

When, from accident or disease, this fibro-cartilage gets detached from the radius, the consequence is a preternatural projection of the lower end of the ulna.

The *synovial membrane* of this joint is distinct from that of the wrist, except in the case of a perforation through the fibro-cartilage. On account of its great looseness, necessary for the free rotation of the radius, it is called ' *membrana sacciformis.*'

Connection of the carpal bones with each other. The bones of the carpus are arranged in two rows, an upper and a lower, adapted to each other, so as to form between them a joint, connected by anterior, posterior, internal, and external lateral ligaments.

The bones, constituting each row, are united by ligaments placed on their palmar and dorsal surfaces, and by others, placed between the bones, and hence called interosseous. Their contiguous surfaces (those of the pisiform and cuneiform excepted) are covered by the reflections of one synovial membrane.

The *upper row* is united by *transverse* ligaments proceeding from the scaphoid to the semilunar bone, and from the semilunar to the cuneiform, both on their dorsal and palmar surfaces: also by *interosseous* ligaments, proceeding from the semilunar to the bones on either side of it (fig. 57).

The *pisiform bone* is articulated to the palmar surface of the cuneiform bone, to which it is united by a fibrous capsule. Inferiorly it is attached by two strong ligaments, the one to the unciform bone, the other to the carpal end of the fifth metacarpal bone. This articulation has a distinct synovial membrane.

The *lower row* of carpal bones is connected in the same way as the upper. The dorsal and palmar ligaments pass transversely from one to the other. There are only two interosseous ligaments, one on either side of the os magnum; they are thicker and stronger than those of the upper row, and unite the bones more firmly together (fig. 57).

INTERCARPAL JOINT.

The upper row of carpal bones is arranged in the form of an arch, so as to receive the corresponding convex surfaces of the os magnum and unciforme. Externally to the os magnum, the trapezium and trapezoid bones present a slightly concave surface, which articulates with the scaphoid. In this way a joint capable of flexion and extension only is formed between the upper and lower row. It is secured by anterior, posterior, and two lateral ligaments. The anterior ligament consists of strong ligamentous fibres, which pass obliquely from the bones of the upper to those of the lower row. The posterior ligament consists of oblique and transverse fibres, which connect the dorsal surfaces of the bones of the upper with the lower row.

The lateral ligaments connect, externally, the scaphoid and trapezium; internally, the cuneiform and unciform bones (fig. 57).

Divide the ligaments, to see the manner in which the carpal bones articulate with each other. Their surfaces are crusted with cartilage, and have a common *synovial membrane.* This membrane extends, superiorly, between the three bones of the upper row, so as to form two culs-de-sac; inferiorly, it is prolonged into the joint between the carpal and the second and third metacarpal bones.

JOINT BETWEEN TRAPEZIUM AND THE FIRST METACARPAL BONE.

The trapezium presents a cartilaginous surface, convex in the transverse, and concave in the anterior posterior direction (i.e. saddle-shaped), which articulates with a cartilaginous surface on the metacarpal bone of the thumb, concave and convex in the opposite directions. This peculiar adaptation of the two surfaces permits the several movements of the thumb, viz., flexion, extension, abduction and adduction; consequently circumduction. Thus we are enabled to oppose the thumb to all the fingers. The joint is surrounded by a fibrous capsule sufficiently loose to admit free motion, and stronger on the dorsal than on the palmar aspect. The security of the joint is increased by the muscles which surround it. It has a separate synovial membrane.

CARPO-
METACARPAL the second row of the carpal bones by ligaments upon
JOINTS. their *palmar* and *dorsal* surfaces.

           The metacarpal bones of the fingers are connected to

The *dorsal* ligaments are the stronger. The metacarpal bone
of the fore-finger has two ; one from the trapezium, another from
the trapezoid bone. That of the middle finger has also two, proceeding from the os magnum, and the os trapezoides. That of the
ring finger has also two, proceeding from the os magnum, and the
unciform bone. That of the little finger has one only, from the
unciform bone.

The *palmar* ligaments are arranged nearly upon a similar plan.
The metacarpal bone of the fore-finger has one, from the trapezoid
bone. That of the middle finger has three, proceeding from the
trapezium, the os magnum, and the unciform bone. Those of the
ring and little fingers have each one, from the unciform bone.

Besides the preceding ligaments, there is another of considerable
strength, called the *interosseous*. It proceeds from the adjacent sides
of the os magnum and the os unciforme, descends vertically, and
is fixed into the radial side of the metacarpal bone of the ring
finger (fig. 57). This ligament isolates the synovial membrane of
the two inner metacarpal bones from the common synovial membrane of the carpus.

Separate the metacarpal bones from the carpus, and observe the
relative form of their contiguous surfaces. The metacarpal bones
of the fore and middle fingers are adapted to the carpus in such
an angular manner as to be almost immovable. The metacarpal
bone of the ring finger, having a plane articular surface with the
unciform bone, admits of more motion. But still greater motion
is permitted between the unciform and the metacarpal bone of
the little finger; the articular surfaces of each being slightly concave and convex in opposite directions. The greater freedom of
motion of the metacarpal bone of the little finger is essential to
the expansion and contraction of the palm.

The *carpal extremities of the metacarpal bones of the fingers*
are connected with each other by transverse ligaments, both on
their dorsal and their palmar surfaces. They are also connected

by interosseous ligaments, which extend between the bones, immediately below their contiguous cartilaginous surfaces.

The *digital extremities* of these bones are loosely connected on their palmar aspect by the transverse metacarpal ligament.

SYNOVIAL MEMBRANES OF THE WRIST.

There are six distinct synovial membranes, proper to the lower end of the radius, and the several bones of the carpus: see the diagram (p. 302).

a. One between the lower end of the radius and the ulna.

b. One between the radius and the first row of carpal bones.

c. One between the trapezium and the metacarpal bone of the thumb.

d. One between the cuneiform and pisiform bones.

e. One between the first and second rows of carpal bones (the intercarpal joint). This extends to the metacarpal bones of the fore and middle fingers.

f. One between the unciform bone and the metacarpal bones of the little and ring fingers.

FIRST JOINT OF THE FINGERS.

The first phalanx of the finger presents a shallow oval cavity, crusted with cartilage, with the broad diameter in the transverse direction, to articulate with the round cartilaginous head of the metacarpal bone, of which the articular surface is elongated in the antero-posterior direction, and of greater extent on its palmar than its dorsal aspect. This formation of parts permits flexion of the finger to a greater degree than extension; and also a slight lateral movement.

Each joint is provided with two strong *lateral*, and a *palmar* or *glenoid* ligament.

The *lateral* ligaments arise from the tubercles on either side of each metacarpal bone, and inclining slightly forward, are inserted into the sides of the base of the first phalanx of the finger.

The *palmar* or *glenoid* ligament. This is a thick, compact, fibro-cartilaginous structure, which extends over the palmar surface of the joint. Its lower end is firmly attached to the base of the first phalanx of the finger; its upper end is loosely adherent to the rough surface above the head of the metacarpal bone. On either side it is inseparably connected with the lateral ligaments, so that with them it forms a strong capsule over the front and sides of the joint. Its superficial surface is slightly grooved, to receive the flexor tendons; its deep surface is adapted to cover the head of the metacarpal bone. Two sesamoid bones are found in the glenoid ligament belonging to the joint between the metacarpal bone and the first phalanx of the thumb.

The glenoid ligaments have a surgical importance for the following reason :—In dislocation of the fingers, the facility of reduction mainly depends upon the extent to which the glenoid ligament is injured. If it be much torn there is but little difficulty : if entire, the reduction is tedious and sometimes impracticable.

These joints are secured on their dorsal aspect by the extensor tendon, and the expansion proceeding from it on either side. Their synovial membranes are loose, especially beneath the extensor tendons.

SECOND AND LAST JOINT OF THE FINGERS.
The corresponding articular surfaces of the phalanges of the fingers and thumb are so shaped as to form a hinge-joint, and, therefore, incapable of lateral movement. The ligaments connecting them are similar in every respect to those between the metacarpal bones and the first phalanges. The glenoid ligament of the last joint of the thumb generally contains a sesamoid bone.

DISSECTION OF THE ABDOMEN.

Arbitrary division into regions. We divide the abdomen into arbitrary regions, that the situation of the viscera contained in it may be more easily described. For this purpose we draw the following imaginary lines: one horizontal across the abdomen on a level with the cartilages of the ninth ribs; another on a level with the anterior spines of the ilia. These lines form the boundaries

Fig. 58.

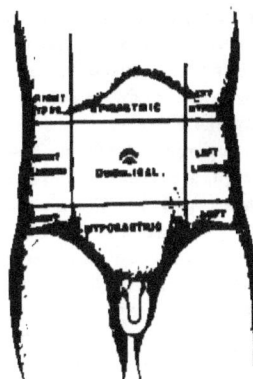

of three spaces, each of which is subdivided into three regions by a vertical line drawn on each side from the cartilage of the eighth rib to the middle of Poupart's ligament. Thus, we have a central and two lateral regions in each space. The central region of the upper space is termed the *epigastric* or *scrobiculus cordis*, the central one of the middle space is called the *umbilical* region, and the central of the inferior space, the hypogastric region. The lateral regions of the spaces from above downwards are termed the right and left hypochondriac, the right and left lumbar, and the right and left inguinal or iliac regions, respectively.

The abdomen should be distended with air, by means of a blowpipe inserted into the abdominal cavity at the umbilicus.

An incision should be made from the sternum to the pubes, another from the anterior spine of the ilium to a point midway between the umbilicus and pubes, and a third from the ensiform cartilage, transversely outwards towards the axilla as far as the angles of the ribs. The skin should then be dissected from the subjacent adipose and areolar tissue, called the 'superficial fascia.'

Superficial fascia.
The subcutaneous tissue of the abdomen presents the same general characters as that of other parts, and varies in thickness in different individuals. At the lower part of the abdomen, it admits of separation into two layers, between which are found the subcutaneous blood vessels, the absorbent glands, the ilio-inguinal nerve, and the hypogastric branch of the ilio-hypogastric nerve.

Respecting the superficial layer, observe that it contains the fat, and is continuous with the superficial fascia of the thigh, the scrotum, and the perineum. The deeper layer is intimately connected with Poupart's ligament and the linea alba; but it is very loosely continued over the spermatic cord and the scrotum, and becomes identified with the deep layer of the superficial fascia of the perineum. These points deserve attention, since they explain how urine, extravasated into the perineum and scrotum, readily makes its way over the spermatic cord on to the surface of the abdomen; but from this it cannot travel down the thigh, on account of the connection of the fascia with Poupart's ligament.

Superficial blood-vessels and glands.
Between the layers of the superficial fascia on the groin and upper part of the thigh, are several absorbent glands and small blood vessels (fig. 59). The glands are named, according to their situation, inguinal and femoral. The inguinal, from three to four in number, are often small, and escape observation. They are of an oval form, with their long axis corresponding to the line of the crural arch (represented by the dark line in fig. 59). They receive the absorbents from the lower part of the wall of the abdomen, from the scrotum and penis, and are therefore generally affected in venereal disease. The lymphatics from the upper part of the abdominal parietes terminate in the lumbar glands.

The *superficial arteries* in the neighbourhood arise from the femoral. One, the *epigastric*, ascends over Poupart's ligament and ramifies over the lower part of the abdomen, inosculating with the deep epigastric artery; another, *the pudic*, crosses the spermatic cord, and is distributed to the skin of the penis and scrotum; a third, the *circumflexa ilii*, ramifies towards the spine of the ilium. These subcutaneous arteries, the pudic especially, often occasion a free hæmorrhage in the operation for strangulated hernia.

The corresponding *veins* join the saphena vein of the thigh. Under ordinary circumstances they do not appear in the living sub-

Fig. 59.

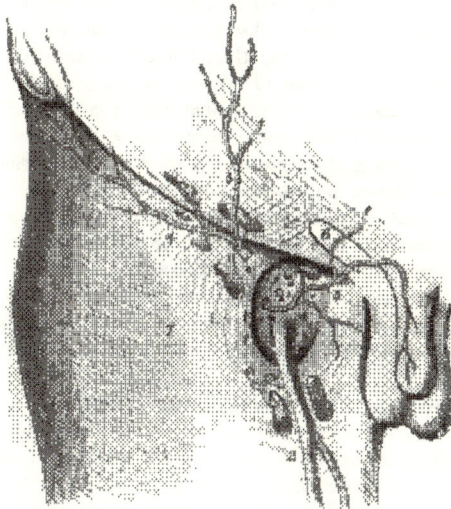

SUPERFICIAL VESSELS AND GLANDS OF THE GROIN.

1. Saphenous opening of the fascia lata.   5. Superficial pudic a.
2. Saphena vein.   6. External abdominal ring.
3. Superficial epigastric a.   7. Fascia lata of the thigh.
4. Superficial circumflexa ilii a.

ject; but, when any obstruction occurs in the inferior vena cava, they become enlarged and tortuous, and constitute the chief channels through which the blood would be returned from the lower limbs.*

* A cast, in illustration of this, is preserved in the Museum of St. Bartholomew's Hospital.

The skin of the abdomen is supplied with nerves after
the same plan as the chest; namely, by lateral and
anterior branches derived from the lower intercostal
nerves.

a. The *lateral cutaneous nerves* come out between the digitations of the external oblique muscle, in company with small arteries, and divide into anterior and posterior branches; the anterior supply the skin as far as the rectus; the posterior, the skin over the latissimus dorsi. Observe, that the lateral branch of the twelfth dorsal nerve is larger than the others, and that it passes over the crest of the ilium to the skin of the buttock. The corresponding branch of the first lumbar has a similar distribution.

b. The *anterior cutaneous nerves* come with small arteries through the sheath of the rectus. They are not only smaller than the lateral nerves, but their number and place of exit is less regular. That which comes through the external abdominal ring (*ilio-inguinal*), as well as that which comes through the wall of the abdomen just above it (the *hypogastric* branch of the *ilio-hypogastric*), are derived from the first lumbar nerve. These, however, are but repetitions of the others, and supply the skin of the groin and scrotum in the male, and the labium pudendi of the female.[*]

The deep layer of the superficial fascia should now be removed from the external oblique, by commencing at the fleshy portion of the muscle, and working in the course of its fibres. Care must be taken not to remove any of its aponeurosis, which is very thin. The digitations of this muscle with the serratus magnus and latissimus dorsi must also be made out.

Muscles of the abdominal wall.
The abdominal muscles, three on each side, are arranged in strata, named, after the direction of their fibres, the 'external oblique,' 'internal oblique,' and 'transversalis.' They terminate in front in strong aponeuroses, arranged so as to form a sheath for a broad muscle, called the

---

[*] A third small nerve, namely, the genital branch of the genito-crural, comes through the external ring. It lies behind the cord close to the outer pillar.

'rectus,' which extends perpendicularly on each side the linea alba
from the sternum to the pubes (fig. 60, p. 314).

External
oblique.

This muscle *arises* from the eight or nine lower ribs,
by as many pointed bundles, called '*digitations.*' The
upper five of these fit in with similar bundles of the
serratus magnus, and are obvious during life; the three lower correspond in like manner with the origin of the latissimus dorsi; but
they cannot be seen unless the body be turned on the side. The
upper part of this muscle descends obliquely forwards, and terminates on the aponeurosis of the abdomen; the lower proceeds
almost perpendicularly from the last ribs, and is *inserted* into the
outer lip of the anterior two-thirds of the crest of the ilium.[*]

The *aponeurosis* of the external oblique increases in strength,
breadth, and thickness, as it approaches the lower margin of the
abdomen, this being the situation where the greater pressure of
the viscera requires the most effective support. Its tendinous
fibres take the same direction as the muscle, and form the '*linea
alba,*' by their decussation in the middle line from the ensiform
cartilage to the pubes.

Poupart's
ligament or
crural arch.

Along the line of junction of the abdomen with the
thigh, the aponeurosis extends from the anterior spine
of the ilium to the spine of the pubes, and forms an
arch over the intermediate bony excavation (p. 317). This, which
is termed the *crural arch*, or, more commonly, *Poupart's ligament,*[†] transmits the great vessels of the thigh, with muscles and
nerves. Near the pubes is an opening in the aponeurosis for the
passage of the spermatic cord in the male, and the round ligament
in the female. It is called the '*external abdominal ring.*' Of
this, as well as of the crural arch, you must postpone the more
particular examination till the dissection of the parts concerned in
inguinal hernia. The external oblique should be carefully detached

---

[*] From its position and the direction of its fibres, it is manifest that the external
oblique represents, in the abdomen, the external intercostal muscles of the chest.

[†] This was first described by Fallopius, an Italian anatomist, in his 'Observationes
Anatomicæ,' published in 1561. It was subsequently described by Poupart in 1705,
in the 'Mem. de l'Acad. de Paris,' and is now commonly called 'Poupart's ligament.'

from the ribs and the crest of the ilium, and turned forwards as
far as this can be done without injuring its aponeurosis or the
crural arch. The second muscular stratum will thus be exposed,
and recognised by the difference in the direction of its fibres which
pass upwards and inwards.

Internal
oblique.
This muscle *arises* from the outer half of the crural
arch, from the anterior two-thirds of the middle lip of
the crest of the ilium, and from the fascia lumborum.
The fibres ascend obliquely, and are *inserted* partly into the
abdominal aponeurosis, partly into the cartilages of the three or
four lower ribs.*

The internal oblique should be detached from the ribs, and from
the crest of the ilium, and turned forwards ; but that portion of it
connected to the crural arch must not be disturbed. In removing
the internal oblique, we are apt to cut away the transversalis. To
avoid this mistake, dissect near the crest of the ilium, and endeavour
to find an artery which runs between the muscles, and nerves as a
guide. This artery, called the deep '*circumflexa ilii*,' proceeds
from the external iliac, and supplies the abdominal muscles. Beneath the internal oblique the continuations of the intercostal nerves
and vessels are brought into view. These must be preserved.

Transversalis.
This muscle *arises* from the outer third of the crural
arch, from the anterior two-thirds of the crest of the
ilium, from a fascia attached to the transverse processes of the
lumbar vertebræ, and, lastly, from the inner surfaces of the six or
seven lower costal cartilages, by digitations which correspond with
those of the diaphragm. From this origin the fibres proceed horizontally forwards, and terminate in the abdominal aponeurosis.
Some of its fibres arch downwards, and are attached conjointly with
fibres of the internal oblique into the pubes.

Rectus.
This muscle lies perpendicularly along the front of
the abdomen, and is enclosed in a sheath formed by the
aponeuroses of the lateral muscles of the abdomen. To expose it,
therefore, slit up its sheath along the middle, and reflect the two

* The internal oblique represents in the abdomen the internal intercostal muscles
of the chest.

halves. It *arises* by two tendons, the *inner* of which is attached to the symphysis, the *outer*, to the crest of the pubes. It is inserted into the fifth, sixth, and seventh costal cartilages. Notice the tendinous intersections across the muscle called '*lineæ transversæ*,' which are only incomplete repetitions of the ribs in the wall of the abdomen.* Their number varies from three to five, but there are always more above than below the umbilicus. These tendinous intersections adhere closely to the sheath in front, but not behind; consequently, matter formed between the front of the rectus and its sheath would be confined by two intersections; not so on the back of the muscle, for matter might travel down the entire length of it.

The sheath of the rectus is composed in front by the aponeurosis

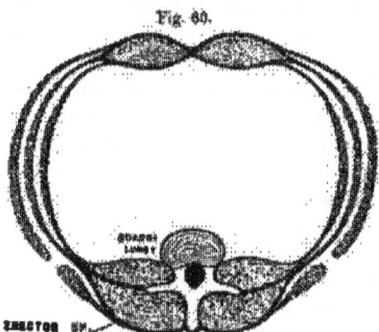

Fig. 60.

DIAGRAM OF A TRANSVERSE SECTION THROUGH THE ABDOMINAL MUSCLES.

of the external oblique, and half the thickness of that of the internal oblique; † while the back of the sheath comprises the aponeurosis of the transversalis, and the other half of the internal oblique (fig. 60). This, however, applies only to the upper three fourths of the muscle; the lower fourth has no sheath behind, for all the aponeuroses pass in front of it.

Pyramidalis. This small triangular muscle is situated near the pubes, close to the linea alba, and has a sheath of its own. It *arises* from the upper part of the pubes in front of the rectus, and terminates in the linea alba about midway between the

* Some animals—e.g. the crocodile—have bony abdominal ribs.
† The line where the internal oblique splits—namely, along the outer border of the rectus—is called the *linea semilunaris.*

pubes and the umbilicus. It is said to be of use in tightening the
linea alba, but it does not appear to have any special purpose
in the human subject, for it is sometimes deficient on one or even
both sides.

Linea alba. Along the middle line of the abdomen the several
aponeuroses decussate so as to form a white tendinous
line extending from the sternum to the pubes. This is the 'linea
alba:' it is but a continuation of the sternum deprived of its
earthy matter, in adaptation to the functions of this part of the
body. A little below the middle of it, is situated what was in the
foetus the opening for the passage of the umbilical vessels. After
birth, the vessels being no longer required, the opening gradually
closes, and becomes plugged by their fibrous remains.

Since the linea alba is the thinnest part of the abdomen, and is
free from blood vessels, it is chosen as a safe line for tapping in
dropsy, and for puncturing the bladder in retention of urine.

By dividing the rectus transversely near the umbilicus, and
raising it from its position, we have a complete view of the manner
in which the sheath is formed; we observe, too, that this is very
indistinct behind the lower fourth of the muscle. Ramifying in
the substance of the muscle is a large artery, called the 'epigastric,'
a branch of the external iliac; also the continuation of the internal
mammary, which descends from the subclavian.

Nerves of the These nerves are the continuations of the six lower
abdominal intercostal nerves, and of the first lumbar. They have
wall. the same general course and distribution. They run
forwards between the internal oblique and transversalis towards
the rectus. They furnish branches to the abdominal muscles,
and each gives off its lateral and anterior cutaneous branches,
described p. 311.

Action of the In consequence of their stratified arrangement, and
abdominal the different direction of their fibres, the abdominal
muscles. muscles answer many important purposes:—1. The
abdominal muscles maintain a gentle but effective pressure upon
the viscera, and serve to shield them from injury. The pressure is
proved by the fact that the bowels are almost sure to protrude

through a wound of the abdominal wall. The protection is proved
by the hard blow which the abdomen will stand provided its muscles
are on their guard; 2. They are the principal muscles concerned
in forcible expiration; 3. By compressing the viscera in conjunction
with the diaphragm, they are the chief agents in the expulsion of
the fæces and urine, also in vomiting, sneezing, laughing, coughing; 4. They act, each in its own way, as movers of the trunk;
e. g. the right external oblique, co-operating with the left internal
oblique, can draw the trunk towards the left side, and *vice versâ.*
The recti raise the body from the horizontal position, as any one
may ascertain by laying the hand on the abdomen while rising
from the ground.

EXAMINATION OF THE PARTS CONCERNED IN INGUINAL HERNIA.

General idea
of the sub-
ject.   Having proceeded so far in the examination of the
abdominal wall, now turn your attention to the anatomy
of the parts concerned in inguinal hernia.

The testicle, originally formed in the loins, passes, about the
eighth month of fœtal life, from the abdomen into the scrotum,
through an oblique canal in the wall of the abdomen, called the
'*inguinal canal.*' A portion of peritoneum is pouched out before
the testicle, and constitutes the tunica vaginalis testis. The blood
vessels, nerves, and excretory duct are drawn down after the
testicle and form the spermatic cord. The inguinal canal is
valvular and runs obliquely, so that the abdominal wall may the
better resist protrusion of the viscera.

The wall of the abdomen, as previously stated, is composed of
strata of different structures, and we shall presently find that the
spermatic cord, as it passes through each stratum, derives from
each a covering similar in structure to the stratum itself. Of these
strata there are three: the first—that is, the aponeurosis of the
external oblique—is called the ' aponeurotic stratum ;' the second—
that is, the internal oblique and transversalis muscles—is called the
' muscular stratum ;' the third—namely, the fascia transversalis,

which lines the under aspect of the transversalis muscle—is called the 'fascial stratum.' The most intelligible way of investigating the subject is to examine each stratum as it appears on dissection, and then to consider the inguinal canal as a whole. First, then, of the aponeurotic stratum.

Aponeurotic stratum, and external abdominal ring.   The lower border of the aponeurosis of the external oblique, extending from the spine of the ilium to the spine of the pubes, constitutes Poupart's ligament, or the crural arch. Above, and somewhat to the outer side of the spine of the pubes, is situated an opening in the aponeurosis called the '*external abdominal ring*,' which varies in size

Fig. 61.

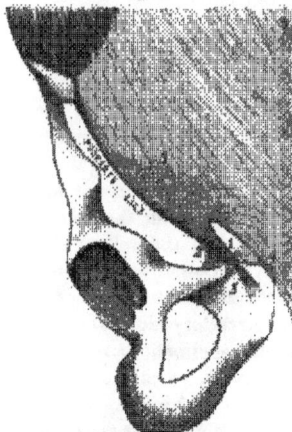

1. External abdominal ring.
2. Gimbernat's ligament.
3. Poupart's ligament, or outer pillar of the ring.

4. Internal pillar of the ring.
5. Position of the internal ring, in dotted outline.

DIAGRAM OF POUPART'S LIGAMENT, OF THE APONEUROSIS OF THE EXTERNAL OBLIQUE, AND OF THE EXTERNAL ABDOMINAL RING.

and shape in different individuals. In the male it is a triangular opening about an inch long, with its base towards the pubes, and will admit the passage of a finger. In the female it is smaller, and transmits the round ligament of the uterus. It is bounded above and below by the free margins of the aponeurosis, which are called its 'columns or pillars.' The inner or upper pillar is thin, and is attached to the front of the pubes, and decussates with its fellow of the opposite side in front of the symphysis. The outer pillar is thicker and stronger, and has three attachments; one to the spine of the pubes (Poupart's ligament), another for nearly an inch along the linea ilio-pectinea (Gimbernat's ligament), and a third (triangular ligament) consists of a few fibres which pass upwards and inwards beneath the inner pillar as far as the linea alba, where they are continuous with the aponeurosis of the opposite side. At the lower part of the aponeurosis of the external oblique, there are a number of arched fibres called ' intercolumnar bands,' which are strongest at its lowest part, above the external ring. Their purpose is to strengthen the opening and prevent the ring from enlarging.

Attached to the margin of the external ring is a thin fascia, the intercolumnar or spermatic fascia, which is prolonged over the spermatic cord, and forms a thin covering over it extending down into the scrotum. The spermatic cord in its passage through the ring rests upon the external pillar.

Muscular stratum and cremaster.   To examine the muscular stratum, the aponeurosis of the external oblique must be reflected. This is to be done by making a transverse incision through it, from the spine of the ilium to the linea alba and another at right angles to it, along the linea alba to the pubes. The triangular flap of aponeurosis is to be reflected and turned downwards, without injuring the external ring or the crural arch. The muscular stratum is now fairly exposed. This stratum consists of the combined fibres of the internal oblique and transverse muscles: these, so far as our present subject is concerned, may be considered as one, having the same origin, direction, and insertion. Their origin is from the outer half of the crural arch; their direction is transversely towards the mesial line, and they terminate upon a thin aponeurosis termed the 'conjoined tendon,' which is inserted into the upper part of the pubes and the linea alba (fig. 62). This tendon is situated immediately behind the external ring, for the purpose of strengthening the abdominal wall just at a part where, without such provision, the liability to hernia would have been very great.

From the middle of the crural arch, and from the lower part of the internal oblique, arises the 'cremaster muscle,' which is thin and pale, or the reverse, according to the condition of the subject. Its fibres descend in front of the cord, and then arch up again towards the pubes, forming a series of loops of different

Fig. 62.

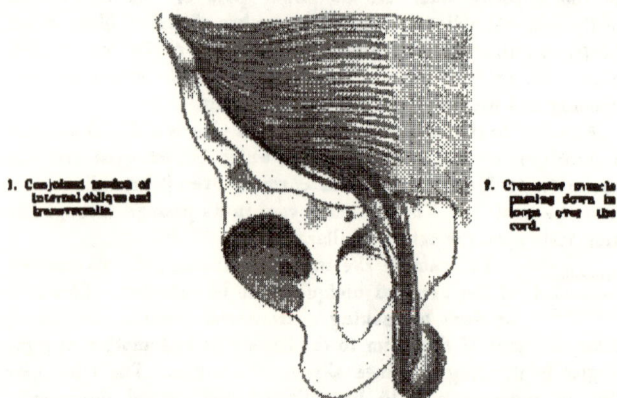

1. Conjoined tendon of internal oblique and transversalis.

2. Cremaster muscle passing down in loops over the cord.

DIAGRAM OF THE LOWER FIBRES OF THE INTERNAL OBLIQUE AND TRANSVERSALIS, WITH THE CREMASTER MUSCLE.

lengths; some, reaching only as low as the external ring, others lower still, whilst the lowest cover the tunica vaginalis of the testicle. Its nerve comes from the genital branch of the genito-crural, and its artery from the deep epigastric. The internal oblique and transversalis must now be reflected, by making incisions similar to those for the reflection of the aponeurosis of the external oblique: this must be done carefully, so as to disturb as

little as possible the transversalis fascia, which lies immediately
behind.

Fascial
stratum.
The third and last stratum is the fascia, which lies
behind the transversalis muscle. It is attached, below,
to the crural arch, thence ascends, and gradually
diminishing in thickness, is lost on the under surface of the
transversalis muscle. Its inner border is connected to the margin
of the rectus, to the lower margin of the conjoined tendon, and

Fig. 83.

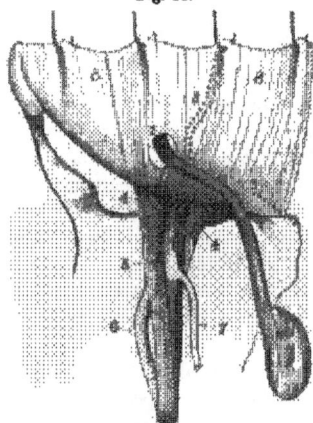

1. Internal abdominal
   ring.
2. Position of the ex-
   ternal abdominal
   ring, in dotted
   outline.
3. Epigastric a. in dot-
   ted outline.

4, 4. Sheath of the femo-
   ral vessels, con-
   tinued from the
   fascia transver-
   salis.
5. Femoral a.
6. Profunda a.
7. Saphena v.
8, 8. Fascia transver-
   salis.

DIAGRAM OF THE FASCIA TRANSVERSALIS SEEN FROM THE FRONT.

also to the pubes. This fascia is strongest just behind the external
ring, and but for it and the conjoined tendon, there would be a
direct opening into the cavity of the abdomen through the external
ring. The outer half of the fascia is very firmly connected to the
crural arch, and also to the fascia iliaca; but the inner half is
loosely connected with the crural arch, and passes down under it,
over the femoral vessels into the thigh, and forms what is called
' the sheath of the femoral vessels.'

Internal abdominal ring. The opening in the fascia transversalis through which the spermatic cord passes, is called the ' internal abdominal ring."[*] It corresponds to a point midway between the anterior superior spine of the ilium and the symphysis pubis, and about two-thirds of an inch above the crural arch. It is oval in shape, with the long diameter directed nearly vertically; its margin is well defined on the pubic side, but not on the iliac, and from its border is continued forwards a funnel-shaped prolongation over the cord as it passes through the opening. This covering, thin and delicate, is termed the ' *infundibuliform fascia.*' (This is not seen in the diagram.) Close by the inner border of the internal ring, the epigastric artery will be found ascending to enter the substance of the rectus.

To see that part of the peritoneum concerned in inguinal hernia, the fascia transversalis must be removed by incisions similar to those recommended before. The fascia is easily separable from the peritoneum, which is situated immediately behind it. The peritoneum at the inner ring presents a well-marked depression, which varies, however, considerably; in some being scarcely visible; in others, being continued downwards into the inguinal canal, in the form of a pouch. In some instances, a communication will be found still existing between the general cavity of the peritoneum and the tunica vaginalis testis.

Inguinal canal. Having examined the several strata through which the spermatic cord passes, replace them in their natural position, and examine the inguinal canal as a whole. You will perceive that its direction is obliquely downwards and inwards. Its length in a well-formed adult male is from one and a half to two inches. It is bounded in front by the aponeurosis of the external oblique; behind, by the fascia transversalis and the conjoined tendon of the internal oblique and transversalis; above, by the lower fleshy fibres of the internal oblique and transversalis; below by the crural arch

---

[*] Or the inner aperture of the inguinal canal.

Y

Course and relations of the epigastric artery. In a surgical point of view this is one of the most important arteries in the body. It arises from the external iliac, just before this vessel passes under the crural arch. It ascends inwards between the fascia transversalis and the peritoneum, forms a gentle curve round the inner side of the internal abdominal ring, and consequently on the inner side of the spermatic cord, and then enters the rectus muscle, in which it is gradually lost.

The artery is accompanied by two veins, of which the larger is constantly found on the inner side of it. They terminate by a single trunk in the iliac vein.

Branches of the epigastric. Of the branches of the epigastric artery the most important is the *'pubic.'* It runs inwards, behind the crural arch, towards the pubes, and derives its chief practical interest from the fact that it is liable to be wounded in dividing the stricture in femoral hernia.[*] But its size varies in different subjects, and is sometimes so small as to escape observation. The second branch is the *'cremasteric.'* It supplies the coverings of the cord, and chiefly the cremaster muscle. After giving off other unnamed muscular branches, the main trunk terminates in the rectus by minute inosculations with the internal mammary.

Such is an outline of the anatomy of the parts concerned in inguinal hernia. The description applies equally to the female, provided the round ligament be substituted for the spermatic cord. Of course the inguinal canal is proportionably smaller, and there is no cremaster.

Nomenclature of the several kinds of inguinal hernia. When a piece of intestine escapes through the inner ring, along the inguinal canal with the cord, and protrudes through the outer ring, it is called an *external*[†] or *oblique* inguinal hernia. If the intestine stop in the

---

[*] There is a preparation (No. 83, Ser. 17) in the Museum of St. Bartholomew's Hospital quite to the point. The patient had profuse haemorrhage, which commenced five hours after the operation. He died with peritonitis.

[†] A hernia is sometimes called external or internal, according to the relationship of the protrusion to the epigastric artery; thus, an oblique inguinal hernia which first protrudes through the inner ring is called an external hernia, and *vice versa*.

inguinal canal, it is called an incomplete inguinal hernia; such an one is generally of small size, and sometimes difficult of detection. Lastly, if a portion of intestine escape at once through the external ring, then it is called an *internal* or *direct* inguinal hernia.

Coverings of the different the cord. Beneath the skin, therefore, and the sub-hernia. cutaneous tissue there will be—

1. The spermatic fascia, derived from the aponeurosis of the external oblique.

2. The cremaster muscle, derived from the internal oblique and transversalis.

3. The infundibuliform fascia, derived from the fascia transversalis.

The incomplete inguinal hernia will be covered by—

1. The aponeurosis of the external oblique.
2. The cremaster.
3. The infundibuliform fascia.

The direct inguinal hernia will be covered by—

1. The spermatic fascia.
2. The fascia transversalis.*

In all cases, or at any rate with very few exceptions, the immediate investment of the intestine is the peritoneum. This constitutes the sac of the hernia. The opening of the sac, communicating with the abdomen, is called its mouth, then comes the neck, and, lastly, the body or expanded part of the sac.

Congenital There are two varieties of oblique inguinal hernia, and infantile termed the 'congenital' and the 'Infantile,' to which a hernia. passing allusion must be made. The *congenital* †

---

* What becomes, it may be asked, of the fibres of the conjoined tendon of the internal oblique and transversalis? They are either protruded before the peritoneum, or permit the hernia to slip between them.

† The term 'congenital' applied to this form of hernia is apt to suggest the idea that it occurs at birth. But this is not of necessity so. Although the state of parts favourable to its occurrence exists at birth, the hernia itself may not take place till many years afterwards; in fact, at any period of life.

Y 2

variety occurs when a protrusion of intestine takes place through
the narrow canal, which in some cases persists between the general
cavity of the peritoneum and the tunica vaginalis testis, in consequence of the non-obliteration of the original communication
between them. In this variety, the intestine surrounds the testicle, and the hernial sac is formed by the tunica vaginalis testis
(fig. 64). The *infantile* variety is rare, and occurs when the
original peritoneal canal alluded to, is only partially obliterated.
The result of which is, that the tunica vaginalis testis may reach
as high as the external or even the internal abdominal ring. Now
in this variety of hernia, the intestine protrudes a sac behind the
almormal extension of the tunica
vaginalis; so that, in front of
the hernia there are three layers
of peritoneum; namely, two
formed by the tunica vaginalis
testis, and one by the hernial
sac (fig. 64).

Fig. 64. *

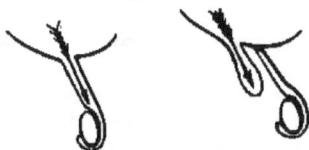

Position of
spermatic
cord in refer-
ence to the
hernia.

The spermatic cord is generally situated behind and
on the outer side of a hernial sac. In some cases, however, the hernia separates the constituents of the cord,
so that one or other of these may lie on the front of
the protrusion.

Seat of
stricture.

The stricture may be seated either at the external
ring, the internal ring, or at any intermediate part.
Sometimes there is a double stricture, one at the external ring, the other at the internal.

The stricture, however, may be caused by the mouth of the sac
itself, independently of the parts outside it; for the peritoneum
may become thickened and indurated, and sufficiently unyielding
to strangulate the protruded parts.

Direction in
which the
stricture
should be
divided.

We cannot do better than adhere to the golden rule
laid down by Sir A. Cooper; namely, to divide the
stricture, in all cases, directly upwards. In this direction, we are least likely to wound the epigastric artery.

* Fig. 64. The arrows denote the course of the hernia.

Changes produced by an old and large hernia. Whoever has the opportunity of dissecting an old hernia, of some size, will observe that the obliquity of the inguinal canal is destroyed. The constant dragging of the protruded viscera gradually brings the internal ring nearer to the external, so that at last the one gets quite behind the other, and there is a direct opening into the abdomen. But the position of the epigastric artery with regard to the sac remains unaltered. It is still on the inner side of the neck of the sac.

In hernia of long standing, all its coverings undergo a change. They become thickened and hypertrophied to such an extent, and so altered from what they once were, that they scarcely look like the same parts.

Expose the contents of the abdomen, by an incision from the ensiform cartilage to the pubes a little to the left side of the linea alba, so as to preserve a ligament, 'ligamentum teres,' which passes from the umbilicus to the liver, and also a cord, 'the urachus,' which ascends in the middle line from the bladder to the umbilicus; then make another incision transversely on a level with the umbilicus, and turn the flaps outwards.

Urachus. On the under surface of the lower right flap, the peritoneum is raised into a fold by a fibrous cord, passing from the bladder to the umbilicus; this is the '*urachus*,' which in fœtal life is a tube connecting the bladder with the allantois. On either side of the urachus are two other folds inclosing cords which ascend obliquely towards the umbilicus: these are the impervious remains of the umbilical arteries.

Take now a survey of the viscera before they are disturbed from their relative positions.

What is seen on opening the abdomen. In the right hypochondrium the liver is seen projecting more or less below the cartilages of the ribs, and the fundus of the gall-bladder below the edge of the liver, near the end of the ninth costal cartilage. In the left hypochondrium is seen more or less of the stomach. Across the umbilical region extends a broad fold of the peritoneum containing fat, the great omentum, which descends from the lower border of

the stomach to the pelvis, forming a curtain over the convolutions
of the small intestines. The breadth of this fold varies in different
instances, sometimes being so shrunk and crumpled as to be scarcely
visible. The lower part of the belly and part of the pelvis are
occupied by the small intestines. The urinary bladder is not
apparent, unless distended sufficiently to rise out of the pelvis.
In the right iliac fossa is the 'caput coli,' the commencement of
the large intestine; but the ascending part of the large intestine
in the right lumbar region, and the descending part of it in the
left, are not visible unless distended: they lie contracted at the
back of the abdomen. These are the viscera usually seen on
opening the abdomen; but a certain latitude is to be allowed, as
sometimes more of one organ is seen and less of another, according
as this or that is distended or hypertrophied. Much also depends
upon the amount of pressure which the ribs have undergone during
life.

Particular position of each viscus. The position of each viscus should now be examined
separately, and first that of the stomach.

The stomach. The stomach is irregularly conical in shape. Its
great end is situated in the left hypochondrium; its
narrow or pyloric end extends obliquely across the epigastrium into
the right hypochondrium, where it is overlapped by the liver.
The relative position and size of the stomach vary according to the
amount of distention; when much distended the anterior surface,
owing to the greater mobility of the great curve and the pyloric
end of the stomach, is turned upwards, and the lower border,
forwards.

Duodenum. The first part of the intestinal canal is termed 'intestinum duodenum,' because it is about twelve inches
long. Commencing at the pyloric end of the stomach (p. 338), the
duodenum ascends as high as the neck of the gall-bladder; then,
suddenly bending, it descends in front of the right kidney; lastly,
making another bend, it crosses the spine obliquely towards the
left side of the second lumbar vertebra: here the intestinum
'jejunum' begins, and this part of the canal may be seen by
raising the transverse colon. Thus then, the 'duodenum' describes

a kind of horse-shoe curve, of which the concavity is towards the left, and embraces the large end or head of the pancreas. For convenience of description, the duodenum is divided into an ascending, a descending, and a transverse portion. The first is completely surrounded by a peritoneal covering; the second and third are only covered by peritoneum in front, and are fixed to the back of the abdomen. The relative anatomy of the duodenum will be more fully seen hereafter.

Pursuing its course from the left side of the second *Jejunum and ileum.* lumbar vertebra, the intestinal canal forms a number of convolutions, which are loosely connected to the spine by a broad peritoneal fold termed the '*mesentery.*' Of these convolutions, the upper two-fifths constitute the '*intestinum jejunum;*' the lower three-fifths the '*intestinum ileum.*' This is an arbitrary division. There is no definite limit: the character of the bowel gradually changes—that is, it becomes less vascular, has fewer folds of the lining membrane, and its coats are therefore less substantial to the feel.

Commence-ment of large intestine. In the right iliac fossa, the small intestine opens into the left side of the colon, which is easily recognised by its sacculated appearance: here the large intestine begins: here is the ilio-cæcal valve (fig. 65). Immediately below the junction, the large intestine is expanded into a blind pouch, called the *cæcum* or *caput coli.* Into the back part of this pouch opens a little tube closed at the other end, called the '*appendix vermiformis.*' This tube is generally three inches long, about as thick as a tobacco-pipe, and is either coiled up behind the cæcum, or connected to it by a peritoneal fold, so as to hang loose in the pelvis. The commencement of the large intestine is generally confined by the peritoneum to the iliac fossa, in which it lies.* Tracing it from this point, it ascends through the right lumbar region in front of the right kidney; then, crossing the umbilical

* * But this is not invariably so. The bowel is, in some subjects, connected to the fossa by a fold of peritoneum or a '*meso-cæcum.*' I have often seen this fold sufficiently loose to allow the caput coli to travel over to the left iliac fossa.

region towards the left side,* it descends in front of the left
kidney † down the left lumbar region into the iliac fossa, where it
curves like the letter S. These successive portions of the large
intestine are termed, respectively, the ascending, transverse, descending, and sigmoid parts of its course. Lastly, the bowel enters
the pelvis on the left side of the sacrum, and here takes the name
of ' rectum.' This term, so far as concerns the human subject, is

Fig. 65.

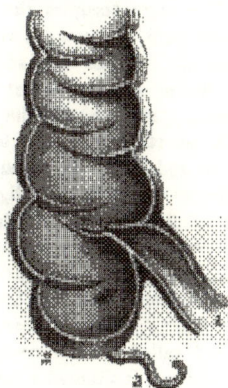

1. Ileum.
2. Cæcum or cæcal cæll.
3. Appendix vermiformis.

SECTION THROUGH THE JUNCTION OF THE LARGE AND SMALL INTESTINE TO SHOW THE
ILEO-CÆCAL VALVE.

misapplied ; the canal runs anything but a straight course through
the pelvis, for it curves so as to adapt itself to the sacrum.

Looking at the entire course of the colon, observe that it forms

* This transverse part of the colon, in some instances, makes a coil behind the
stomach to the diaphragm ; such a state of things, when the bowel happens to be distended, is apt to give rise to symptoms of diseased heart. See some observations in
point by Dr. Copland, in Lond. Med. Gaz. 1847. vol. v. p. 660.

† The contiguity of the ascending and descending colon to the right and left kidney
respectively, explains the occasional bursting of renal abscesses into the intestinal
canal.

an arch, of which the concavity embraces the convolutions of the small intestines.

Length of the alimentary canal.   The small intestines, including the duodenum, vary from sixteen to twenty-four feet in length, and the large intestines from five feet to five feet and a half; these measurements are subject to some variation according to the height of the individual. In round numbers, we may say that the small and large intestines are from five to six times the length of the body.

The liver.   The *liver* occupies the whole of the right hypochondrium, and extends over the epigastric region mor or less into the left. Unless the individual be very corpulent, we can ascertain during life the extent to which the liver projects below the costal cartilages, and the general dimensions of the organ may be tolerably well told by percussion. Its anterior border is sharp and thin; its posterior is broad and connected to the diaphragm by peritoneal ligaments. Its under surface overlays part of the stomach, of the duodenum, of the right kidney, of the transverse colon, and of the suprarenal capsule: its upper surface is convex, and accurately adapted to the arch of the diaphragm. To this muscle the liver is connected by folds of peritoneum, called 'ligaments.' One of these, nearly longitudinal in direction, and called the '*suspensory*,' or, from its shape, the '*falciform*' ligament, is situated a little to the right of the mesial line. The free edge of it in front contains the impervious remains of the umbilical vein, called the '*round*' ligament. The suspensory ligament, traced backwards, leads to another broad fold extending horizontally from the diaphragm to the posterior border of the liver; this constitutes the '*lateral*' ligament, right or left, according as we trace it on one or other side of the falciform ligament.

The junction of the lateral and falciform ligaments is described by some authors as the *coronary* ligament.

Gall-bladder.   The gall-bladder is the reservoir for the bile, and is closely confined by the peritoneum in a slight depression on the under surface of the liver. Its lower end or fundus

projects beneath the cartilage of the ninth rib. This is important
practically. It sometimes happens that the gall-bladder, in consequence of some obstruction to its duct, becomes unusually distended,
and occasions a swelling below the margin of the ribs, which might
be mistaken for an hepatic abscess.* The close proximity of the
gall-bladder to the duodenum and the transverse colon explains the
occasional evacuation of gall-stones by ulceration into the intestinal canal.†

The spleen.
  The spleen is deeply situated in the left hypochondrium, between the stomach and the ninth, tenth,
and eleventh ribs. Its outer surface is smooth and convex, to
correspond with the diaphragm and the ribs; its inner surface;
where its great vessels enter, is concave and connected to the
great end of the stomach by a peritoneal fold called the 'gastro-
splenic omentum.' Generally, too, the spleen is connected by a
small peritoneal fold, the suspensory ligament, to the under
aspect of the diaphragm.‡

Pancreas.
  This is the salivary gland of the abdomen. It lies
behind the stomach, transversely across the spine, about
the level of the first lumbar vertebra. Its right end or head is contained within the curve of the duodenum : its left end or tail
extends as far as the spleen. The further connections and relations
of the pancreas cannot in this stage of the dissection be satisfactorily seen.

Kidneys.
  The kidneys are situated in the lumbar region,
nearly opposite the two lower dorsal and the two upper
lumbar vertebræ; the right being a little lower than the left.
They lie imbedded in fat, partly upon the quadratus lumborum,
partly upon the psoas. In contact with the right kidney, we have
the liver, the second part of the duodenum, and the ascending
colon; in contact with the left, are the spleen, the end of the
pancreas, and the descending colon.

* See cases in point recorded by Andral, Clin. Méd. tom. iv.; and Graves, Dublin
Hospital Report, vol. iv.
† See preparations in the Museum, Ser. 16, No. 84.
‡ Every now and then we find in the gastro-splenic omentum one or more little
spleens in addition to the large one.

This body is situated at the top of the kidney. It
Renal capsule. lies upon the crus of the diaphragm. You will see
the right renal capsule by lifting up the liver; the left, by lifting
up the spleen, and the great end of the stomach.

A certain range of motion being necessary to the
Peritoneum. abdominal viscera, they are provided with a serous
membrane, called the 'peritoneum.' This membrane is, like other
serous membranes, a closed sac, one part of which lines the containing cavity, the other is reflected over the contained viscera.
These are respectively termed the *parietal* and the *visceral* layers.
In the female, however, it is not, strictly speaking, a closed sac,
since it communicates with the cavity of the uterus through the
Fallopian tubes. The internal surface of the peritoneum is smooth
and polished, and lined by squamous epithelium : the external
surface, the *subperitoneal tissue*, is composed of areolar tissue
which connects the internal layer to the invested viscus or
abdominal parietes. There is nothing between the parietal and
the visceral layers, in other words, inside the sac, but just sufficient
moisture to lubricate its smooth and polished surface. The viscera
are all, more or less, outside the sac; some lie altogether behind
it, as the pancreas, kidneys, and renal capsules; others, as the lower
parts of the duodenum, cæcum, ascending and descending colon,
are only partially covered by it; while others, as the stomach,
liver, jejunum, ileum, and some parts of the large intestine, are
completely invested by it : these latter push the visceral layer
before them, and so give rise to membranous folds ; the larger the
fold, the freer is the mobility of the viscus which occasions it.

Now trace the peritoneum as a continuous membrane.
Course of the Since the peritoneum is a perfect sac, it matters not
peritoneum. where we begin, for we must come back to the starting
point.

Supposing, then, a longitudinal section to be made through the
viscera in the middle of the body, one might trace the peritoneum
thus—beginning at the diaphragm, and taking, for brevity's sake,
two layers at a time (fig. 66).

From the diaphragm two layers of peritoneum proceed to the

liver, forming its lateral ligaments; they separate to inclose the
liver, meet again on its under aspect, and pass on, under the name
of the gastro-hepatic omentum, to the small curve of the stomach.
Separating here they embrace the stomach, and meeting again at
its greater curve, pass down as a
curtain over the small intestines
to form the great omentum. At
the lower margin of the great
omentum, they are reflected upwards (so that the great omentum
consists of four layers), to the front
of the colon, which they inclose,
and after joining again at the back
of the colon, proceed to the spine,
forming the transverse meso-colon.
At this situation the two layers diverge, the upper one ascends in
front of the pancreas, and the
crura of the diaphragm to its
under surface, at which point we
started.*

The lower layer is reflected from
the spine over the small intestines
back again to the spine, to form
the mesentery. From the root of
the mesentery it descends into
the pelvis, and invests the upper
two-thirds of the rectum. From
the rectum, in the male, it is reflected to the posterior part of the
bladder, forming the recto-vesical

Fig. 65 a.

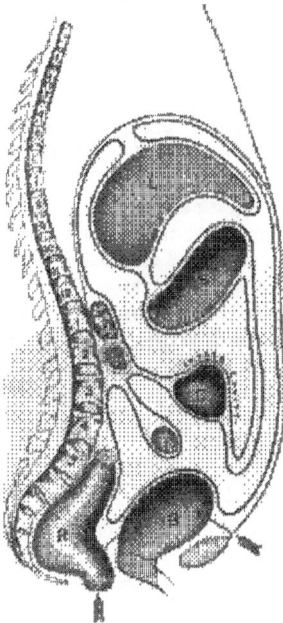

DIAGRAM OF THE PERITONEUM.

* In fœtal life, the ascending layers of the great omentum may be traced back to the
spine near the pancreas; and here the layers diverge from each other. The upper
layer ascends in front of the pancreas to the diaphragm; the lower layer proceeds over
the arch of the colon, and then back to the spine, thus forming the transverse meso-
colon. Its reflections afterwards are the same as in the adult. As the fœtus grows,
the great omentum becomes adherent to the arch of the colon.

pouch, and thence to the wall of the abdomen, along which we trace it up to the diaphragm. In the female, it is reflected from the rectum on to about one inch of the posterior wall of the vagina, constituting the recto-vaginal pouch, and thence over all the back, but only about half-way down the front of the uterus, to the posterior wall of the bladder; after which its reflections are the same as in the male.

Such is the course of the peritoneum as seen in a longitudinal section, but there are certain lateral reflections which cannot be seen except in a transverse section: thus, from the great end of the stomach, two layers proceed to the spleen, forming the gastro-splenic omentum; from the transverse meso-colon it is reflected on either side over the ascending and descending colon.

The following parts of the alimentary canal are only partially covered by peritoneum: the descending and transverse portions of the duodenum, the cæcum, the ascending and descending colon, (with exceptional cases) the lower part of the rectum.

Anatomists speak of the *lesser* cavity of the peritoneum as distinguished from the greater. This lesser cavity, or sac of the omentum, is situated behind the stomach and the descending layers of the great omentum. If air be blown through the foramen of Winslow (which is the constricted communication between the greater and lesser cavities of the peritoneum), we distend the lesser cavity; it is bounded, in front, by the lesser omentum, the stomach, and the descending layers of the great omentum: behind, by the ascending layers of the great omentum, the colon, and the transverse meso-colon; above, by the liver.

Foramen of Winslow. This foramen is the narrow circular opening between the greater and lesser cavities of the peritoneum, through which the two cavities communicate. It is situated behind the right edge of the gastro-hepatic, or lesser omentum. By passing your finger into it, you will find the foramen bounded *above* by the lobulus Spigelii of the liver, *below*, by the commencement of the duodenum, *in front* by the lesser omentum, and *behind* by the vena cava inferior.

The several folds, formed by the reflections of the peritoneum,

which connect the viscera either to each other or to the back of
the abdomen, have now to be examined.

Mesentery.   This is the fold which suspends the small intestines
from the back of the abdomen. To see it, raise the
great omentum and the transverse arch of the colon. Its attached
part or root extends from the left side of the second lumbar
vertebra obliquely across the spine to the right iliac fossa. The
loose part of the mesentery curves as it were like a ruffle, and
incloses the small intestines from the beginning of the jejunum to
the end of the ileum. Between its layers the mesenteric vessels,
nerves, glands. and lymphatics must be made out.

Transverse meso-colon.   This broad fold connects the transverse colon to the
back of the abdomen. It forms a sort of partition
dividing the abdomen into an upper compartment,
containing the stomach, liver, and spleen; and a lower, containing
the convolutions of the small intestines. As regards the cæcum,
the ascending and descending portions of the colon, they, as a
general rule, are bound down by the peritoneum in their respective
situations. It covers only two-thirds or thereabouts of their anterior surface; the rest is connected by loose cellular tissue to the
back of the abdomen.*

Great omentum.   This broad peritoneal fold is composed of four layers,
and proceeds from the lower border of the stomach,
like a curtain over the convolutions of the small intestines. Its thickness varies considerably, in thin subjects it is
often transparent, while in fat persons, on the other hand, it is
loaded with fat, and contributes in great measure to the size of the
abdomen. Its length also varies. In some bodies we find it extending far into the pelvis, in others, small and crumpled.

Gastro-hepatic or lesser omen-tum.   This fold passes from the transverse fissure on the
under surface of the liver to the upper aspect of the
stomach. It is composed of two layers; and between
them, we find the vessels and nerves going to, and the

---

* In some (rare) cases, the ascending and descending colon are *completely* surrounded by peritoneum, and connected to the lumbar regions, respectively, by a right
and left lumbar meso-colon.

duct coming from the liver. The right border of this reflected
fold is free, while the left passes on to the œsophagus. In this
fold the bile-duct lies to the right, the hepatic artery to the left,
and the vena portæ behind and between them. If the finger be
introduced behind the right border, it passes through the foramen
of Winslow into the lesser cavity of the peritoneum.

Gastro-splenic omentum. This fold proceeds from the great end of the stomach
to the spleen, and is continuous below with the great
omentum. It contains between its layers, the 'vasa

Fig. 66.

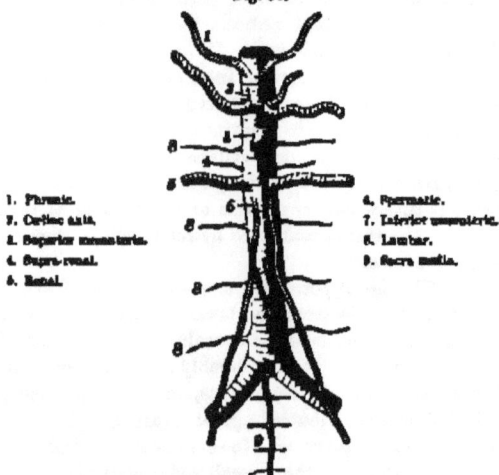

1. Phrenic.
2. Cœliac axis.
3. Superior mesenteric.
4. Supra-renal.
5. Renal.

6. Spermatic.
7. Inferior mesenteric.
8. Lumbar.
9. Sacra media.

BRANCHES OF THE ABDOMINAL AORTA.

brevia,' branches which proceed from the splenic artery to the
great end of the stomach.

Branches of the abdominal aorta. Our next object should be the examination of the
arteries which supply the viscera. The aorta enters
the abdomen between the pillars of the diaphragm,
and then descending a little to the left side of the front of the

spine, divides opposite the fourth lumbar vertebra into the two
common iliac arteries. In this course it gives off its branches in
the following order (fig. 66).

1. The *phrenic*, for the supply of the diaphragm.

2. The *cœliac axis*, a short thick trunk which immediately
subdivides into three branches for the supply of the stomach, the
liver, and the spleen.

3. The *superior mesenteric*, for the supply of all the small intestines and the upper half of the large.

4. 5. The *supra-renal* and the *renal* arteries.

6. The *spermatic*, for the testicles in the male, and the ovaries
in the female.

7. The *inferior mesenteric*, for the supply of the lower half of
the large intestine.

8. The *lumbar*, a series of branches, analogous to the intercostals,
for the supply of the back part of the abdomen.

9. The *arteria sacra media*, which is given off at the bifurcation of the aorta, and runs down in front of the sacrum.

These branches are to be traced throughout in the order most
convenient. Take the cœliac axis first. To dissect this artery and its
branches, the liver must be well raised, as in fig. 67, and a layer of
peritoneum removed from the gastro-hepatic omentum. There is
a close network of very tough tissue about all the visceral branches
of the aorta. This tissue consists almost entirely of plexuses of
nerves, derived from the sympathetic system. Of these plexuses,
the largest surrounds the cœliac axis like a ring. This is the solar
plexus, or more appropriately, the brain of the abdomen, and is
formed by the junction of the two semi-lunar ganglia (see dissection
of thorax, p. 126). From this, as from a root, other secondary
plexuses branch off, and surround the following arteries :—the
phrenic, coronary, hepatic, splenic, superior mesenteric, inferior
mesenteric, and renal : the plexus receiving the name of the arteries
around which they twine. It requires a very lean subject, and
great anatomical dexterity to trace them.

PLAN OF THE BRANCHES OF THE CÆLIAC AXIS.

	Coronaria ventriculi.		
Cæliac axis . .	Splenic	pancreatic branches. gastro-epiploica sinistra. vasa brevia to stomach.	
	Hepatic	pyloric. gastro-epiploica dextra. cystic.	pancreatico-duodenalis. omental.

Cæliac axis and its branches. The cœliac axis arises from the front of the aorta, between the pillars of the diaphragm, just above the upper border of the pancreas. It is a very thick, short trunk, which after a course of about half an inch divides into three branches—the coronaria ventriculi or gastric, the splenic, and the hepatic.

The *coronaria ventriculi*, the smallest of the three, ascends a little to the left towards the œsophageal end of the stomach, where it gives off branches to the œsophagus, which inosculate with the œsophageal offsets of the thoracic aorta. It then curves along the upper border of the stomach towards the pylorus, to anastomose with the pyloric branch of the hepatic artery.

The *hepatic* artery ascends to the right between the layers of the lesser omentum to the transverse fissure of the liver, where it divides into two branches, right and left, for the supply of the respective lobes of the liver.

In its course to the liver, it lies to the left of the bile duct, and in front of the portal vein; all three are contained in the right border of the lesser omentum. The hepatic gives off—

a. The *pyloric*, which runs along the upper curve of the stomach from right to left, and inosculates with the coronaria ventriculi.

b. The *gastro-epiploica dextra*, which runs behind the duodenum, then along the great curve of the stomach, from right to left, and inosculates directly with the gastro-epiploica sinistra, a branch of the splenic. It gives off: 1. The pancreatico duodenalis, which runs down between the head of the pancreas and the descending part of the duodenum. It supplies branches to each, and

z

inosculates frequently with a similarly named branch of the superior mesenteric artery. 2. Branches which descend to supply the great omentum.

Fig. 67.

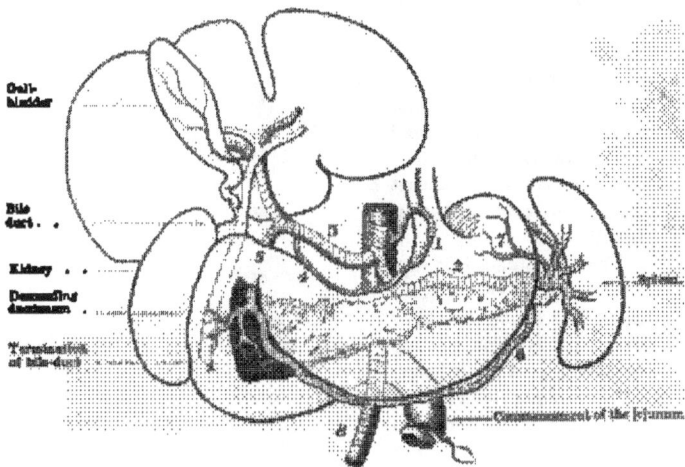

Gall-bladder

Bile duct . .

Kidney . .

Descending duodenum

Termination of bile-duct

Commencement of the jejunum.

DIAGRAM OF THE BRANCHES OF THE CŒLIAC AXIS.

(Pancreas in dotted outline behind the stomach.)

1. Coronaria ventriculi.	5. Gastro-epiploica dextra.
2. Splenic a.	6. Gastro-epiploica sinistra.
3. Hepatic a.	7. Vasa brevia.
4. Pyloric a.	8. Superior mesenteric a.

c. The *cystic*, commonly a branch of the right hepatic, ramifies on the under surface of the gall-bladder, supplying its coats.

The *splenic*, the largest of the three, proceeds tortuously towards the left side, along the upper border of the pancreas to the spleen, which it enters by numerous branches.

It gives off: 1. Several small branches to the pancreas, *pancreaticœ parvœ*. One, rather larger than the rest, which accompanies the pancreatic duct, is called *pancreatica magna*. 2. The *gastro-epiploica sinistra*, which runs to the right along the great curve of the stomach, and inosculates with the gastro-epiploica dextra. 3. *Vasa brevia*, which proceed between the layers of the *gastro-splenic* omentum, to the great end of the stomach, where they communicate with branches from the coronaria ventriculi.

Thus the stomach is supplied with blood by four channels, which by their inosculations form a main artery along its lesser curve, another along its greater; from these, numerous branches are furnished to both sides of the stomach. The artery of the greater curve also sends down numerous branches to the omentum, which form a beautiful network between its layers. The advantage of this free inosculation of arteries about the stomach must be apparent.

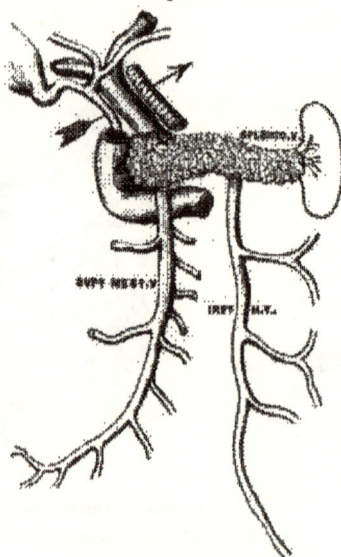

Fig. 68.

DIAGRAM OF THE VENA PORTÆ.
(The arrow is introduced behind the free border of the lesser omentum.)

Vena portæ: its peculiarities. The veins which return the blood from the abdominal portion of the alimentary canal, the pancreas, and the spleen, have this peculiarity, that they do not empty themselves into the vena cava, but all unite into one great vein, called the 'vena portæ,' which ramifies throughout the liver, and

z 2

secretes the bile. The trunk of the vena portæ itself is from three to four inches long. By tracing it downwards you find that it is formed behind the great end of the pancreas, by the confluence of the splenic and superior mesenteric veins (fig. 68). In its passage to the liver, the vena portæ is accompanied by the hepatic artery and the common bile-duct, lying behind and between them. Traced upwards you find that at the transverse fissure of the liver it divides into two branches corresponding to the two great lobes of the organ. The vein ramifies in the substance of the liver like an artery, and is inclosed with branches of the hepatic artery and duct in a sheath called ‘ *Glisson's capsule*.’ The vena portæ may, then, be compared to the stem of a tree, of which the roots arise in the digestive organs, and the branches spread out in the liver. After receiving the veins corresponding to the branches of the hepatic artery, the vena portæ returns its blood into the inferior vena cava through the venæ cavæ hepaticæ.

The veins which empty themselves into the vena portæ are also peculiar, in that they have no valves. Therefore, if any obstruction arise in the venous circulation through the liver, the roots of the portal vein are apt to become congested: this is a common cause of hæmorrhoids, diarrhœa, hæmorrhage from the bowels, and ascites. Leeches applied to the anus have been long recognised as beneficial in congestion of the liver.

Bile-duct.   The hepatic duct is composed of two trunks, one from the right lobe and the other from the left: it is soon joined by the cystic or the duct from the gall-bladder. The common duct, ‘ *ductus communis choledochus*,’ thus formed, passes along the right edge of the lesser omentum, then behind the first portion of the duodenum, and opens obliquely into the back part of the second portion (p. 338). This common duct is from three to four inches long, and, if distended, would be about the size of a small writing quill.

The great omentum, with the arch of the colon, must now be turned up over the chest, and the small intestines should be pushed towards the left side. Then, by removing a layer of peritoneum from the mesentery, we expose the mode in which the superior

mesenteric artery ramifies so as to supply the small intestines. In
making this dissection, the mesenteric glands immediately attract
notice. They lie in great numbers between the layers of the
mesentery, and vary considerably in size. The fine tubes, called
lacteal vessels, which traverse the glands, are too thin and trans-

Fig. 69.

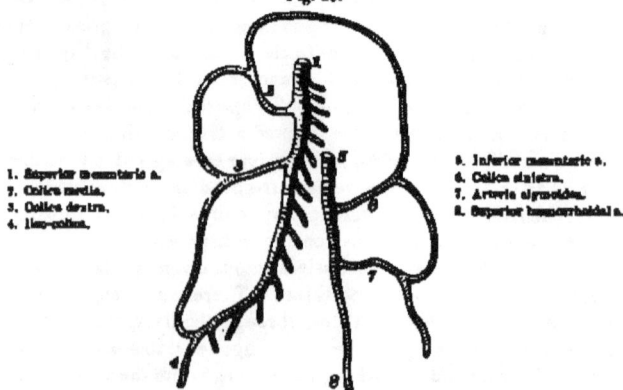

1. Superior mesenteric a.　　　　　　　　　　　5. Inferior mesenteric a.
7. Colica media.　　　　　　　　　　　　　　　6. Colica sinistra.
3. Colica dextra.　　　　　　　　　　　　　　　7. Arteria sigmoidea.
4. Ileo-colica.　　　　　　　　　　　　　　　　8. Superior hæmorrhoidal a.

PLAN OF THE MESENTERIC ARTERIES, AND THEIR COMMUNICATION.

parent to be seen under ordinary circumstances. But in cases
where sudden death has taken place during digestion, they are
found distended with chyle, and can be traced into the glands from
all parts of the small intestines.* After traversing the glands,
they all eventually empty their contents into the receptaculum
chyli (p. 122).

Superior
mesenteric
artery and
branches.

This large artery descends beneath the pancreas, over
the transverse part of the duodenum (p. 338), and then
runs between the layers of the mesentery towards the
right iliac fossa, where it terminates in branches for the

* The arrangement of the chyliferous vessels is extremely well displayed in the
beautiful plates of Mascagni.

supply of the cæcum. Thus its course describes a gentle curve
from left to right. It gives off the following branches: 1, the
pancreatico duodenal branch, given off close to its origin, runs up
to inosculate with a similar named branch of the hepatic artery;
2, branches to the small intestines from ten to sixteen in number
are given off from the left or convex side of the curve; while from
the concave side come, 3, the ileo-colic; 4, the right colic; and 5,
the middle colic arteries for the supply of the upper half of the
large intestines.

The student should now trace the branches to the small intestines, in order to see the beautiful series of arches which they form
by their mutual inosculations. There are three or four tiers of
them, each tier composed of smaller and more numerous branches
than the preceding. The ultimate branches ramify in circles
round the intestine. This circular arrangement of the vessels in
the coats of the bowel is practically interesting, because it enables
one in almost all cases to distinguish the intestine from the hernial
sac.

The *colic* branches of the superior mesenteric are the *ileo-colic*,
which is the continuation of the main trunk, and divides into two
branches; one supplies the lower part of the ileum, and the other
the cæcum:—the *right colic*, which proceeds towards the ascending
colon, and the *middle colic*, which ascends between the layers of the
meso-colon to the arch. They are arranged after the same plan as
those of the small intestines; that is, they inosculate so as to form
a series of arches which successively decrease in size and finally terminate in circles round the bowel.

The superior mesenteric vein joins the splenic behind the pancreas, and forms the vena portæ (p. 339).

Inferior me-
senteric artery
and branches.
 To trace this artery, the small intestines must be drawn
over towards the right side, and the peritoneum covering
the artery removed. It is given off about two inches
above the bifurcation of the aorta. Descending into the pelvis over
the left common iliac artery, it passes between the layers of the
meso-rectum, and, taking the name of superior hæmorrhoidal, is
finally distributed to the upper part of the rectum. Its branches

are: 1, The *colica sinistra*, which crosses over the left kidney and supplies the descending colon; 2, the *sigmoidea*, which is distributed to the sigmoid flexure; and 3, the *superior hæmorrhoidal*, which supplies the rectum, and will be dissected with the side view of the pelvis.

These inosculate in the form of arches. The colica sinistra, too, forms a large arterial arch with the colica media, so that there is a chain of arterial communications from one end to the other of the intestinal canal (fig. 69).

The inferior mesenteric vein joins the splenic behind the pancreas.

To see the relations of the duodenum and the pancreas, two ligatures about an inch apart should be placed on the upper end of the jejunum, and two others at a similar distance apart on the lower end of the sigmoid flexure of the colon. The intestines should be cut through between each set of ligatures, and the intermediate portions of the small and large intestines removed. By turning up the stomach we expose at once the horse-shoe course of the duodenum round the great end of the pancreas.

The duodenum (p. 338) commences at the pyloric end of
Duodenum. the stomach, and terminates on the left side of the second lumbar vertebra. It is divided into three parts, an ascending, descending, and transverse.

The first portion ascends obliquely as high as the neck of the gall-bladder; then making a sudden bend, it descends in front of the right kidney as low as the third lumbar vertebra. Lastly, making another bend it ascends obliquely across the spine to the left side from the third to the second lumbar vertebra: here the canal takes the name of jejunum.

Thus the duodenum describes a horse-shoe curve, the concavity of which is towards the left side, and embraces the head of the pancreas. The first part of the duodenum is completely invested by peritoneum, and is comparatively loose, that the movements of the stomach may not be restricted. The second and third parts are only covered by peritoneum in front. Into the descending portion, the common bile duct and the pancreatic duct empty themselves, either by separate or conjoined openings.

Pancreas.   This great salivary gland of the abdomen is situated immediately behind the stomach (p. 338). It is of an elongated form, and is placed transversely across the spine ; its larger end, or head, is embraced by the duodenum ; its lesser is in contact with the spleen. The splenic artery and vein run along the upper border of the gland ; the lower border is in relation with the transverse portion of the duodenum, from which it is separated by the superior mesenteric vessels. Posteriorly the pancreas rests upon the inferior vena cava, the left kidney, the left supra-renal capsule, and the commencement of the vena portæ. Its duct runs from left to right near the lower border and anterior surface of the gland, and empties itself into the back part of the descending portion of the duodenum, conjointly with, or close to, the opening of the common bile duct. It receives numerous branches from the splenic artery, which runs along its upper border ; some from the superior mesenteric, which lies immediately beneath it, and others from the gastro-epiploica dextra.

The liver, stomach, duodenum, pancreas, and spleen, should now be collectively removed. For this purpose it is necessary to cut through the ligaments of the liver, the venæ cavæ hepaticæ, and the branches of the cœliac axis. These viscera, with the remainder of the intestinal canal, should be macerated in water, while you examine all that is to be seen at the back of the abdomen ; namely, the deep-seated muscles, the aorta, the inferior vena cava, the kidneys, the lumbar plexus of nerves, and the sympathetic nerve.

Kidneys and ureter.   The kidneys are placed in the lumbar region, one on each side of the spine. They lie imbedded in more or less fat, on the quadratus lumborum, and psoas muscles, nearly opposite the two lower dorsal and the two upper lumbar vertebræ. On the top of each is situated a little body, called the supra-renal capsule. The excretory duct of the kidney, or ureter, descends almost vertically on the psoas muscle, enters the pelvis over the division of the common iliac artery, and empties itself into the lower part of the bladder after running obliquely through its coats.

In front of the right kidney is the liver, the ascending colon, and the vertical portion of the duodenum; in front of the left, the descending colon, part of the spleen, and pancreas. This explains how it is that a renal abscess or calculus is sometimes evacuated by the rectum.

The kidneys and supra-renal capsules must be removed and reserved for further examination.

Two large ganglia, the *semilunar*, are now to be searched for in the solar plexus. They are situated on each side of the cœliac axis, in the neighbourhood of the supra-renal bodies; that on the

Fig. 70.

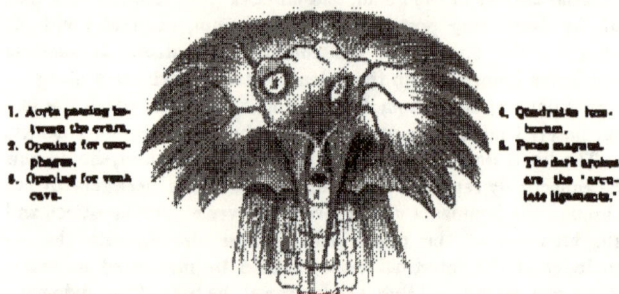

1. Aorta passing between the crura.
2. Opening for œsophagus.
3. Opening for vena cava.

4. Quadratus lumborum.
5. Psoas magnus. The dark arches are the 'arcuate ligaments.'

DIAGRAM OF THE DIAPHRAGM, THE OPENINGS IN IT, AND THE PHRENIC ARTERIES.

right side will be found lying under the vena cava inferior. They are more or less oval, and filaments are distributed to the supra-renal and renal plexuses, and to the plexuses which surround the branches of the abdominal aorta. Above it is connected with the great splanchnic nerve (p. 126).

Diaphragm.   This is a partly muscular and partly tendinous arch, so constructed as to form a complete movable partition between the chest and the abdomen; a floor for the one, and a roof for the other. Its upper or thoracic surface is convex; its lower or abdominal, concave. To see the structure of the arch, its peritoneal lining must be removed. We then observe that there is a broad tendon in the centre, and that muscular fibres converge to it from all sides (fig. 70). The diaphragm arises, 1. From the ensiform cartilage; 2. From the inside of the cartilages of the six lower ribs by as many digitations, which correspond with those of the transverse muscle of the abdomen; 3. In the interval between the last rib and the spine, it arises from two thin tendinous arches, called respectively, the *ligamenta arcuata* (externum and internum). The external arch extends from the last rib to the transverse process of the first lumbar vertebra, and arches over the quadratus lumborum; the internal passes from the transverse process of the first lumbar vertebra to the body of the same vertebra, and arches over the psoas; lastly, it arises from the front of the bodies of the lumbar vertebra by two elongated bundles, called the *crura* of the diaphragm. Both crura have tendinous origins; the right crus is, however, a little longer than the left; for the former arises from three or four upper lumbar vertebræ and their intervening cartilages, whereas the left does not descend so low by one vertebra. Between the two crura, the aorta enters the abdomen.

From these various origins the fibres ascend, at first nearly vertically, and then all arch inwards, and converge to be *inserted* into the central tendon.

The *central tendon* is nearly the highest part of the diaphragm. It presents a beautiful glistening surface, owing to the crossing of its fibres; and its shape may be rudely compared to that of a trefoil leaf. The chief point of interest about the tendon is, that, in consequence of its connections with the pericardium, beneath which it lies (p. 115), it is always maintained nearly on the same level; so that it helps to support the heart, and serves as a fixed point for the insertion of the muscular fibres of the diaphragm.

There are three large openings in the diaphragm for the transmission of the aorta, the oesophagus, and the inferior vena cava respectively. The aortic opening lies between the crura in front of the spine; it transmits, also, the vena azygos and the thoracic duct, both of which lie rather to the right side of the aorta. Trace the crura upwards, and ob-

Openings in the diaphragm.

serve that the inner fibres of each cross each other in front of the
aorta, somewhat like the letter X.* Just above the crossing, and
a little towards the left side of it, is the œsophageal opening; this
is entirely muscular, and transmits the œsophagus and the pneumogastric nerves. The opening for the vena cava is situated in the

central tendon, rather to the
right of the middle line:
observe that the vein is intimately connected to its
margin, so that it may be
kept permanently open.
Lastly, there pass through
the crus, on each side, the
sympathetic, the greater and
lesser splanchnic nerves.

Fig. 71.

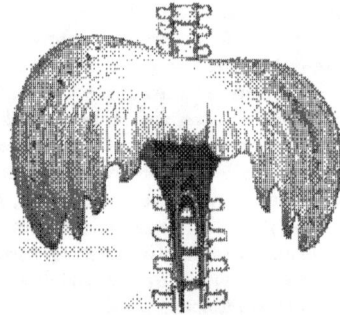

DIAPHRAGM FROM ITS UPPER SURFACE.
(The dotted lines show how much it descends
when it contracts.)

The nerves of the dia-
phragm are the phrenic
(p. 111), and the five or six
lower intercostal nerves on
each side. Its blood vessels
are the two phrenic, derived
from the aorta, the internal
mammary (p. 103), and the
lower intercostal.

Function of
the dia-
phragm.

The diaphragm is the great muscle concerned in inspiration. Truly it may be said with Haller, that it is
'musculus post cor nobilissimus.' During inspiration the
muscular sides of the diaphragm contract, and become less arched
(as shown by the dotted line in fig. 71); the floor of the chest
sinks in consequence, and more room is made for the expansion of
the lungs. During expiration the diaphragm relaxes, and the air
is expelled partly by the elasticity of the lungs and the thoracic
walls; partly by muscular action. This alternate falling and rising

* This decussation is not invariable. But the right crus always crosses more or
less over the left, so that the crura are never strictly parallel.

of the diaphragm constitutes the mechanical part of the breathing. But the diaphragm conduces to the performance of many other functions. Acting in concert with the abdominal muscles, it assists in the expulsion of the fæces and the urine, also in parturition and in vomiting: for in all these operations, we first take in a deep breath, that the diaphragm may be in a state of contraction, and so form a resisting surface, against which the viscera may be compressed by the abdominal muscles. Moreover, by its rapid or spasmodic contractions it is one of the chief agents concerned in laughing, sneezing, coughing, hiccough.

The muscles and nerves at the back of the abdomen must be carefully cleaned; also, the abdominal aorta, and vena cava inferior in front of the spine, without injuring the sympathetic nerves, situated on each side of the bodies of the vertebræ. The sheath which invests the psoas should be examined, and the branches of the lumbar plexus preserved as they emerge from the outer part of the muscle.

The sheath of the psoas is attached to the sides of the vertebræ, the brim of the pelvis, and above to the ligamentum arcuatum internum. It is this sheath which determines the ordinary course of a psoas abscess, namely, beneath the crural arch into the upper part of the thigh; for it is a rare exception when the matter travels into the pelvis.

Psoas magnus.
This long muscle arises from the bodies and transverse processes of the last dorsal and the lumbar vertebræ, and their intervening fibro-cartilages; but observe, only from the projecting borders of the vertebræ, not from the central grooved part: here the fibres arise from a tendinous arch thrown over the lumbar vessels. The muscle descends vertically along the brim of the pelvis, beneath the crural arch into the thigh, and is inserted by a strong tendon into the back part of the lesser trochanter of the femur.

As it passes under the crural arch, the tendon of the psoas lies immediately over the capsule of the hip-joint, and there is a large bursa between them to facilitate the play of the tendon. It should be borne in mind, that occasionally, even in young subjects, but more frequently in old ones, in consequence of wear and tear, this bursa communicates with the capsule of the hip-joint. The fact is interesting; for it explains how a psoas abscess sometimes makes its way into the hip-joint; a result almost always fatal.

Psoas parvus. Once in about eight or ten subjects there is a small muscle called the *psoas parvus*. It arises from the last dorsal and the first lumbar vertebra, and the intervening cartilage; thence descending in front of the great psoas, it soon ends in a long flat tendon, which spreads out, and is inserted into the brim of the pelvis.

Iliacus internus and iliac fascia. This muscle occupies the iliac fossa, and is covered by a fascia. This *iliac fascia*, as it is called, is attached to the crest of the ilium, and indirectly to the brim of the pelvis through its connection with the sheath of the psoas. But its most important attachment is to the outer half of the crural arch; here it is directly continuous with the fascia transversalis (p. 320), so that together they present an effectual barrier to the escape of intestine beneath this part of the arch.*

To return to the muscle. It arises from the iliac fossa, from the ilio-lumbar ligament,† also from the capsule of the hip-joint. The fibres pass beneath the crural arch, and are inserted into the outer side of the tendon of the psoas. Thus the two muscles, so far as their action goes, may be considered as one.

The combined *action* of the psoas and iliacus is to assist in raising the body from the recumbent position, and to fix the pelvis steadily on the thigh: this supposes the fixed point to be at the trochanter minor. But supposing the fixed point to be at the spine, then the muscle can raise and rotate the femur outwards.

---

* The iliac fossa are very liable to be the seat of suppuration, and the course which the matter takes depends upon its position with regard to the iliac fascia. If the matter be seated in the loose cellular tissue between the peritoneum and the fascia, it usually advances just above the crest of the ilium, or else towards the groin through the inguinal canal; but, if seated beneath the fascia, the chances are that the matter will make its way under the crural arch towards the upper and outer part of the thigh.

† This ligament extends from the transverse process of the last lumbar vertebra to the ilium.

It is this action which is so troublesome to counteract in fractures
of the upper third of the femur.

Quadratus
lumborum
and its
sheath.

This muscle extends from the crest of the ilium to
the last rib, and is contained in a sheath formed for it
by the aponeurotic origin of the transversalis (p. 314).
The anterior layer of its sheath is attached to the roots
of the *transverse* processes of the lumbar vertebræ, and the posterior layer to their summits. The muscle, broader below than
above, arises from about an inch and a half of the crest of the
ilium and from the ilio-lumbar ligament: it ascends nearly perpendicularly, and is inserted into the last rib, and into the front
of the transverse processes of the four upper lumbar vertebræ
by as many tendinous slips. In addition to these, a few fibres
frequently take origin from the transverse processes, and run
up to the last rib, crossing the front of the other part of the
muscle. The principal use of the muscle is to steady the
spine; it also steadies the last rib, and enables it to serve as a
fixed point for the action of the intercostal muscles and the
diaphragm.*

By raising the quadratus, we observe the aponeurotic origin of
the transversalis from the summits of the transverse processes:
this constitutes the posterior part of its sheath, and separates the
muscle from the erector spinæ.

Before examining the course of the aorta and its great primary
divisions, notice that a chain of absorbent glands extends along
the brim of the pelvis and the bodies of the lumbar vertebræ,
following nearly the course of the great blood vessels. Generally
speaking they are small; only one here and there attracts observation. They transmit the lymphatics from the lower limbs, the
abdominal wall, and the testicle; and all eventually lead to the

---

* The respective attachments of the quadratus lumborum, the crossing of its fibres,
and its mode of action, lead to the inference that it is a large intercostal muscle. It
is worth remembering that the outer edge of the quadratus lumborum, in a well-grown
adult, is about three inches from the spines of the lumbar vertebræ, and midway between the last rib and the crest of the ilium. It is just outside the edge of this muscle
that we can cut down to open the large bowel without wounding the peritoneum.

receptaculum chyli, or the beginning of the thoracic duct (p. 122). This is usually found on the right of the aorta, close to the second lumbar vertebra.

Relations of the abdominal aorta.
The aorta enters the abdomen between the crura of the diaphragm about the last dorsal vertebra, and descends a little to the left side of the mesial line in front of the spine, as low as the fourth lumbar vertebra, where it divides into the two common iliac arteries. The exact point of division cannot be specified with precision, because it varies in different subjects. But for all practical purposes it is sufficient to know that its division takes place about the level of the highest point of the crest of the ilium. The aorta is crossed in front by the splenic vein, the pancreas, the transverse portion of the duodenum, and the left renal vein. To the right side of it lie the vena cava inferior, the thoracic duct, and the vena azygos. On each side are situated the sympathetic nerves.

The branches of the aorta still to be examined, arise from it in pairs—namely, the phrenic, capsular, renal, spermatic, and lumbar. See diagram (p. 335).

Phrenic arteries.
These arteries supply the diaphragm, and arise separately, or by a common trunk, from the aorta as soon as it comes through the pillars (p. 345). The right phrenic passes outwards, behind the vena cava, the left behind the œsophagus, and both ascend to ramify extensively on the under aspect of the diaphragm. Their first branches are to the suprarenal capsules; after which, each divides into two branches: an internal, which supplies the anterior part of the diaphragm; and an external, distributed to the outer part of it. They inosculate with each other, with the internal mammary, and the intercostal arteries. The right phrenic vein terminates in the inferior vena cava; the left, in the renal vein, when not in the vena cava.

The *capsular* arteries proceed to the renal capsules. The capsular veins terminate on the right side in the vena cava; on the left in the renal.

Renal arteries and veins. The renal arteries arise from the aorta at right angles, and run transversely to the kidneys. Both are covered by their corresponding veins. The right is necessarily longer than the left, and passes beneath the vena cava. Each, after sending a small branch to the supra-renal body, enters its kidney, not as one trunk, but by several branches, corresponding to the original lobes of the organ. The renal veins lie in front of the arteries, and join the vena cava at right angles. The left is longer than the right, and crosses over the aorta; it receives the spermatic, capsular, and sometimes the phrenic veins of its own side.

Spermatic arteries and veins. The spermatic arteries arise from the front of the aorta, a little below the renal. They descend along the psoas, behind the peritoneum, and then through the inguinal canal to the testicle. In the female, the corresponding arteries proceed between the layers of the broad ligament to the ovaries. Each artery is accompanied by two very tortuous veins, which unite and then empty themselves, on the right side, into the vena cava; on the left, into the renal vein.

Lumbar arteries and branches. There are five of these arteries on either side: four arise from the aorta, the fifth comes from the arteria sacra media. They are strictly repetitions of the intercostal arteries on a small scale, so that 'lumbar intercostals' would be an appropriate name for them. They proceed outwards over the bodies of the vertebræ towards the intervertebral foramina, and then, like the thoracic intercostals, divide into dorsal and abdominal branches.

The *dorsal* branches pass between the transverse processes accompanied by the posterior branches of the corresponding nerves, and are of a size proportionate to the large development of the muscles of the back which they supply. They also send arteries into the spinal canal, some of which are distributed to the cauda equina, and others to the bodies of the lumbar vertebræ.

The *abdominal* branches all run outwards behind the quadratus lumborum, except the last, which usually runs in front. After supplying the quadratus and psoas, they are lost in the wall of the abdomen.*

The lumbar veins empty themselves into the vena cava inferior.

The *arteria sacra media*, a diminutive continuation of the aorta, proceeds from its bifurcation, and runs down in front of the sacrum to the coccyx. In animals it is the artery of the tail. It sends off the fifth lumbar artery, and lateral branches, which anastomose with the lateral sacral arteries; it also supplies small vessels to the posterior part of the rectum. Its vein empties itself either into the left common iliac vein, or into the inferior vena cava.

Vena cava inferior. The vena cava inferior is formed by the junction of the two common iliac veins. It ascends on the right of the aorta, close to the spine in the greater part of its course. As it approaches the diaphragm, the vena cava passes off a little to the right, to go through its tendinous opening in the diaphragm, and reach the right side of the heart. Its relations, beginning from below, are—in front, the mesentery, the third part of the duodenum, the pancreas and liver; behind, the right renal artery, the right lumbar arteries, and part of the sympathetic of the right side. It receives the lumbar veins, the right spermatic (the left joins the renal), the renal, the capsular, the right phrenic, and the hepatic veins.

Common iliac arteries and veins. The two common iliac arteries resulting from the bifurcation of the aorta opposite the fourth lumbar vertebra, diverge from each other at an acute angle, towards the sacro-iliac symphysis, and after a course of about two inches, divide into the external and internal iliac. They lie close to the vertebræ, and each, at or near its point of division, is crossed by the ureter; the left is crossed by the colon, and by the inferior mesentery artery.

* Just as the thoracic intercostals, by communicating with the internal mammary, form a vascular ring round the chest, so do the lumbar, by communicating with the epigastric, form a vascular ring, though less perfect, round the walls of the abdomen.

A A

The right lies upon the right and left common iliac veins, and is in relation also with the inferior vena cava.

The relations of these arteries are interesting in a practical point of view; and the most important one is their position with regard to their corresponding veins. By reason of the close connections of the right iliac artery with the right and left iliac veins, it is easier to pass a ligature round the left artery than the right.

With the parts before you, consider what would be the easiest way of performing this operation. Several modes have been recommended. Upon the whole, the best authorities* agree that the artery is most accessible from behind. An incision should be made perpendicularly from the end of the last rib to the ilium; another transversely along the margin of this bone nearly to its spine. We then cut, layer after layer, through the abdominal muscles till the peritoneum is exposed; this is easily raised from the iliac fascia, and with it the ureter is raised too. The application of the ligature is, after all, the most delicate part of the operation. It ought to be placed, as near as possible, midway between the origin and the division of the artery, so that there may be room enough for the formation of a clot on either side.†

This artery passes along the brim of the pelvis, on EXTERNAL ILIAC ARTERY. the inner side of the psoas, and then running under the crural arch about midway between the spine of the ilium and the symphysis pubis, takes the name of femoral. The corresponding vein lies close to its inner side, and on a posterior

---

* Consult some observations in point by Sir P. Crampton, in Med. Chir. Trans. vol. xvi.

† It is important to be aware that the length of the common iliac artery is apt to vary in different persons. I have seen it from three-fourths of an inch to three and a half inches long. These varieties may arise either from a high division of the aorta, or a low division of the common iliac, or both. It is impossible to ascertain, beforehand, what will be its length in a given instance, for there is no necessary relation between its length and the height of the adult individual. It is often very short in men of tall stature, and vice versâ. Anatomists generally describe the left as rather longer than the right; but, from the examination of 100 bodies, I conclude that their average length is the same.

plane. The artery, with its vein, is bound down upon the psoas by a thin layer of fascia derived from the iliac. There are two other circumstances of practical interest respecting this artery: 1. A slender nerve, the genito-crural, runs close to its outer side; 2. Just before it leaves the pelvis it is crossed by the circumflexa ilii vein. The branches given off by this artery are:—

The *epigastric*, already described (p. 322).

The *circumflexa ilii*, which arises just above the crural arch, and running towards the spine of the ilium in a sheath formed for it by the fascia iliaca, subsequently perforates the transversalis muscle.* In the dissection of the abdominal muscles (p. 313), the continuation of it was seen skirting the crest of the ilium between the internal oblique and the transversalis, and sending a branch upwards between these muscles for their supply. The main trunk, much reduced in size, inosculates with the ilio-lumbar derived from the internal iliac.

How to tie the external iliac. The easiest way of tying the external iliac is to make a curved incision at the lower part of the abdomen, beginning a little above the middle of the crural arch, and ending a little beyond the spine of the ilium. The strata of the abdominal muscles, with the fascia transversalis, should then be divided to the same extent; after which, the peritoneum must be separated by the fingers from the iliac fossa. It is necessary to make a small incision through the sheath of the vessel, to facilitate the passage of the needle. Remember that the vein is closely connected to its inner side,† and that the genito-crural nerve is not far off.

* The course of this artery should be borne in mind in opening iliac abscesses.

† This relative position of the vessels must not always be taken for granted. In old subjects, less frequently in adults, it is sometimes found that the external iliac artery runs very tortuously, instead of nearly straight, along the brim of the pelvis. But the vein does not follow the artery in its windings, and may possibly lie outside the artery just where we propose to place the ligature.

The mode of performing the operation described in the text is recommended by Sir A. Cooper. Mr. Abernethy, however, who first set the example of tying this artery, in 1796, adopted a somewhat different proceeding. He says: 'I first made an incision about three inches in length through the integuments of the abdomen, in

A A 2

The general plan upon which the sympathetic nerve
SYMPATHETIC is arranged, has been noticed in the dissection of the
NERVE. neck (p. 99). The lumbar portion of it must now be
examined.

The abdominal part of the sympathetic descends on either side,
in front of the bodies of the lumbar vertebræ, along the inner
border of the psoas. The nerve has a ganglion opposite each
lumbar vertebra, so that there are five on each side. These
ganglia are connected with one another by small filaments, and
each ganglion receives two branches from the corresponding spinal
nerve, just as in the chest. They give off filaments, of which
some twine round the aorta, and accompany the inferior mesenterio
and spermatic arteries to the large intestine and the testicle; but
the greater number terminate in the hypogastric plexus.

The hypogastric plexus is situated between the com-
Hypogastric mon iliac arteries, on the last lumbar and first sacral
plexus. vertebræ. It consists of an inextricable interlacement
of nerves, partly sympathetic, and partly spinal, and is a sort of
nerve centre for the supply of the pelvic viscera. Tracing it forwards, you find that it is continued on in two divisions, one for
each side of the pelvis. The minute filaments proceeding from
each division accompany the visceral branches of the internal iliac
artery of their respective sides, and supply the bladder, prostate
gland, and rectum; and in the female, the uterus and vagina.
Thus we have the vesical, hæmorrhoidal, uterine, and vaginal
plexuses. Of these, however, none are seen in an ordinary dissection. No ganglia are found in the hypogastric plexus.

LUMBAR This plexus is formed by the union of the anterior
PLEXUS OF branches of the four upper lumbar nerves. The fifth
NERVES. lumbar does not form part of this plexus, but joins

the direction of the artery, and thus laid bare the aponeurosis of the external oblique
muscle, which I next divided from its connection with Poupart's ligament, in the
direction of the external wound, for the extent of about two inches. The margins of
the internal oblique and transversalis muscles being thus exposed, I introduced my
finger beneath them for the protection of the peritoneum, and then divided them.
Next, with my hand, I pushed the peritoneum and its contents upwards and inwards,
and took hold of the artery.'

the sacral plexus under the name of the lumbo-sacral cord. The plexus lies over the transverse processes of the corresponding vertebræ, embedded in the substance of the psoas, so that this muscle must be dissected away before it can be seen. Like the brachial plexus, the nerves composing it successively increase in size from above. Its branches are five in number, and generally arise in the following order (fig. 72).

The *first lumbar* nerve generally divides into two branches; the upper being commonly the *ilio-hypogastric*, the lower, the *ilio-inguinal*. They cross obliquely over the quadratus lumborum to the crest of the ilium, and then separate. The ilio-hypogastric passes through the transversalis, and divides into its two terminal branches; the *iliac* branch, which supplies the skin over the glutæal region, and the *hypogastric* branch, which runs forwards between the transversalis and internal oblique, and then perforates the aponeurosis of the external oblique in the hypogastric region to supply the skin. The ilio-inguinal perforates the transversalis and internal oblique, comes out through the external abdominal ring in front of the spermatic cord, and supplies the skin of the penis and scrotum in the male, and the labium in the female.

The *external cutaneous nerve of the thigh* is generally derived from the second lumbar. It runs through the psoas, then, crossing obliquely over the iliacus towards the spine of the ilium, passes beneath the crural arch, and is finally distributed to the skin on the outside of the thigh. If the external cutaneous be not found in its usual situation, look for it as a distinct branch of the anterior crural, nearer the psoas muscle.

The *genito-crural nerve* is of small size, and generally comes from the second lumbar. After perforating the psoas, it runs down along the outer side of the external iliac artery, and near the crural arch divides into the *genital* branch (*g*), which runs through the inguinal canal, on the under aspect of the spermatic cord, and supplies the cremaster; and the *crural* (*e*), which proceeds under the crural arch, and is lost in the skin of the upper part of the thigh, where it communicates with the middle cutaneous nerve.

The *anterior crural* (*d*), the largest and most important branch, is generally formed by the union of the third and fourth lumbar. It descends in a groove between the psoas and the iliacus, supplies both these muscles, and then, passing under the crural arch, is finally distributed to the extensor muscles, to the sartorius and pectineus, and the skin of the thigh.

Fig. 72.

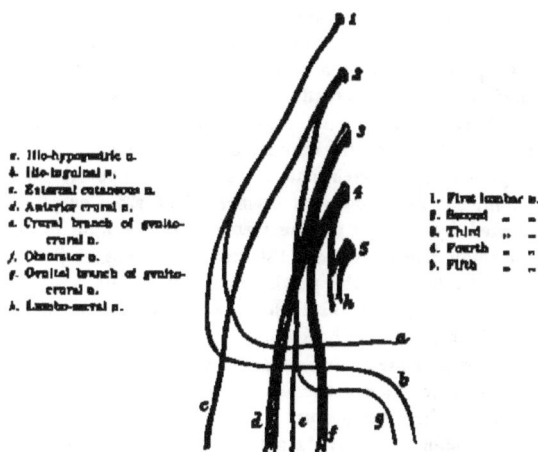

a. Ilio-hypogastric n.
b. Ilio-inguinal n.
c. External cutaneous n.
d. Anterior crural n.
e. Crural branch of genito-crural n.
f. Obturator n.
g. Genital branch of genito-crural n.
h. Lumbo-sacral n.

1. First lumbar n.
2. Second „ „
3. Third „ „
4. Fourth „ „
5. Fifth „ „

PLAN OF THE LUMBAR PLEXUS AND BRANCHES.

The *obturator nerve* (*f*) is next in size to the anterior crural. It proceeds from the third and fourth lumbar nerves, descends along the brim of the pelvis to the obturator foramen, and is distributed to the adductor muscles of the thigh.

The *accessory obturator nerve* is by no means a constant branch, but when present, comes from the obturator or third and fourth lumbar nerves. It descends over the horizontal ramus of the pubes, and supplies the pectineus on its under aspect.

Postponing the minute anatomy of the abdominal viscera, begin the examination of the contents of the pelvis.

DISSECTION OF THE PELVIS.

The purposes of the pelvis are to protect its own viscera; to support those of the abdomen; to give attachment to the muscles which steady the trunk; to transmit the weight of the trunk to the lower limbs, and to give origin to the muscles which move them. In adaptation to these functions, the form of the pelvis is that of a perfect arch, with broadly expanded wings at the sides, and projections in appropriate situations to increase the leverage of the muscles. The sacrum, impacted between the ilia, represents the key-stone of the arch, and is capable of supporting not only the trunk, but great burdens besides. The sides or pillars are represented by the ilia; these transmit the weight to the heads of the thigh bones, and are thickest and strongest just in that line, i.e. the brim of the pelvis, along which the weight is transmitted. Moreover, to effect the direct transmission of the weight, the plane of the arch is oblique. This obliquity of the pelvis, its hollow expanded sides, its great width, the position and strength of the tuberosities of the ischia, are so many proofs that man is adapted to the erect posture.

The general conformation of the pelvis in the female is modified, so as to be adapted to utero-gestation and parturition. Its breadth and capacity are greater than in the male. Its depth is less. The alæ of the iliac bones are more expanded. The projection of the sacrum is less perceptible, and consequently the brim is more circular. Above all, the span of the pubic arch is wider. The bones, too, are thinner, and the muscular impressions less strongly marked.

The cavity of the pelvis being curved, the axis, or a central line drawn through it, must be curved in proportion. For all practical purposes, it is sufficient to remember that the axis of the pelvis corresponds with a line drawn from the anus to the umbilicus.*

Contents of the male pelvis. The male pelvis contains the last part of the intestinal canal, named the 'rectum,' the bladder with the prostate gland at the neck, and the vesiculæ seminales. If the bladder be empty, some of the small intestines will be in the pelvis; not so if the bladder be distended.

Course of the rectum. The rectum enters the pelvis on the left side of the sacrum, and, after describing a curve corresponding with the concavity of the sacrum, terminates at the anus. In the first part of its course, it is loosely connected to the back of the pelvis by a peritoneal fold, called the 'meso-rectum;' between the layers of this fold the terminal branches (superior hæmorrhoidal) of the inferior mesenteric vessels with nerves and absorbents run to the bowel.

It is worth remembering that the rectum does not take this course in all cases; sometimes it makes one, or even two lateral curves. In some rare cases it enters the pelvis on the right side instead of the left. Since these variations from the usual arrangement cannot be ascertained during life, they should make us cautious in the introduction of bougies.†

Recto-vesical pouch. Whilst the parts are still undisturbed, introduce the finger into what is called the recto-vesical peritoneal pouch (fig. 73). This is a cul-de-sac formed by the peritoneum in passing from the front of the rectum to the lower and back part of the bladder. In the adult male subject, the bottom of this pouch is about one inch distant from the base of the

---

* In a well-formed female the base of the sacrum is about four inches higher than the upper part of the symphysis pubis, and the point of the coccyx is rather more than half an inch higher than the lower part of the symphysis.

The obliquity of the pelvis is greatest in early life. In the fœtus, and in young children, its capacity is small; and the viscera, which subsequently belong to it, are situated in the abdomen.

† In old age the rectum has sometimes a zig-zag appearance immediately above the anus. These lateral inclinations are probably produced by the enormous distentions to which the bowel has been occasionally subjected.

prostate gland : * therefore part of the under surface of the bladder
is not covered by peritoneum ; and since this part is in immediate
contact with the rectum, it is practicable to tap the distended
bladder through the front of the bowel without injuring the
peritoneum. The operation has, of late years, been revived, and
with great success.† It is easily done, and not attended with risk,
provided all the parts be in their regular position. But this is
not always the case. It sometimes happens that the peritoneal

Fig. 73.

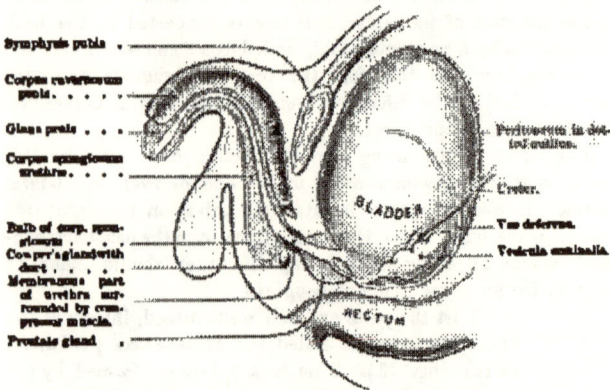

DIAGRAM OF THE RELATIVE POSITION OF THE PELVIC VISCERA.

pouch comes down nearer to the prostate than usual—we have
seen it in actual contact with the gland ; so that in such a case it
would be almost impossible to tap the bladder from the rectum
without going through the peritoneum. In children the peritoneum comes down lower than it does in the adult, because the
bladder in the child is not a pelvic viscus.

The recto-vesical pouch is permanent. But there is another

* The bottom of the pouch is from three to four inches distant from the anus.
† See a paper in the Med. Chir. Trans. vol. xxxv. by Mr. Cock.

peritoneal pouch on the front part of the bladder, which is only
produced when the bladder is distended. To produce it, the
bladder should be blown up through one of the ureters. It soon
fills the pelvis, and then, rising into the abdomen, occasions the
pouch in question between it and the abdominal wall. At first,
the pouch is shallow, but it gradually deepens as the bladder rises.
Now, if the bladder be distended half way up to the umbilicus,
which is commonly the case when it has to be tapped, we find that
the bottom of the pouch would be about two inches from the symphysis pubis (fig. 73). Within this distance from the symphysis,
the bladder may be tapped in the linea alba, without risk of
wounding the peritoneum. Thus, the surgeon has the choice of
two situations in which he may tap the bladder—above the pubes,
or from the rectum. Which of the two be the more appropriate,
must be decided by the circumstances of the case.

DISSECTION OF THE MALE PERINEUM.

Before dissecting the perineum, it is expedient first to examine
the osseous and ligamentous boundaries of the lower aperture of

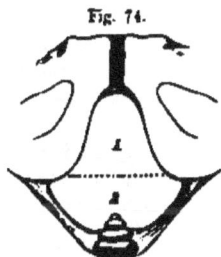

Fig. 74.

DIAGRAM OF THE FRAMEWORK
OF THE PERINEUM.

the pelvis. Looking at the male pelvis
(with the ligaments preserved), we observe that this aperture is of a lozenge
shape; that it is bounded in front by
the symphysis of the pubes, laterally by
the rami of the pubes and ischium; behind, by the coccyx and the great sacro-
ischiatic ligaments.

This space, for convenience of description, we divide into two by an imaginary
line drawn from one tuber ischii to the
other. The anterior forms a nearly equi-
lateral triangle, of which the sides are
from three to three and a half inches long; and since it transmits the urethra, it is called the urethral division of the perineum.

The posterior, containing the anus, is called the anal division (fig. 74).*

The subject is to be placed in the usual position for lithotomy, with a full-sized staff in the bladder, the rectum moderately distended with tow, and the scrotum raised by means of hooks. Observe that a central ridge, named the 'raphé,' extends from the anus, along the perineum, scrotum, and under surface of the penis. Between the tuberosities of the ischia and the anus are two depressions, marking out the ischio-rectal fossæ, which are found immediately beneath the skin, filled with fat. In the lateral operation of lithotomy, the incision should commence an inch and a quarter above the anus, close to the left side of the raphé; it should be carried downwards and outwards for three inches, to a point midway between the tuber ischii and the anus. In the bilateral operation, the incision is semi-lunar, the horns being made on either side between the tuber ischii and the anus, equidistant from these points respectively; while the centre of the incision runs about three-quarters of an inch above the anus.

Anal glands.   At the anus the skin becomes finer and more delicate, forming a gradual transition towards mucous membrane: during life it is drawn into wrinkles by the permanent contraction of the cutaneous sphincter. Moreover, the skin at the margin of the anus is richly provided with minute glands,† which secrete an unctuous substance to facilitate the passage of the fæces. When this secretion becomes defective or vitiated, the anal cutaneous folds are apt to become excoriated, chapped, or fissured; and then defæcation becomes exceedingly painful.

Subcutaneous tissue.   The skin should be reflected, by making an incision along the raphé, round the margin of the anus to the coccyx. Two others must be made on each side at right

---

* It is well to bear in mind, that the dimensions of the lower outlet of the pelvis are apt to vary in different subjects, and the lithotomist must modify his incisions accordingly.

† These glands are the analogues of the anal glands in some animals, e.g. the dog and the beaver. They are found not only about the anus, but also in the subcutaneous tissue of the perineum, a fact for the demonstration of which we are indebted to Professor Quekett. They are large enough to be seen with the naked eye.

angles to the first, the one at the upper, and the other at the lower
end of it. The skin of the perineum must then be reflected outwards. In reflecting the skin, we have to notice the characters of
the subcutaneous structure.* Its characters alter in adaptation to
the exigencies of each part. On the scrotum the fat constituent
of the tissue is entirely, and for obvious reasons, absent; while the
fibro-cellular element is most abundant, and during life elastic
and contractile. But, as we recede from the scrotum, and approach the anus, the fat accumulates more and more,
and on either side of the rectum it is found in the shape

Fat in ischio-
rectal fossæ.

of large masses, filling up what would otherwise be two
deep hollows in this situation—namely, the ischio-rectal fossa.
These fossæ are triangular, with their bases towards the skin, and
their apices at the divergence of the obturator internus and levator
ani. They are about two inches in depth, and are much deeper
posteriorly than in front. The purpose of this accumulation of fat
on each side of the anus, is to permit the easy distention and contraction of the lower end of the bowel during and after the passage
of the fæces.† Over the tuberosities of the ischia, we meet with
large masses of fat, separated by tough, fibrous septa, passing from
the skin to the bone, so as to make an elastic padding to sit upon.
Occasionally, too, there are one or more large bursæ, interposed
between this padding and the bone.

So much respecting the general characters of the subcutaneous
tissue of the perineum. Some anatomists describe it as consisting
of three, four, or even more layers, but in nature we do not find
it so. It may, indeed, be divided into as many layers as we please,
according to our skill in dissection; but this only complicates
what is, in itself, simple.

* The probable thickness of this subcutaneous tissue is a point which ought to be
determined by the lithotomist in making his first incision. Its great thickness in
some cases explains the depth to which the surgeon has to cut in letting out matter
from the ischio-rectal fossa.

† It is this fat in the ischio-rectal fossæ which renders them so liable to the occurrence of peculiarly fœtid gangrenous abscesses. These should be opened as early as
possible, lest they burst into the rectum; and one sees how deep the knife must be
introduced, in order to reach the seat of the mischief.

The cutaneous sphincter ani must now be cleaned; care being taken not to remove any of its fibres. Posteriorly, the lower border of the glutæus maximus must be displayed, and the vessels and nerves crossing the perineum, towards the anus, carefully dissected.

Cutaneous sphincter ani. The cutaneous sphincter of the anus arises from the point of the coccyx, and from the ano-coccygeal ligament. The muscular fibres surround the anus, and are inserted in a pointed manner in the tendinous centre of the perineum (p. 367). It is called the cutaneous sphincter, to distinguish it from a deeper and more powerful band of muscular fibres which surrounds the last inch or more of the rectum, and is situated nearer to the mucous membrane.

Cutaneous vessels and nerves. The cutaneous vessels and nerves of the perineum come from the internal pudic artery and nerve, and chiefly from that branch of it called the ' *superficialis perinei.*' This will be traced presently. Besides this, a cutaneous nerve is distributed to these parts from the lesser ischiatic, called the *long pudendal nerve* (p. 367). It comes through the muscular fascia of the thigh a little above the tuber ischii, and ascends, dividing into filaments, which supply the skin of the perineum and scrotum.

Crossing transversely through the ischio-rectal fossa, from the ramus of the ischium towards the anus, are the *external* or *inferior hæmorrhoidal arteries.* These come from the pudic (which may be felt on the inner side of the ischium), and running inwards, supply the rectum, levator ani, and sphincter ani. The nerve which accompanies the artery comes from the pudic, and supplies the sphincter ani and the skin of the perineum.

Superficial or muscular fascia of the perineum. The subcutaneous fascia of the perineum is composed of a *superficial* and a *deep* layer. The *superficial* layer contains more or less fat, and is continuous with that of the scrotum, the thighs, and the posterior part of the perineum. The *deeper* layer is best demonstrated by blowing air beneath it with a blow-pipe; its connections are as follow: — It is attached on either side to the anterior lip of the ramus of the pubes and ischium; traced forwards, it is directly continuous with the *tunica dartos* of the scrotum; traced backwards, we find that at the base of the urethral triangle it is reflected beneath the transversus perinei muscle, and joins the '*deep perineal fascia*' or '*triangular ligament.*' These connections explain the reason why urine effused into the perineum, does not make its way into the ischio-rectal fossæ, or down the thighs.

Remove the fascia to see the muscles which cover the bulb of the urethra and the crura of the penis. The bulb of the urethra lies in the middle of the perineum, and is covered by a strong muscle, called 'accelerator urinæ.' The crura penis are attached, one to each side of the pubic arch, and are covered each by a muscle, called 'erector penis.' A narrow slip of muscle, called 'transversus perinei,' extends on either side from the tuber ischii to the *central tendinous point* of the perineum. This point is about one inch and a quarter in front of the anus, and serves for the attachment of muscular fibres from all quarters of the perineum.

Thus the muscles of the perineum describe on each side a triangle, of which the sides are formed by the accelerator urinæ and the crus penis respectively, and the base by the transversus perinei. Across this triangle run up from base to apex the superficial perineal vessels and nerves. External to the ramus of the ischium is seen a nerve, the *long pudendal*, a branch of the lesser ischiatic, perforating the muscular fascia of the thigh.

Superficial perineal vessels and nerves.　The *superficial perineal* artery proceeds from the internal pudic as it runs up the inner side of the tuber ischii. Though the main trunk cannot be seen, it can be easily felt by pressing the finger against the bone. The artery comes into view a little above the level of the anus, and then passes up the perineal triangle, distributing branches to all the muscles, and is finally lost on the scrotum. The only named branch is a muscular one, called '*transversalis perinei*' (p. 367). This is given off near the base of the triangle, and runs with the transversus perinei muscle towards the central point of the perineum. It is necessarily divided in the first incision in lithotomy, and deserves attention, because it is sometimes of considerable size.

The artery is accompanied by two veins, which are frequently dilated and tortuous, especially in diseased conditions of the scrotum.

The nerves, two in number, are derived from the internal pudic, follow the course of their corresponding arteries, and give off

Fig. 75.

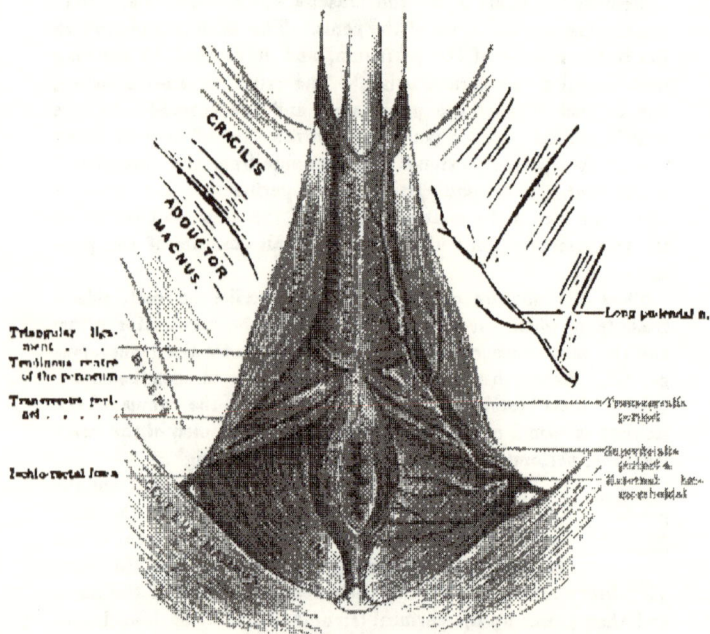

MUSCLES, WITH SUPERFICIAL VESSELS AND NERVES, OF THE PERINEUM.

similar branches. They not only supply the skin of the perineum and scrotum, but each of the perineal muscles.

The *long pudendal nerve*, a branch of the lesser ischiatic, makes its exit through the muscular fascia of the thigh, a little above the tuber ischii. It ascends nearly parallel to the ramus of the ischium and pubes, and dividing into filaments, supplies the skin of the perineum and scrotum.

Accelerator urinæ. This muscle embraces the bulb of the urethra. It arises from a fibrous median raphé beneath the bulb, and from the tendinous centre of the perineum. Starting from this origin, the fibres diverge and are inserted as follows: —The upper ones proceed on either side round the corpus caver-

Fig. 76.

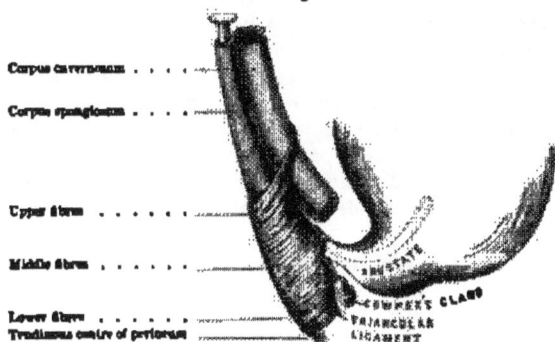

Corpus cavernosum . . . . .
Corpus spongiosum . . . . .
Upper fibres . . . . . .
Middle fibres . . . . . .
Lower fibres . . . . . .
Tendinous centre of perineum . . .

PROSTATE
COWPER'S GLAND
TRIANGULAR LIGAMENT

DIAGRAM TO SHOW THE ACCELERATOR URINE IN PROFILE.

nosum penis, like the branches of the letter V, and are fixed on its upper surface: the middle completely embrace the bulb, like a ring, and meet in a tendon on the upper surface of the urethra; the lower are fixed to the anterior surface of the deep perineal fascia (fig. 76).

Thus, the entire muscle acts as a powerful compressor of the bulb, and expels the last drops of urine from this part of the urethra. By dividing the muscle along the middle line and turning back each half, its insertion, as above described, can be clearly made out.

Erectores penis. These muscles are moulded, one upon each crus of the penis. Each muscle *arises* from the inner surface of the tuber ischii; the fibres ascend, completely covering the crus, and terminate on a strong aponeurosis, which is *inserted* into the external and inferior aspect of the crus. The *action* of these muscles is to compress the root of the penis, and so to contribute to the erection of the organ.

Transversi perinei. These muscles are of insignificant size, and sometimes absent. They arise, one on each side, from the tuber ischii, and proceed towards the central point of the perineum, where they are blended with the fibres of the accelerator urinæ. This muscle with its artery is divided in lithotomy.

The next stage of the dissection consists in reflecting and removing the accelerator urinæ from the bulb of the urethra, the erector penis with the crus penis from the rami of the pubes and ischium, and the transversi perinei muscles. This done, the *triangular ligament* or 'deep perineal fascia' is fairly exposed.

Triangular ligament of the urethra. Understand that the 'triangular ligament of the urethra' and the deep perineal fascia are synonymous terms.

The triangular ligament, shown in fig. 77, is a strong and resisting membrane stretched across the upper part of the pubic arch. On each side it is firmly attached to the *posterior* lip of the rami of the pubes and ischium; superiorly, i.e. towards the symphysis of the pubes, it is connected with the sub-pubic ligament; inferiorly, it does not present a free border, but is connected to the tendinous centre of the perineum, and becomes identified with the deep layer of the superficial perineal fascia under the transversus perinei muscle (p. 367). This ligament, by most anatomists, is described as composed of two layers, an anterior and a posterior, between which the membranous portion of the urethra is situated. The anterior layer becomes continuous below with the superficial perineal fascia; the posterior is a part of the pelvic fascia, and is lost upon the prostate.

The membranous part of the urethra runs through the triangular ligament about one inch below the symphysis pubis. The aperture for it does not present a distinct edge, because the ligament is prolonged forwards over the bulb, and serves to keep it in position.

Fig. 77.

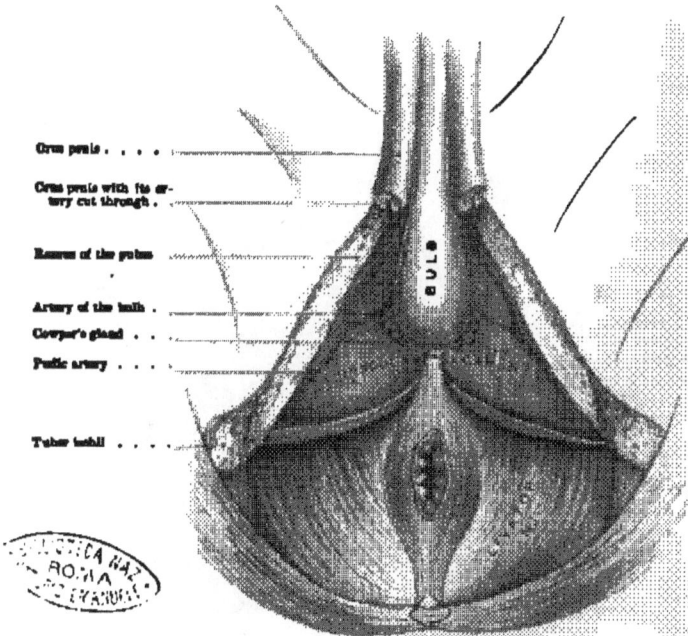

Crus penis . . . .

Crus penis with its artery cut through .

Ramus of the pubes

Artery of the bulb .

Cowper's gland . .

Pudic artery . . .

Tuber ischii . . .

BULB

DIAGRAM TO SHOW THE TRIANGULAR LIGAMENT OF THE URETHRA.

Points of surgical interest. The triangular ligament is very important surgically for these reasons :—

1. Here we meet with difficulty in introducing a catheter, unless we can hit off the right track through the ligament. The soft and spongy tissue of the bulbous part of the urethra in front of

the ligament readily gives way, if violence be used, and a false
passage results.

Fig. 78.

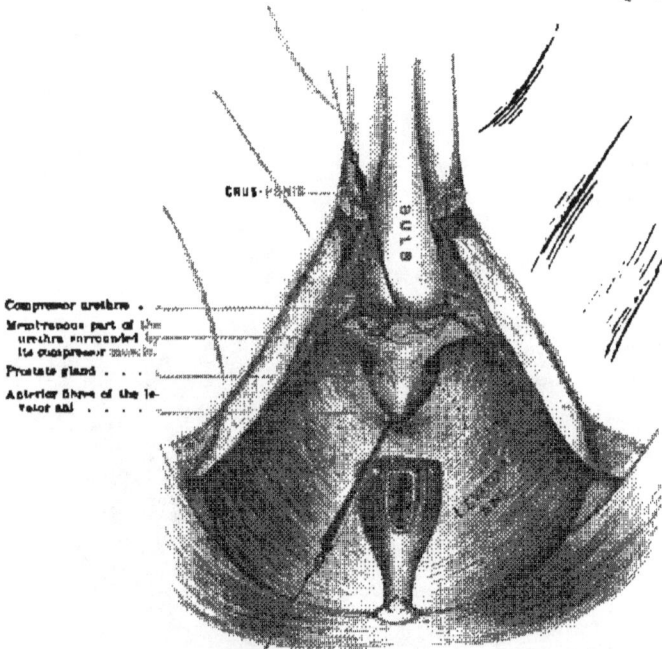

DIAGRAM OF THE PARTS BEHIND THE TRIANGULAR LIGAMENT OF THE URETHRA.

(The anterior fibres of the levator ani are hooked down to show part of the prostate;
the rest is tracked by a dotted line.)

2. By elongating the penis, we are much more likely to hit off
the proper opening through the ligament.

3. When, in retention of urine, the urethra gives way *anterior*

to this ligament, it is this which prevents the urine from travel-
ling into the pelvis. Its connection with the superficial perineal
fascia prevents the urine from getting into the ischio-rectal fossa:
nor can the urine make its way into the thighs. The only outlet
for it is into the cellular tissue of the scrotum and penis.

4. When suppuration takes place *behind* the ligament, the
matter is pent up and should be speedily let out; if not, it will
find its way into the cellular tissue of the pelvis and may burst
into the urethra or the rectum.

5. The ligament is partially cut through in lithotomy.

The parts divided in the lateral operation of lithotomy are: the
skin, the superficial fascia, the transverse perineal muscle, vessels
and nerve; the accelerator urinæ, the anterior fibres of the levator ani, the compressor urethræ, the triangular ligament, the membranous and prostatic parts of the urethra, and a small portion of
the prostate.

The anterior layer of the triangular ligament must
What lies
between the
layers of the
triangular
ligament. now be cut away to see what lies behind it. These parts
are shown in fig. 78; namely: 1, the membranous part of
the urethra, surrounded by, 2, the compressor urethræ
muscle; 3, Cowper's glands; 4, the pudic artery and
its three terminal branches, i.e. the artery of the bulb, the artery
of the crus, and the dorsal artery of the penis.

To obtain the best perineal view of the compressor urethræ
muscle, cut through the spongy part of the urethra about three
inches above the end of the bulb, and dissect it from the corpus
cavernosum. Thus, the upper fibres of the constrictor will be
exposed; to see the lower, it is only necessary to raise the bulb.
The most perfect view, however, of the muscle is obtained by
making a transverse section through the rami of the pubes, so as
to get at the muscle from above, as shown in fig. 79.

This muscle surrounds and supports the urethra in
Compressor
urethræ. its passage beneath the pubic arch. It arises from the
ramus of the pubes on either side; from thence its
fibres pass, some above, some below the urethra, along the whole
length of its membranous part. It forms a complete muscular

covering for the urethra between the prostate and the bulb. It is chiefly through its agency that we retain the urine. This muscle is the chief cause of spasmodic stricture of the urethra.[*]

Fig. 79.

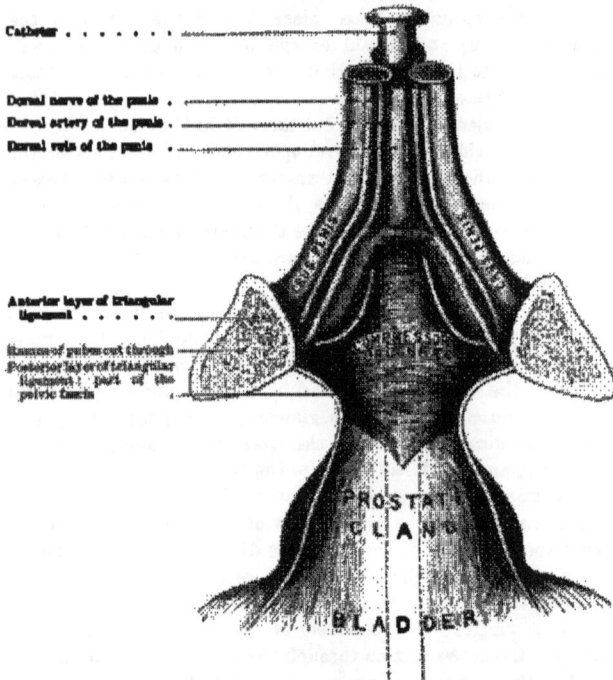

Catheter . . . . . .

Dorsal nerve of the penis .
Dorsal artery of the penis .
Dorsal vein of the penis .

Anterior layer of triangular ligament . . . . . .

Ramus of pubes cut through
Posterior layer of triangular ligament : part of the pelvic fascia

PROSTATE GLAND

BLADDER

DIAGRAM OF THE RELATIONS OF THE COMPRESSOR URETHRÆ SEEN FROM ABOVE.

[*] The compressor urethræ was first accurately described and delineated by Santorini (septemdec. tabulæ), and afterwards by Müller in his monograph (Ueber die organ. Nerv. der männlich. Geschlechtsorgane).

These glands are imbedded, one on either side, immediately behind the bulb, in the substance of the compressor urethræ. Each consists of a cluster of little glands. Their collective size is about that of a pea, but it varies in different individuals. From each a slender duct runs forwards, and, after a course of about one inch, opens into the under surface of the bulbous part of the urethra (p. 377). Their use is to furnish a secretion accessory to generation.

The pudic artery is a branch of the internal iliac. It leaves the pelvis through the great ischiatic notch, winds round the spine of the ischium, re-enters the pelvis through the lesser ischiatic notch, and then runs along the inner side of the tuber ischii up towards the pubic arch. About an inch and a half above the tuber ischii, we can *feel* the trunk of the pudic artery; but we cannot see it, nor draw it out, for it is securely lodged in a fibrous canal formed by the obturator fascia. Traced upwards, it runs between the two layers of the triangular ligament, and divides into three principal branches; the artery of the bulb, the artery of the crus, and the dorsal artery of the penis (fig. 78). The external hæmorrhoidal and superficial perineal branches have already been described (p. 366).

The *artery of the bulb* is of considerable size, and passes transversely inwards; it runs through the substance of the compressor urethræ, and before it enters the bulb divides into two or three branches. It also sends a small branch to Cowper's gland. From the direction of this artery it will at once strike the attention that there is great risk of dividing it in lithotomy. If the artery run along its usual level, and the incision be not made too high in the perineum, then indeed it is out of the way of harm. But, supposing the reverse, the artery cannot escape; and its size is such that it might occasion alarming hæmorrhage. If it be asked, how often does the artery run along a dangerous level? about once in twenty subjects; and there is no possibility of ascertaining this anomaly beforehand.

The *artery of the crus penis* is given off after that of the bulb.

It ascends for a short distance under cover of the arch, but soon enters the crus.

To see the *dorsal artery* of the penis, the penis must be dissected from its attachment to the symphysis pubis. The artery should be traced running upon the dorsum of the penis down to the glans. It forms a complete arterial circle round the corona glandis, and gives numerous ramifications to the papillæ on the surface.

Pudic nerve. The pudic nerve comes from the sacral plexus, and corresponds both in its course and branches with the artery. It gives off its external or inferior hæmorrhoidal, and its superficial perineal branches—a small one to the bulb, and another to the crus penis; but the main trunk of the nerve runs with the artery along the dorsum of the penis to the glans (p. 373). In its passage it supplies the integuments of the penis, and sends one or two branches into the corpus cavernosum. This part of the penis also receives nerves from the sympathetic system.

Ischio-rectal fossa. This is the deep hollow on each side between the anus and the tuber ischii. When all the fat is removed from it, observe that it is lined on all sides by fascia. Introduce the finger into it to form a correct idea of its extent and boundaries. Externally, it is bounded by the tuber ischii and the fascia covering the obturator internus muscle; internally, by the rectum, levator ani and coccygeus; posteriorly, by the glutæus maximus; anteriorly, by the transversus perinei. The fossa is crossed by the external hæmorrhoidal vessels and nerves.

These deep recesses on each side of the rectum explain the great size which abscesses in this situation may attain. The matter can be felt only through the rectum. Nothing can be seen outside. Perhaps nothing more than a little hardness can be felt by the side of the anus. These abscesses should be opened early; else they form a large cavity, and may burst into the rectum.

ANATOMY OF THE SIDE VIEW OF THE PELVIC VISCERA.

To make a side view of the pelvic viscera, the left innominate bone should be removed thus:—Detach the peritoneum and the levator ani from the left side of the pelvis; saw through the pubes about two inches external to the symphysis, and cut through the sacro-iliac symphysis; now draw the legs apart, and saw through the base of the spine of the ischium; after cutting through the pyriformis, the great sacro-ischiatic ligament and ischiatic nerves, the innominate bone can be easily detached. This done, the rectum should be distended with tow, and the bladder blown up through the ureter. A staff should be passed through the urethra into the bladder.

You have already seen how the peritoneum passes from the front of the rectum to the lower part of the bladder (forming the recto-vesical pouch), and thence over the back of the bladder to the wall of the abdomen. You see where the distended bladder is bare of peritoneum, and that it can be tapped either through the rectum or above the pubes without injury to the serous membrane, as shown by the arrows in fig. 80.

False ligaments of the bladder.   The peritoneal connections of the bladder are called its false ligaments; *false* in contradistinction to the *true*, which are formed by the fascia of the pelvis, and really *do* fasten the neck of the bladder in its proper position. The false ligaments are five in number, two posterior, two lateral, and one superior. The *posterior* are produced by two peritoneal folds, one on either side the recto-vesical pouch, over the fibrous remains of the umbilical arteries; the *two lateral* by reflections of the peritoneum from the side of the pelvis to the side of the bladder; the *superior* is produced by the passage of the peritoneum to the abdominal wall, and contains the *urachus* and obliterated umbilical arteries.

Pelvic fascia.   To expose the *pelvic fascia*, the peritoneum must be removed from that side of the pelvis which has not been disturbed : in doing so, notice the abundance of loose cellular tissue interposed between the peritoneum and the fascia, to allow the bladder to distend with facility.   Whenever urine gains access to this cellular tissue, it is sure to produce the most disastrous consequences; therefore in all operations on the perineum, it is of the utmost importance not to injure this fascia.

Fig. 80.

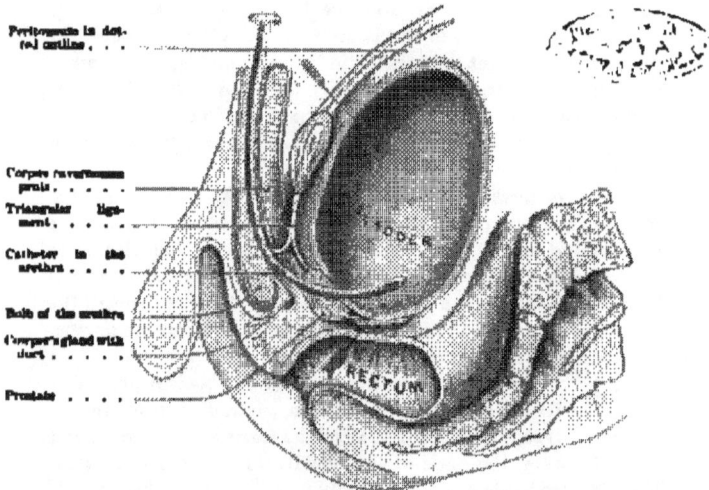

Peritoneum in dot-
ted outline . . .

Corpus cavernosum
penis . . . . .

Triangular liga-
ment . . . .

Catheter in the
urethra . . . .

Bulb of the urethra

Cowper's gland with
duct . . . . .

Prostate . . . . .

VERTICAL SECTION THROUGH THE PERINEUM AND PELVIC VISCERA.

The pelvic fascia is a thin but strong membrane, and constitutes the true ligaments of the bladder, and the other pelvic viscera, supporting and maintaining them in their proper position.

Examine first, to what parts of the pelvis the fascia is attached; secondly, the manner in which it is reflected on the viscera.

Beginning, then, in front (fig. 81), the fascia is attached to the body of the pubes; thence, we trace its attachment along the side

of the pelvis, just above the obturator foramen, to the greater
ischiatic notch: here it becomes gradually thinner, covers the
pyriformis muscle, and is lost on the sacrum.   From this attachment the fascia descends as far as a line drawn from the spine of
the ischium to the symphysis pubis.   Along this line, which corre-

Fig. 81.

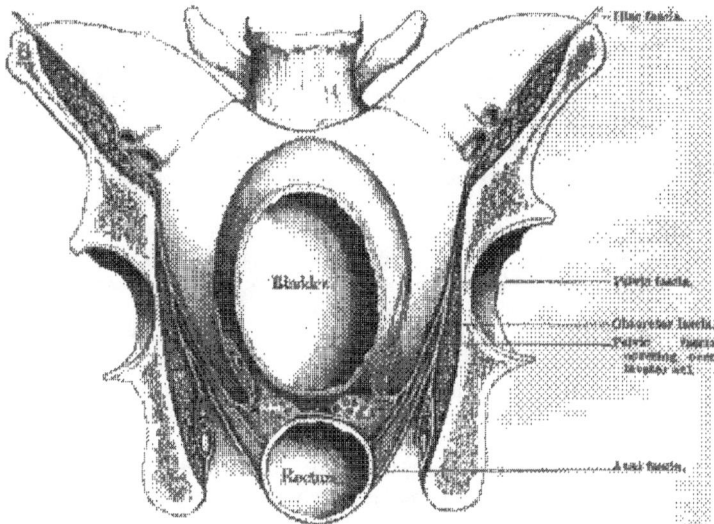

TRANSVERSE SECTION OF THE PELVIS, TO SHOW THE REFLECTIONS OF
THE PELVIC FASCIA.   (*After Gray.*)

sponds with the origin of some of the fibres of the levator ani, the
fascia divides into two layers, an inner, called the *recto-vesical
fascia*; an outer, called the *obturator fascia.*

The *obturator fascia* is the continuation of the pelvic fascia,
and runs down on the inner surface of the obturator internus,

forming, at the same time, a sheath for the pudic vessels and nerve. It is attached to the arch of the pubes, and to the tuberosities of the ischia. From this fascia is derived the *anal fascia* which lines the lower surface of the levator ani, and is subsequently lost upon the rectum.

The *recto-vesical fascia* descends on the upper or internal surface of the levator ani to the bladder and prostate. From the pubes it is reflected over the prostate and the neck of the bladder, to form, on either side of the symphysis, two well-marked bands— the *anterior true ligaments* of the bladder. From the side of the pelvis it is reflected on to the side of the bladder, constituting the *lateral true ligaments* of the bladder, and incloses the prostate and the vesical plexus of veins. A prolongation from this ligament incloses the vesicula seminalis, and then passes between the bladder and the rectum, to join its fellow from the opposite sides.

GENERAL POSITION OF THE PELVIC VISCERA IN THE MALE.

The pelvic viscera are so surrounded by veins and loose areolar tissue, that he who dissects them for the first time will find a difficulty in discovering their definite boundaries. The rectum runs at the back of the pelvis. The bladder lies in front of the rectum, immediately behind the symphysis pubis. At the neck of the bladder is the prostate gland through which the urethra passes. In the cellular tissue, between the bladder and the rectum, there is, on each side, a convoluted tube called the ' vesicula seminalis; ' and on the inner side of each vesicula, is the seminal duct or vas deferens. Before describing these parts in detail, it is necessary to say a few words about the large tortuous veins which surround them.

Plexus of veins about prostate and neck of bladder.

Beneath the pelvic fascia about the prostate and the neck of the bladder, are large and tortuous veins, which form the prostatic and the vesical plexuses. They empty themselves into the internal iliac. In early life they are not much developed, but as puberty approaches, they gradually increase in size; and one not familiar with the anatomy of these parts would hardly credit the volume which they sometimes attain in old persons. They communicate

freely with the inferior hæmorrhoidal plexus, or veins about the
anus, and they receive the blood returning from the penis through
the large veins which pass under the pubic arch.   This is one of
the reasons why the prostatic plexus is so capacious.

Fig. 82.

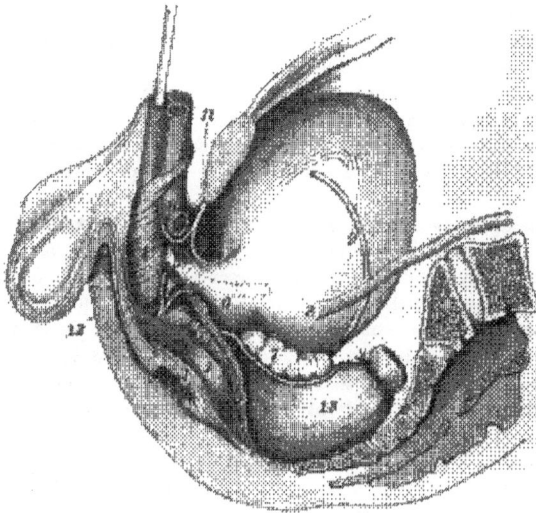

SIDE VIEW OF THE PELVIC VISCERA.

(Taken from a Photograph.)

1. External sphincter.
2. Internal sphincter.
3. Levator ani cut through.
4. Accelerator urinæ.
5. Membranous part of the urethra, surrounded by compressor muscle.
6. Prostate gland.
7. Vesicula seminalis.
8. Ureter.
9. Vas deferens.
10. Crus penis divided.
11. Triangular ligament.
12. Superficial perineal fascia.
13. Rectum.

If, in lithotomy, the incision be carried beyond the limits of
the prostate, the great veins around it must necessarily be divided:
these, independently of any artery, are quite sufficient to occasion
serious hæmorrhage.

Rectum
intestinum
and its
relations.

The rectum enters the pelvis on the left of the sacrum, and describes a curve corresponding to the axis of the pelvis. Before its termination, the bowel curves downwards so that the anal aperture is dependent. The rectum is not throughout of equal calibre. Its capacity becomes greater as it descends into the pelvis; and, immediately above the sphincter, it presents a considerable dilatation (fig. 80). This dilatation is not material in early life, but it increases as age advances. An adequate idea of it cannot be formed unless the bowel be fully distended. Under such circumstances the rectum loses altogether its cylindrical form, and bulges up on either side of the prostate and the base of the bladder. For this reason the rectum should always be emptied before the operation of lithotomy.

The upper part of the rectum is connected to the sacrum by a fold of peritoneum termed 'meso-rectum.' In this fold, the terminal branch of the inferior mesenteric artery with its vein runs up to supply the bowel. Below the meso-rectum, the gut is connected to the sacrum and coccyx by loose cellular tissue, which allows its easy distention. The rectum is supported by the levatores ani, the larger portions of which are inserted into its side.

The relations of the front part of the rectum,—that, namely, included between the recto-vesical pouch and the anus—are most important. Supposing the forefinger to be introduced into the anus, and a catheter in the urethra, the first thing felt through the front wall of the bowel is the membranous part of the urethra (fig. 82). It lies just within the sphincter, and is about ten lines in front of the gut. About one and a half or two inches from the anus the finger comes upon the prostate gland; this is in close contact with the gut, and is readily felt on account of its hardness; by moving the finger from side to side we recognise its lateral lobes. Still higher up, the finger goes beyond the prostate, and reaches the 'trigone' of the bladder: the facility with which this can be examined depends not only upon the length of the finger and the amount of fat in the perineum, but upon the degree of distention of the bladder; the more distended the bladder, the

better can the prostate be felt.   These several relations are practically important.   They explain why, with the finger in the rectum,
we can ascertain whether the catheter is taking the right direction,
—whether the prostate be enlarged or not.   We might even raise
a stone from the bottom of the bladder so as to bring it in contact
with the forceps.   The rectum is supplied with blood by the
superior, middle, and inferior hæmorrhoidal arteries.   The superior
come from the inferior mesenteric (p. 341); the middle and inferior from the pudic artery.   The superior and middle hæmorrhoidal veins join the inferior mesenteric, and consequently the
portal system; the inferior hæmorrhoidal veins join the internal
pudic.   They are very large and form a very tortuous plexus about
the lower part of the rectum.   Having no valves, they are liable
to become dilated and congested from various internal causes;
hence the frequency of hæmorrhoidal affections.

Bladder.   This viscus, being a receptacle for the urine, must
necessarily vary in size, and accordingly the nature of
its connections and coats are such as to permit this variation.
When contracted, the bladder sinks into the pelvis behind the
pubic arch, and is completely protected from injury.   But, as it
gradually distends, it rises out of the pelvis into the abdomen,
and, in cases of extreme distention, may reach nearly up to the
umbilicus.[*]   Its outline can then be easily felt through the walls
of the abdomen.   The form [†] of the distended bladder is oval, and
its long axis, if produced, would pass superiorly through the
umbilicus, and inferiorly through the end of the coccyx.   The

---

[*] When the bladder is completely paralysed it becomes like an inorganic sac, and
there seems to be no limit to its distention.   Haller found in a drunkard the bladder
so dilated that it would hold twenty pints of water.   (Elem. Phys. art. Vesica.)
Frank saw a bladder so distended as to resemble ascites, and evacuated from it twelve
pounds of urine.   (Oratio de Signis morborum, &c. &c. Ticini, 1788.)

[†] W. Hunter, in his Anatomy of the Gravid Uterus, has given the representation of a
bladder distended nearly as high as the ensiform cartilage.

[†] In all animals with a bladder, the younger the animal the more elongated is the
bladder.   This is indicative of its original derivation from a tube, i.e. the urachus.
In the infant, the bladder is of a pyriform shape, as it is, permanently, in the quad-
ruped; but as we assume more and more the perpendicular attitude, the weight of the
urine gradually makes the lower part more capacious.

axis of a child's bladder is more vertical than in the adult; for in children, the bladder is not a pelvic viscus. This makes lithotomy in them so much more difficult.

The quantity of urine which the bladder will hold without much inconvenience varies. As a general rule it may be stated at about a pint. A good deal depends upon the habits of the individual; but some persons have, naturally, a very small bladder, and are obliged to empty it more frequently.

In young persons the lowest part of the bladder is the neck, or that part which joins the prostate. But as age advances, the

Fig. 83.

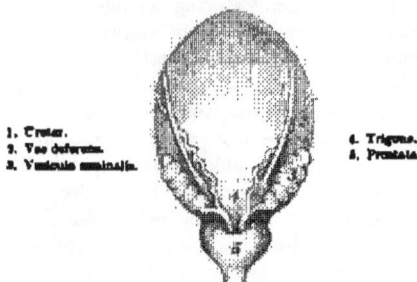

1. Crura.
2. Vas deferens.
3. Vesicula seminalis.

4. Trigone.
5. Prostate.

POSTERIOR VIEW OF THE BLADDER.

bottom of the bladder gradually deepens so as to form a well or pouch behind the prostate. In old subjects, more particularly if the prostate be enlarged, this pouch becomes of considerable depth, and renders micturition tedious. It sometimes happens that a stone in the bladder cannot be felt; the reason of which may be that the stone, lodged in such a pouch below the level of the neck of the bladder, escapes the detection of the sound. Under these circumstances, if the patient be placed on an inclined plane with the pelvis higher than the shoulders, the stone falls out of the pouch, and is easily recognisable.

Ureter.   This tube, about eighteen inches long, conveys the urine from the kidney to the bladder. In the dissection of the abdomen we saw it behind the peritoneum, descending along the psoas muscle, and crossing the division of the common iliac arteries. Tracing it downwards, in the posterior false ligament of the bladder, we find that it runs along the bladder, external to the vas deferens, and enters it about an inch and a half behind the prostate, and about two inches from its fellow of the opposite side (fig. 82). It perforates the bladder very obliquely, so that the aperture, being valvular, allows the urine to flow into, but not out of the organ. The narrowest part of the ureter is at the vesical orifice; here, therefore, a calculus is more likely to be detained than at any other part of the canal.

Vas deferens.   This tube conveys the seminal fluid from the testicle into the prostatic part of the urethra. It ascends at the back part of the spermatic cord through the inguinal canal into the abdomen; then leaving the cord at the inner ring, it curves downwards over the side of the bladder, gradually approaching nearer the middle line. Before it reaches the prostate it passes between the bladder and the ureter; then, becoming very tortuous, it runs internal to the vesicula seminalis, and is joined by the duct of this vesicle. The common duct thus formed (*ductus communis ejaculatorius*) terminates in the lower part of the prostatic portion of the urethra (fig. 73, p. 361). In point of size and hardness, the vas deferens has very much the feel of whipcord.[*]

Vesiculæ seminales.   These are situated, one on either side, between the bladder and the rectum (fig. 82). Each is a tube, but so convoluted that it looks like a little sacculated bladder. When rolled up, the tube is about two and a half inches long; when unravelled, it is more than twice that length, and about the size of a small writing quill. Several blind tubes, or cæcal prolongations, proceed from the main one, after the manner

---

[*] The description in the text presumes the bladder to be distended. But when the bladder is empty the vas deferens runs down upon the side of the pelvis. In this course it may be seen, through the peritoneum, crossing—1, the external iliac vessels; 2, the remains of the umbilical artery; 3, the obturator artery and nerve; 4, the ureter.

of a stag's horn.   The vesiculæ seminales do not run parallel, but
diverge from each other posteriorly, like the branches of the letter
V; and each lies immediately on the outer side of the vas deferens,
into which it leads.   The function of the vesiculæ seminales is to
serve as reservoirs for the semen.

They contain a brownish-coloured fluid, presumed to be in
some way accessory to the function of generation.[*]

Prostate
gland.

The prostate gland is situated at the neck of the
bladder, and surrounds the first part of the urethra
(p. 394).   In the healthy adult it is about the size and
shape of a chesnut.   Its apex is directed forwards.   It is surrounded by a plexus of veins (p. 379), and is maintained in its
position by the pelvic fascia (p. 378).   Its upper surface is about
three-quarters of an inch below the symphysis pubis: its apex is
about one inch and a half from the anus; the base is about two
and a half.

Above the prostate are the anterior ligaments of the bladder,
with the dorsal vein of the penis between them; below, and in
contact with it, is the rectum; on each side of it is the levator
ani; in front of it we have the membranous part of the urethra
(surrounded by its compressor muscle), and the triangular ligament; behind, are the neck of the bladder and the vesiculæ
seminales with the ejaculatory ducts.

The transverse diameter is about one inch and a half; the
vertical is about half an inch less.   But the gland varies in size
at different periods of life.   In the child it is not developed, or at
all events is very small: it gradually grows towards puberty, and
generally increases in size with advancing age.

To ascertain the size and condition of the prostate during life,
the bladder should be at least half full: the prostate is then
pressed down towards the rectum, and more within reach of the
finger.

Anatomy of
the urethra

The urethra is a canal about eight inches in length,
and leads from the bladder to the end of the penis.

---

[*] The vesiculæ seminales are imperfectly developed till the age of puberty.   In a
child of three years of age they can hardly be inflated with the blowpipe.

In its passage under the pubic arch. It is divided into three portions—the prostatic, the membranous, and the spongy. At present we can only examine the relations of the *membranous part*, which comprises that part of the canal intermediate between the prostate and the bulb. The urethra in this part is about one inch in length, but somewhat longer on its upper than its lower surface, in consequence of the encroachment of the bulb. In its passage under the arch of the pubes, it is surrounded by the muscular fibres of the compressor urethræ. It traverses the two layers of the triangular ligament, and is about an inch below the symphysis pubis, and nearly the same distance from the rectum; it is not, however, equidistant from this portion of the intestine at all points, because of the downward bend which the rectum makes towards the anus.[*]

The membranous part of the urethra in children is very long, owing to the smallness of the prostate at that period of life; it is also composed of thin and delicate walls, and lies close to the rectum. In sounding a child, therefore, it is very necessary not to use violence, else the instrument is likely to pass through the coats of the urethra and make a false passage.

Levator ani.   This muscle supports the anus and lower part of the rectum like a sling; and, with the coccygeus and compressor urethræ, forms a muscular floor for the cavity of the pelvis. To see it, the pelvic fascia must be reflected from its inner surface. It arises from the ramus of the pubes near the symphysis, from the spine of the ischium, and from a tendinous line extending in a gentle curve between these points of bone; this line being the division of the pelvic fascia (p. 378). From this long origin the fibres descend, and are inserted thus—the anterior, passing under the prostate, meet their fellow in the middle line of the perineum in *front* of the anus (sometimes called levator prostatæ); the middle are inserted into the side of the rectum, while the posterior meet their fellow behind the rectum.

[*] If a clean vertical section were made, we should see that the two canals form the sides of a triangular space, of which the apex is towards the prostate. This is sometimes called the recto-urethral triangle.

The function of the levatores ani is to retract the anus and the rectum after it has been protruded in defæcation by the combined action of the abdominal muscles and the diaphragm.

Coccygeus.   This muscle should be regarded as a continuation of the levator ani. It arises from the spine of the ischium, gradually spreads out, and is inserted into the side of the coccyx, which it serves to support.

At this stage of the dissection, the bladder should be drawn downwards, and the branches of the internal iliac artery and the sacral plexus clearly displayed.

Fig. 84.

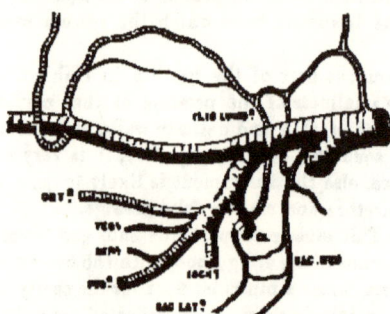

PLAN OF THE BRANCHES OF THE INTERNAL ILIAC.

Internal iliac artery and branches.   From the division of the common iliac artery, the internal iliac descends into the pelvis, and, after a course of about an inch and a half, divides, opposite the great sacro-ischiatic notch, into two large branches, an anterior and a posterior (fig. 84). The artery lies upon the lumbo-sacral cord and the pyriformis muscle; the ureter, inclosed in the posterior false ligament of the bladder, passing in front.

The *posterior* division gives off the ilio-lumbar, lateral sacral, and glutæal arteries; the *anterior* gives off the superior vesical, obturator, inferior vesical, middle hæmorrhoidal, ischiatic and

pudic; also the uterine and vaginal in the female. Such is their
usual order; but these branches, though constant as to their
general distribution, vary as to their origin.

a. The *ilio-lumbar* is analogous to the lumbar branches of the
aorta. It ascends outwards beneath the psoas, sends branches to
this muscle and the quadratus lumborum; then, running near
the crest of the ilium, it supplies the iliacus internus, and finally
inosculates with the circumflexa ilii (p. 354).

b. The *lateral sacral*, usually two in number, descend perpendicularly in front of the sacral foramina, and inosculate on the
coccyx with the middle sacral artery. They give branches to the
pyriformis, the bladder, and rectum, and others which enter the
anterior sacral foramina for the supply of the cauda equina.

c. The *gluteal* is the largest branch. It passes immediately out
of the pelvis through the great ischiatic notch, above the pyriformis
muscle, and then divides into branches for the supply of the great
muscles of the buttock. These will be dissected with the thigh.

d. The *superior vesical* artery comes off from the unobliterated
portion of the hypogastric, and supplies the upper part of the
bladder. It gives off the *middle vesical* artery; and a still smaller
one, the deferential, which accompanies the vas deferens. The
inferior vesical artery ramifies on the under surface of the bladder,
the vesiculæ seminales and the prostate, and gives off the middle
hæmorrhoidal which supplies the rectum.

e. The *obturator* artery runs along the side of the pelvis, below
the corresponding nerve, to the upper part of the obturator foramen, through which it passes to be distributed to the muscles of
the thigh. In the pelvis it gives off a small branch to the iliacus
internus, and another, the *pubic*, which ramifies on the back of
the pubes.

The obturator artery does not, in all subjects, take the course
above stated. It may arise from the external iliac near the crural
arch, or by a short trunk in common with the epigastric.* Under

---

* In most subjects a small branch of the obturator ascends behind the ramus of the
pubes to inosculate with the epigastric. The variety in which the obturator arises in

these circumstances, in order to reach the obturator foramen, it generally descends on the *outer* side of the femoral ring. Instances, however, occasionally occur, where it makes a sweep round the *inner* side of the ring; so that three-fourths of the ring, or, what comes to the same thing, of the mouth of a femoral hernia, would in such a case be surrounded by a large artery.*

f. The *ischiatic* artery is smaller than the gluteal. It proceeds over the pyriformis and the sacral plexus, to the lower border of the great ischiatic notch, through which it passes out of the pelvis to the buttock, where it runs with the great ischiatic nerve. It gives off small muscular branches in the pelvis to the pyriformis and coccygeus.

g. The *pudic* artery supplies the perineum and the penis. It passes out of the pelvis through the great ischiatic notch, below the pyriformis, crosses the spine of the ischium, and re-enters the pelvis through the lesser notch. It then ascends on the inner side of the obturator internus towards the pubic arch, where it gives branches to the several parts of the penis. In its passage over the obturator muscle it is inclosed in a strong tube of fascia (formed by the obturator fascia), and is situated about one inch and a quarter above the tuberosity of the ischium. The branches of the pudic artery were described in the dissection of the perineum (p. 374).

The pudic artery, however, sometimes takes a very different course. Instead of passing out of the pelvis, it may run by the side of the prostate gland to its destination; or, one of the large branches of the pudic may take this unusual course, while the pudic itself is regular, but proportionably small. All practical anatomists are familiar with these varieties, and we seldom pass a

common with the epigastric is but an unusual development of this branch. The branch derives additional interest from the fact, that after ligature of the external iliac it becomes greatly enlarged, and carries blood directly into the epigastric. See a case in Med. Chir. Trans. vol. xx. 1836.

* The Museum of St. Bartholomew's Hospital contains two examples of double femoral hernia in the male, with the obturator arising on each side from the epigastric. In three out of the four ruptures the obturator runs on the inner side of the mouth of the sac. (See Preparations 55, 69, Series 17.)

winter session without meeting with one or two examples of them. It need hardly be said that lithotomy, under such conditions, might be followed by fatal hæmorrhage.

h. The *middle sacral artery* is a very diminutive prolongation of the aorta down to the coccyx. It becomes gradually smaller as it descends, and finally inosculates with the lateral sacral arteries. In animals this is the artery of the tail.

Respecting the *veins* in the pelvis, they correspond with the arteries, and empty themselves into the internal iliac vein. The remarkable plexus of veins about the prostate, neck of the bladder, and rectum, has been described (p. 379).

Nerves of the pelvis.   Those which proceed from the spinal cord should be examined first, afterwards those derived from the sympathetic system.

Sacral nerves and plexus.   Five sacral nerves proceed from the spinal cord through the sacral foramina. The upper four, from their large size, at once attract observation; but the fifth is small, perforates the coccygeus muscle, supplying it and the skin over the coccyx.

The coccygeal nerve is not easily found: it communicates with the fifth sacral nerve, and supplies the same parts as that nerve; namely, the coccygeus and the skin over the coccyx.

The three upper sacral nerves, and part of the fourth, with the lumbo-sacral cord, form the sacral plexus. The great nerves of the plexus lie on the pyriformis muscle, beneath the branches of the internal iliac artery, and coalesce to form the *great ischiatic* nerve, which passes out at the back of the pelvis, for the supply of the flexor muscles of the inferior extremity. The other branches of the plexus are as follow:—

a. Muscular branches distributed to the levator ani, the coccygeus, the cutaneous sphincter of the anus, the pyriformis, gemelli, quadratus femoris, and obturator internus. The nerve to the last-named muscle (sometimes derived from the pudic) leaves the pelvis with the pudic artery, and re-enters with it to reach the muscle.

b. The *superior gluteal* nerve proceeds from the lumbo-sacral, leaves the pelvis above the pyriformis with the glutæal artery, and supplies the glutæus medius and minimus, and the tensor fasciæ femoris.

c. The *lesser ischiatic* supplies the glutæus maximus, the skin of the buttock, the perineum, and the back of the thigh.

Fig. 85.

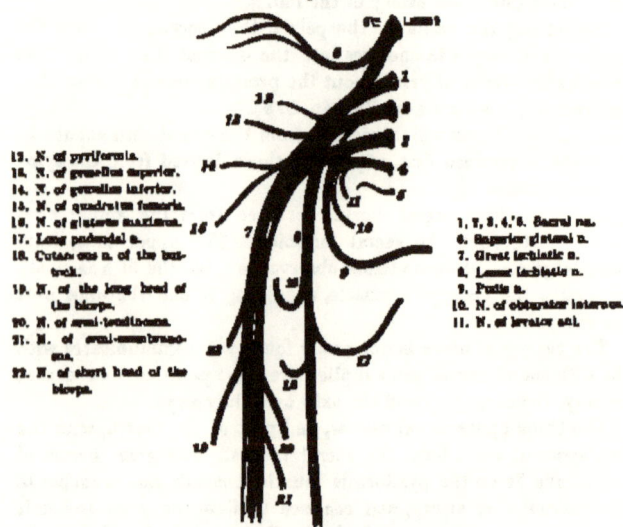

13. N. of pyriformis.
14. N. of gemellus superior.
15. N. of gemellus inferior.
16. N. of quadratus femoris.
17. N. of glutæus maximus.
18. Long pudendal n.
19. Cutaneous n. of the buttock.
20. N. of the long head of the biceps.
21. N. of semi-tendinosus.
22. N. of semi-membranosus.
23. N. of short head of the biceps.

1, 2, 3, 4, 5. Sacral nn.
6. Superior glutæal n.
7. Great ischiatic n.
8. Lesser ischiatic n.
9. Pudic n.
10. N. of obturator internus.
11. N. of levator ani.

PLAN OF THE SACRAL PLEXUS AND BRANCHES.

d. The *pudic* nerve runs with the pudic artery, and like it, supplies the rectum, the muscles of the perineum, and the penis.

e. The *branches for the pelvic viscera* are very small. They proceed chiefly from the third and fourth sacral nerves, and form an intricate plexus about the bladder, prostate, and rectum.

Sympathetic nerve.   From the lumbar region the sympathetic nerve descends into the pelvis, along the inner side of the sacral foramina. In this part of its course its ganglia vary in number from three to five. The nerves of opposite sides unite in front of the coccyx, where they form the 'ganglion impar.'

The plan upon which the sympathetic nerves are distributed in the pelvis is similar to that in the abdomen. Each ganglion receives one or two filaments from a spinal nerve, and then gives off its branches to the viscera. The visceral branches are exceedingly delicate, and cannot be traced unless the parts have been previously hardened in spirit. They accompany the arteries supplying the respective organs, and are called the 'vesical,' 'prostatic,' and 'inferior hæmorrhoidal plexuses;' and in the female the 'uterine' and 'vaginal.'

According to the accurate dissections of Müller, the vesical filaments of the sympathetic do not stop at the prostate, but pass on beneath the pubic arch into the corpus cavernosum penis. Thus the erectile tissue of the intromittent organ is brought directly within the influence of the sympathetic system.

STRUCTURE OF THE BLADDER, PROSTATE, URETHRA, AND PENIS.

The parts are presumed to have been collectively taken out from the pelvis, and the partial peritoneal covering of the bladder to have been removed.

Structure of the bladder. The bladder is composed of a partial peritoneal coat, a muscular, and a mucous; these latter are connected by an intermediate layer of cellular tissue, out of which anatomists make a fourth coat, and call it the cellular.

The serous or peritoneal coat invests the posterior, lateral, and superior surfaces of the bladder; being absent on the anterior and inferior aspect.

The muscular is situated beneath the serous, and consists of unstriped or involuntary muscular fibres, which interlace with each other in all directions. Their general arrangement is as follows:—An outer, or longitudinal, layer arises from the upper half of the circumference of the prostate and the neck of the

bladder, and thence its fibres spread out longitudinally over the summit of the bladder, pass round its posterior aspect and base, to be inserted into the prostate in the male, and the vagina in the female. This layer is especially marked on the anterior and posterior surfaces of the bladder. Under this is a layer of *circular fibres*, especially developed near the neck. Towards the sides of the bladder the two sets of fibres have a less definite arrangement, and form a kind of network: these, therefore, are the weakest parts of the bladder, and more liable to the formation of pouches.*
The development and colour of the muscular fibres depend upon whether the subject has suffered from irritation of the bladder, or any obstruction to the expulsion of the urine.

The cellular coat serves to connect the muscular to the mucous, and is composed of ordinary connective tissue. The mucous coat is everywhere loosely connected to the muscular, except opposite the '*trigone*,' where they adhere more firmly.

The bladder must be laid open by an incision along its front surface, to examine its interior. In a recently contracted bladder, the mucous membrane is disposed in irregular folds, which disappear when the bladder is distended. In a healthy state, it is pale; when inflamed it becomes of a bright red. Under the microscope, its surface is seen to be studded with follicles. These follicles secrete the thick ropy mucus in inflammation of the bladder.

The epithelium lining the mucous membrane varies in different parts of the bladder. Part is squamous; part consists of a variety transitional between squamous and columnar.

The *orifice of the urethra* is situated at the lower and anterior part of the bladder, not at the most dependent part, which forms

* These pouches arise in the following manner:—A portion of mucous membrane is protruded through one of the muscular interstices, so as to form a little sac. This is small at first, but gradually increases in size, because, having no muscular coat, it has no power of emptying itself; generally speaking, several such sacs are met with in the same bladder; and they sometimes contain calculi. If a calculus, originally loose in the bladder, happen to become lodged in a pouch by the side of it, a sudden remission of the symptoms may ensue. This explains our inability to detect its presence by a wound.

Fig. 86.

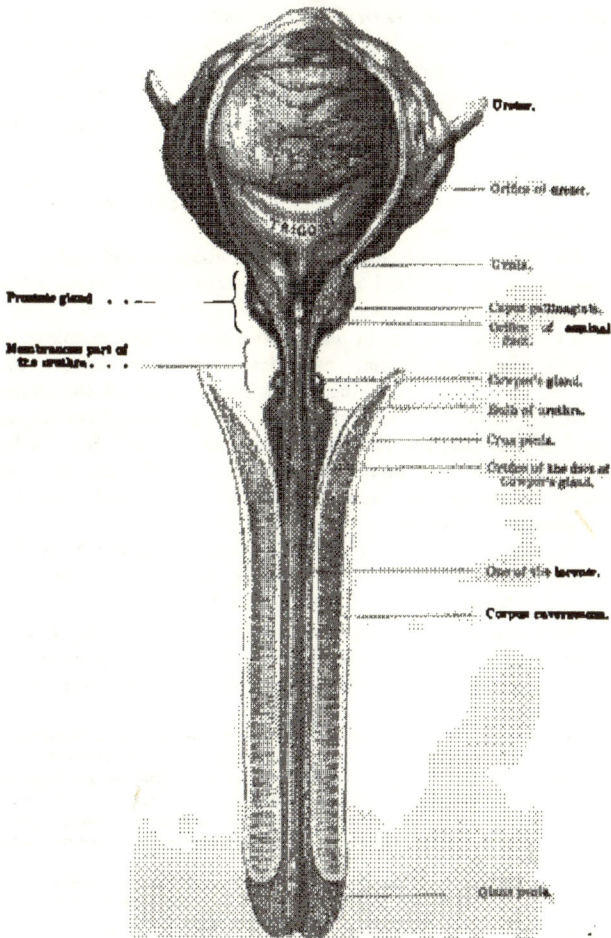

BLADDER AND URETHRA LAID OPEN BY AN INCISION ALONG ITS UPPER SURFACE.

the well behind the orifice, in which urine is apt to accumulate in old persons.   It appears small and contracted in the fresh bladder, but if the little finger be introduced into it, we find that it will dilate to a very considerable size.   Immediately behind the orifice is observed in some bladders a slight elevation, called the ' *uvula*.' It is composed of a portion of the mucous membrane raised up by an accumulation of the submucous tissue, and is rarely of sufficient size to interfere with the passage of the urine.   This elevation must be distinguished from enlargement of the third or middle lobe of the prostate.

The *orifices of the ureters* are situated about an inch and a half behind the urethra, and about two inches apart.   These tubes perforate the coats of the bladder obliquely, and slant towards each other, standing out in relief under the mucous membrane.* A little ridge proceeds from the orifice of each ureter down to the neck of the bladder, looking like a continuation of the ureter itself.   If the mucous membrane be removed from these ridges, we find that they are produced by muscular fibres.   Sir Charles Bell,† who first drew attention to them, believed them to be of use in regulating the orifices of the ureters, and named them ' *the muscles of the ureters.*'

The ridges, converging from the ureters, together with an imaginary horizontal line, drawn between their orifices, include a smooth triangular area, called, by the French anatomists, the ' *trigone vesicale.*'   The mucous membrane of this area is more firmly adherent to the subjacent tissue than in other parts of the bladder, and is therefore perfectly smooth.   It is more richly

---

* This slanting of the ureters serves all the uses of a valve.   The urine enters the bladder, drop by drop, but cannot return, because the internal coat is pressed against the other side of the orifice, so as to stop it.   When the bladder becomes thickened, in consequence of difficulty in passing the water, it sometimes happens that the ureters lose their valvular direction, so that the urine, when the bladder contracts, is partly forced back up the ureters; the result is, that they become dilated, and so does the pelvis of the kidney.

† Med. Chir. Trans. vol. iii.   He says, ' These muscles guard the orifices of the ureters by preserving the obliquity of the passage, and pulling down the extremities of the ureters according to the degree of the contraction of the bladder generally.'

provided with blood vessels and nerves than the rest of the bladder, and is endowed with more acute sensibility. This is the reason why a stone is more painful when the bladder is empty; and in the erect, than in the recumbent position.

The bladder is supplied with blood by the 'superior,' 'middle,' and 'inferior' vesical arteries. The superior comes from the unobliterated portion of the umbilical; the middle from the superior vesical or the internal iliac; the inferior from the anterior division of the internal iliac or the pudic.

The vesical plexus of veins terminates in the internal iliac vein.*

The nerves of the bladder are derived from the hypogastric and sacral plexuses.

Prostate. Having already examined the form, size, and relations of the prostate (p. 385), you have now to make out its two lateral symmetrical lobes. There is, also, a third or middle lobe.† It unites the lateral lobes, and is situated above the seminal ducts. In health, this does not appear like a separate lobe; but when abnormally enlarged, it projects towards the cavity of the bladder, and acts like a bar at the mouth of the urethra.

Make a longitudinal incision through the upper surface of the prostate to expose the urethra. The canal does not run exactly in the centre of the gland, but rather nearer to its upper surface; nor is it of the same calibre throughout. It forms a 'sinus' in the interior of the prostate, described by anatomists as the '*sinus of the prostate.*' Along the floor of the sinus is a longitudinal ridge, about three quarters of an inch in length, broad and elevated behind, but gradually lost forwards in a narrow point. This is

---

* The attention of the student should be directed to the very admirable injections of the veins of the bladder by Pettigrew, in the Museum of the Royal College of Surgeons.

† Attention was first attracted to this middle lobe, in England, by Sir Everard Home, whose account of it is published in the Philos. Trans. for 1806. The preparation prepared by Sir Everard in illustration is preserved in the Museum of the Royal College of Surgeons in London, Physiol. Series, No. 2583 A. But the anatomy and effect of the enlargement of this part of the prostate gland is not a discovery of modern times. It was accurately described by Santorini in 1739, and subsequently by Camper, and is alluded to by Morgagni in the third book of his Epistles.

called the crest of the urethra, and the most prominent part of it is named the 'veru montanum,' or 'caput gallinaginis,' from its supposed resemblance to the head of a woodcock. The seminal ducts open close to each other, one on either side of this prominence (p. 394).

Immediately in front of the caput gallinaginis, precisely in the middle line, is a small opening which will admit a probe. It leads backwards into a little 'cul-de-sac' or pouch in the substance of the prostate. This pouch is described as the analogue of the uterus, and called the 'utriculus' or 'sinus pocularis.' It is of a pyriform shape, with the narrowest part at the orifice, and its length is about five or six lines. Practically it deserves attention, because in some persons it is large enough to catch the end of a small catheter. The minute orifices of the proper ducts of the prostate, from fifteen to twenty in number, are seen opening into the floor of the prostatic sinus.* The whole substance of the gland is permeated by the divisions and subdivisions of the ducts. They are not visible to the naked eye, but if traced out with the microscope, they are seen to terminate in blind sacculated extremities, upon which the capillaries ramify in rich profusion.†

Modern observations prove that the prostate is more of a muscular than a glandular body. Nearly two-thirds of it is made up of muscular fibre of the non-striped variety. The great mass of this muscular fibre is arranged in a circular manner round the urethra, so as to form a sphincter. The prostate is remarkable for its dilatability. If a small incision be made through the anterior part of the gland, the *base being left entire*, the gland may be dilated

* In the ducts of the prostate we often find small calculi, of a brown colour, consisting of phosphate of lime. Cases are sometimes met with in which these calculi by degrees attain a considerable size, and distend the prostate into a kind of sac, which when examined by the rectum feels not unlike a bag of marbles.

† This was first demonstrated by Mr Quekett. The same distinguished anatomist has also discovered that the secreting cells of the gland contain calculi of microscopic minuteness. He finds them, almost without exception, in the prostate at every period of life. For further detail concerning them consult the article 'Prostate' in Todd's Cyclopædia.

by the finger sufficiently to admit the extraction of even large
calculi.

Any change in the dimensions of the prostate must affect the
canal which runs through it, and more or less obstruct the flow of
urine. If the entire gland be uniformly enlarged, the length of
the prostatic urethra will be increased; if the enlargement pre-
ponderate at one part more than another, then the canal will
deviate more or less from its natural track and assume a more
angular or a lateral curve according to the part enlarged. When
the middle lobe becomes enlarged, there arises, at the neck of the
bladder, a growth, which will, in proportion to its size, more or less
obstruct the passage of the urine. In the efforts made to introduce a catheter into the bladder, it sometimes happens that the
end of the instrument is pushed through this hypertrophied lobe.[*]

Vesica
seminales.

The external appearance of these bodies has been
already described (p. 384). Respecting their structure,
we find that they have an external coat derived from
the pelvic fascia; a middle or fibrous, strong and somewhat elastic,
and an internal or mucous. The mucous membrane is lined by a
scaly epithelium, and presents a beautiful honey-comb structure, not
unlike that of the gall-bladder: the purpose of this is to increase
the extent of the secreting surface. According to some anatomists,
muscular fibres are present in the fibrous investment of the vesiculæ
seminales, for the purpose of expelling their contents. The duct
emerges from the anterior part of the vesicula, and joins at an
acute angle the vas deferens behind the prostate, to form the
common ejaculatory duct (p. 361). The function of these bodies
is twofold: they act as reservoirs for the semen, and secrete a fluid
accessory to generation.

Cowper's
glands.

The glands of Cowper have been examined in situ in
the dissection of the perineum (p. 374). We find them
close to the urethra, one on either side, immediately
behind the bulb and between the two layers of the triangular
ligament. They consist of an aggregation of smaller glands, of

* See the Museum of St. Bartholomew's, Prep. 6 and 21, Series xxix.

which the collective size is somewhat larger than a pea. Each pours its secretion by a single and very minute duct about one inch long into the bulbous part of the urethra. The use of these glands appears to be like that of the vesiculæ seminales and the prostate; namely, to pour into the urethra a fluid accessory in some way to generation. They are found in all mammalia, and in some, e.g. the mole, they increase in size periodically with the testicle.

Urethra. The urethra is the tube which leads from the bladder to the end of the penis, and serves not only as the excretory duct of the bladder, but transmits the secretion of the testicles and the several glands accessory to generation. It is surrounded by different structures in different parts of its course. The first inch, or thereabouts, is surrounded by the prostate gland (p. 361); the second inch, which passes under the pubic arch, is surrounded by the compressor urethræ (p. 372); the remainder of its course along the penis is surrounded by erectile tissue, termed 'corpus spongiosum.' Hence it is divided into the prostatic, the muscular or membranous, and the spongy. The length of the whole is about seven or eight inches, but this varies according to the condition of the penis.

The direction of the urethra, when the penis hangs flaccid, is like the letter S reversed; but if the penis be held straight, the canal forms only one curve through the pubic arch, with the concavity upwards. The degree of this curvature varies at different periods of life. In the child, the bladder being more in the abdomen than in the pelvis, the curve forms part of a much smaller circle than in the adult; but it gradually widens as age increases, and catheters are shaped accordingly.[*] However, the parts, when in a sound state, will yield sufficiently to admit the introduction of a straight instrument into the bladder. Aston Key always used a straight staff in lithotomy.

In its contracted state, the sides of the urethra are in close appo-

---

[*] The sharper curve of the urethra in the child was well known to Camper. 'In recenter natis, vesica basi sua elatius sita, pedetentim descendit, unde necessario sequitur curvaturam urethræ majorem esse in junioribus quam in adultis.'—Demon. Anat. Pathol. lib. ii. p. 13.

sition; the appearance it presents on a transverse section differs in
the different parts of its course. Through the glans it is flattened
vertically, its two sides being in contact; through the prostate, also,
it is nearly flat, except at the lower part, where its sides are kept
asunder by the verumontanum, which projects upwards, fitting accurately between them.* But throughout the rest of its course the
lining membrane is disposed in longitudinal folds, which project
into and accurately close the canal, precisely on the same plan as
that by which nature closes the œsophagus (p. 124). These longitudinal folds are plainly seen even when the urethra is slit open;
indeed, they do not disappear unless the canal be forcibly stretched
contrary to their direction.†

The urethra must be laid open from end to end, to see that the
canal is not of uniform calibre throughout. The external orifice
is the narrowest, and the least dilatable part; so that the urine
may be expelled in a jet. Therefore, any instrument which will
enter the meatus ought to pass into the bladder, if there be no
stricture. The junction of the membranous with the bulbous part
is almost as narrow. The centre of the prostatic and the bulbous
parts are the largest. In the centre of the glans penis, the canal
widens into a little sinus, termed 'fossa navicularis.'

The most *dilatable* part of the urethra is the prostatic. Even
the narrowest parts of the canal must admit of considerable dilatation, since calculi of from 3 to 4 lines in diameter have been
known to pass through it.

The seminal ducts open into the prostatic part of the urethra,
by the side of the verumontanum. The ducts of Cowper's glands
open into the bulbous part. Besides these glands, a number of
ducts open into the urethra, proceeding from little glands situated
in the submucous tissue. These ducts, called 'lacunæ,' are large
enough to admit a bristle, and run in the same direction as the

---

* See the transverse sections made by Pettigrew through the prostatic part of the
urethra in the Museum of the Royal College of Surgeons.

† In a well-injected urethra we observe that the ridges of the folds possess very few
blood vessels, while the furrows between them are exceedingly vascular. For the demonstration of this fact the author is indebted to Mr. Quekett.

stream of the urine. Most of them are on the lower surface of the urethra; but one called 'lacuna magna' is on the upper surface about 1½ inch down the canal.

The mucous membrane of the urethra is laid upon a substratum of areolar tissue. Then comes a thin layer of elastic fibrous tissue, of which the fibres are arranged in a longitudinal and a transverse direction—giving the parts that springiness of which we are sensible in introducing the catheter. Outside this is a layer of muscular fibre. It has been demonstrated that the urethra is surrounded throughout its whole course by muscular fibres of the involuntary kind. Therefore, the whole of the canal having a muscular coat, similar to an intestine, any part of it is liable to spasmodic contraction.

The urethra is lined by spheroidal epithelium, and near the glans is provided with papillæ: this, therefore, is the most sensitive part.

Lastly, the urethra is provided with a closely-set network of absorbent vessels,—a fact which has been demonstrated by the beautiful quicksilver injections of Panizza.[*] They run from behind, forwards, and join the absorbents of the glans penis. Eventually, their contents are transmitted down the great trunks on the dorsum penis to the inguinal glands. This explains the pathology of a bubo.

Anatomy of the penis.
The skin of the penis is remarkably thin and extensible, and connected to the body of the organ by loose cellular tissue, destitute of fat. At the extremity, the skin forms the prepuce, or foreskin, for the protection of the glans;[†] and the thin fold which passes from the under surface of

---

[*] Osservazioni antropo-zootom. &c., Pavia, 1830. This anatomist has also displayed by injections an extremely fine network of absorbents which cover the glans penis. The interstices of this network are smaller than the diameter of the tubes.

[†] When the foreskin is, from birth, so tight that the glans cannot be uncovered, such a state is called a 'congenital phimosis.' This condition occasions no inconvenience in childhood, but is apt, after puberty, to become troublesome and painful, so that it may become necessary to slit up the prepuce and set the glans at liberty. In persons who have a tight foreskin, it sometimes happens that, when the glans has been uncovered, the prepuce cannot be again drawn over it: this is called a 'paraphymosis.' The neck of the glans becomes tightly girt; great distension and inflammation are the consequences, and serious results may ensue, unless the foreskin be reduced.

the glans to the prepuce is called '*frenum preputii*.' The skin
is reflected over the glans, to which it adheres closely, and at the
orifice of the urethra is continuous with the mucous membrane.

The surface of the glans is covered, like the end of the finger,
by minute papillæ, which are endowed with keen sensibility by
the dorsal nerves of the penis. Round its margin—termed the
'*corona glandis*'—are a number of minute sebaceous glands,
which secrete a substance called 'smegma preputii.'

The bulk of the penis consists of two cylindrical bodies, of
erectile structure, named from the appearance of their interior
'*corpora cavernosa*.' In a groove along their under surface runs
the urethra, which is itself surrounded by a vascular spongy tissue
called '*corpus spongiosum*;' an expansion of this at the end of
the organ forms the glans. These structures, then—the corpora
cavernosa and the corpus spongiosum—together form the penis;
though the corpus spongiosum appears closely united to the
corpora cavernosa, yet it is quite distinct from them, as shown in
the transverse section (p. 403).

The corpora cavernosa constitute more than two-thirds of the
bulk of the penis. Each commences posteriorly by a gradually
tapering portion, called the '*crus penis*,' which is attached along
a groove in the rami of the ischium and pubes. The crura
converge, come into apposition at the root of the penis, and then
run on, side by side, to form the body of the organ. Anteriorly,
each terminates in a rounded end, received into a corresponding
depression in the glans, which fits on like a cap.

The upper part of the penis is connected to the symphysis pubis
by an elastic triangular ligament, called '*ligamentum suspensorium
penis*.'

In a longitudinal section through the corpus cavernosum, we
observe that its interior is composed of a delicate reticular
structure, surrounded by a thick fibrous coat. This coat is from
half a line to a line in thickness, and is composed of white fibrous
tissue intermingled with yellow elastic fibres. It forms a cylinder
of adequate strength to support the delicate structure within, and
sufficiently elastic to allow the distention of the penis. This coat,

also, forms a median vertical partition between the two corpora cavernosa.

The partition is only complete near the root of the penis; along the rest of the organ there are gaps in it, giving it the appearance of a comb; hence its name '*septum pectiniforme.*' Through this partition the blood vessels on one side communicate freely with those on the other.

Fig. 87.

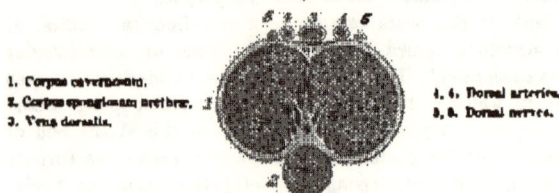

1. Corpus cavernosum.
2. Corpus spongiosum urethrae.
3. Vena dorsalis.

4, 4. Dorsal arteries.
5, 5. Dorsal nerves.

TRANSVERSE SECTION THROUGH THE PENIS.

The interior of each cylinder is occupied by a number of delicate elastic fibrous septa ('trabeculi'), which intersect each other in all directions, and form a multitude of minute cells. These communicate freely with each other, as may be readily ascertained by blowing air into the penis. They are not of equal size throughout the penis; they are smaller, and their component septa thicker at the circumference than in the centre of the corpora cavernosa; at the root, than towards the glans. All the cells communicate freely with the arteries. When the penis is flaccid, they are empty; when it is erect, they are distended with blood.

The arteries of the corpora cavernosa come from the pudic, enter the inner side of each crus, and proceed forwards near the septum, distributing numerous ramifications. These are supported in the middle of the fibrous septa, and end, some in capillaries which discharge their blood at once into the cells, others in tendril-like prolongations with dilated extremities which project into the cavities of the veins. These arteries (called '*helicine*' by Müller) are absent near the glans, and are best marked at the root of the penis.

The blood from the cells of the penis returns partly through veins which pass out on the upper surface of the penis into the great dorsal vein, which joins the prostatic plexus; partly through the deep veins which leave the inner side of each crus, and the bulb, to join the internal iliac.

The corpus spongiosum is the erectile tissue which
Corpus spon-
giosum. surrounds the urethra as it runs along the penis. It
commences in the middle of the perineum, in a bulb-like form, and at the end of the penis it expands to form the glans. This is proved by the fact, that if the spongy body be injected, the glans is filled also; not so, if we inject the cavernous body. The urethra does not pass exactly through the middle of the spongy body, but runs nearer to its upper surface. The bulb hangs more or less pendulous from the urethra (p. 361). In old persons it extends lower down than in children, and is, consequently, more exposed to injury in lithotomy.

The corpus spongiosum has a much thinner external coat than the corpus cavernosum, but resembles it very much in its internal appearance. The reticular structure, however, is somewhat finer and more delicate. Its interior is composed of a plexus of minute tortuous veins. This is easily demonstrated by injecting the dorsal vein of the penis with wax. In this way we not only fill the spongy body, but also the glans and the large veins which form the plexus round the corona glandis.*

The chief nerves of the penis are the pudic. The largest branches run along the dorsum to the outside of the glans: a few only enter the erectile tissue of the organ. This, it has already been mentioned (p. 392), is supplied by filaments of the sympathetic nerve proceeding from the hypogastric plexus.

The absorbent vessels proceeding from the glans and the integument of the penis join the inguinal glands. The absorbents of the glans communicate freely all round it : this explains why a venereal sore on one side, sometimes affects the inguinal glands on the other.

* In the Museum of the Royal College of Surgeons there is a beautiful preparation in which the glans penis is injected with quicksilver, clearly showing it to consist of a plexus of veins.—Physiol. Series, No. 2588 A.

THE DISSECTION OF THE FEMALE PERINEUM.

The *pudenda* in the female consist of folds of the integument, called the labia. Between these is a longitudinal fissure which leads to the orifices of the urinary and genital canals.

Labia
majora. The pubic region is generally covered by an accumulation of fat, called '*mons Veneris.*' From this, two thick folds of skin descend, one on either side, constituting the '*labia majora.*' Their junction, about one inch above the anus, is called the commissure, or '*frenulum labiorum:*' it is generally torn in the first labour. The inner layer of the skin of the labium is thinner, softer, and more like mucous membrane than the outer: for this reason, whenever matter forms in the labium, the abscess bursts on the inner side. Where the labia are in contact, they are provided with small sebaceous glands, of which the minute ducts are observable on the surface. These glands sometimes inflame and secrete an acrid matter which creates great irritation and pruritus of the mucous surface of the vulva, often difficult to allay.

Labia
minora. By separating the external labia, two small and thin folds of integument are exposed, one on either side, termed '*labia minora,*' or, by the old anatomists, '*nymphæ.*' These folds converge anteriorly, and form a hood for the clitoris, called '*preputium clitoridis;*' posteriorly they are gradually lost on the inside of the labia majora. They never contain fat, like the labia majora, but are composed of a minute plexus of veins. Between the nymphæ and about the clitoris, are a number of sebaceous glands.

Between the labia minora, and below the clitoris, is an angular depression called the '*vestibule,*' at the back of which is the orifice of the urethra, or '*meatus urinarius.*' Immediately below this is the vagina, of which the orifice is partially closed in the virgin by a thin fold of mucous membrane called the '*hymen.*'

Clitoris. In form and structure the clitoris resembles the penis on a very diminutive scale; but there is no corpus spongiosum, or urethra. Like the penis, it is attached to the sides of the pubic arch by two crura (fig. 88, p. 407), each of which is grasped by its special *erector clitoridis*. The crura unite to form the body of the organ, which is tipped by a small glans. The glans is provided with extremely sensitive papillæ, and covered by a little prepuce. Its dorsal arteries and nerves are exceedingly large in proportion to its size, and have precisely the same course and distribution as in the penis. Its internal structure consists of a plexus of blood vessels, which freely communicate with those of the labia minora, for one cannot be injected without the other.

Urethra. A smooth channel called the vestibule, three-quarters of an inch in length, leads from the clitoris down to the orifice of the urethra. This orifice is not a perpendicular fissure like that of the penis, but rounded and puckered, and during life it has a peculiar dimple-like feel, which assists us in finding it when we pass a catheter. You should practice the introduction of the catheter in the dead subject, for the operation is not so easy as might at first be imagined, provided the parts are not exposed. The point of the fore-finger of the left hand should be placed at the entrance of the vagina, and the meatus felt for; when the catheter, guided by the finger, slips, after a little manœuvring, into the urethra. The canal is about one inch and a half in length, and runs along the upper wall of the vagina (p. 410). The two canals adhere so closely together that you can feel the urethra through the vagina like a thick cord. The urethra is slightly curved with the concavity upwards; but for all practical purposes it may be considered straight. Its direction, however, is not horizontal. In the unimpregnated state of the parts it runs nearly in the direction of the axis of the outlet of the pelvis; so that a probe pushed on in the course of the urethra would strike against the promontory of the sacrum. But after impregnation, when the uterus begins to rise out of the pelvis, the bladder is more or less raised also in consequence of their mutual connection; therefore the urethra, in the latter months of utero-gestation, acquires a much more perpendicular course.

The female urethra is provided with a 'compressor' muscle,

essentially similar, in origin and arrangement, to that which surrounds the membranous part of the urethra in the male. It also passes through the triangular ligament (fig. 89, p. 410). Though the prostate gland is wanting, yet there are minute glands scattered all round it, especially near the neck of the bladder. In consequence of the wider span of the pubic arch, and the more yielding nature of the surrounding structures, the female urethra is much more dilatable than the male. By means of a sponge tent, it may be safely dilated to admit the easy passage of the fore-finger into the bladder. Advantage is taken of this great dilatability in the extraction of calculi from the bladder.

The mucous coat of the urethra is arranged in longitudinal folds,

Fig. 89.

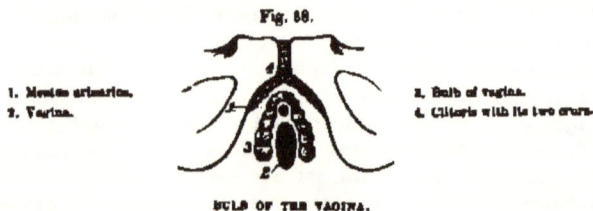

1. Meatus urinarius.
2. Vagina.
3. Bulb of vagina.
4. Clitoris with its two crura.

BULB OF THE VAGINA.

and is lined by squamous epithelium, which changes to the spheroidal variety near the bladder. Next to the mucous coat is a layer of elastic and non-striped muscular fibres intermixed. Outside all is a plexus of veins bearing a strong resemblance to erectile tissue.

Vagina.   The vagina is the canal which leads to the uterus; at present, only the orifice of it can be seen. It is surrounded by a sphincter muscle, easily displayed by removing the integument. The muscle is about three-fourths of an inch broad, and connected with the cutaneous sphincter of the anus in such a manner that they together form something like the figure 8.

Bulb of the vagina.   On each side of the orifice of the vagina, between the mucous membrane and the sphincter, is a plexus of tortuous veins, termed the bulb of the vagina, from its

analogy to the bulb of the urethra in the male. This vaginal bulb
extends across the middle line between the meatus urinarius and
the clitoris, as shown in fig. 88, which was taken from an injected
preparation in the Musée Orfila at Paris.

Hymen.   The hymen is a thin fold of mucous membrane which,
in the virgin, extends across the lower part of the entrance of the vagina, about half an inch behind the fourchette.
In most instances its form is crescent-shaped, with the concavity
upwards. There are several varieties of hymen; sometimes there
are two folds, one on either side, so as to make the entrance of the
vagina a mere vertical fissure; * or there may be a septum perforated by several openings (*Hymen cribriformis*), or by one only
(*Hymen circularis*). Again, there may be no opening at all in it,
and then it is called *Hymen imperforatus*. Under this last
condition no inconvenience arises till puberty. The menstrual
discharge must then necessarily accumulate in the vagina: indeed,
the uterus itself may become distended by it to such an extent as
even to simulate pregnancy.†

The presence of the hymen is not necessarily a proof of
virginity, nor does its absence imply the loss of it. Cases are
related by writers on midwifery in which a division of the hymen
was requisite to facilitate parturition. In Meckel's Museum, at
Halle, are preserved the external organs of a female in whom the
hymen is perfect even after the birth of a seven-months' child.

Bartholin's or Duverney's glands.   At the lower part of the orifice of the vagina is
imbedded, in the loose tissue on either side, a small
gland,‡ which corresponds to Cowper's gland in the
male. Each has a long slender duct, which runs forwards and
opens on the inner side of the nympha. In cases of virulent
gonorrhœa these glands are apt to become diseased, and give rise
to the formation of an abscess in the labium, very difficult to
heal.

The description of the perineal branches of the pudic vessels

* Such an one may be seen in the Museum of the College. Phys. Series, No. 2813.
† See Burns' Midwifery.
‡ See Tiedemann, Von den Duverneyschen Drüsen des Weibs. Heidelberg. 1840.

and nerves, given in the dissection of the male perineum, applies, *mutatis mutandis*, to the female, excepting that they are proportionably small, and that the artery which supplies the bulb of the urethra in the male is distributed to the bulb of the vagina in the female.

DISSECTION OF THE FEMALE PELVIS.

The internal organs of generation, viz., the vagina, uterus, and its appendages, should now be examined.

Their relative position should first be noticed; and afterwards, their special anatomy.

General position of the uterus and its appendages.
The uterus is interposed between the bladder in front, and the rectum behind. From each side of it a broad fold of peritoneum extends transversely to the side of the pelvis, dividing that cavity into an anterior and a posterior part. These folds are called the *broad ligaments* of the uterus (fig. 90, p. 419). On the posterior surface of the ligament are the ovaries, one on each side. They are completely covered by peritoneum, and suspended to the ligament by a small peritoneal fold. Each ovary is attached to the uterus by a round cord termed the '*ligament of the ovary*.' Along the upper part of the broad ligament we find between its layers a tube about four inches long, called the Fallopian tube, which conveys the ovum from the ovary into the uterus. For this purpose, one end of it terminates in the uterus, while that nearer to the ovary expands into a wide mouth, furnished with prehensile fringes—'*fimbriæ*'—which, like so many fingers, grasp the ovum as soon as it is ready to escape from the ovary. One of these fimbriæ is attached to the ovary Lastly, there run up to the ovary, between the layers of the broad ligament, the ovarian vessels and nerves, which arise from the aorta in the lumbar region, like the spermatic arteries in the male, because the ovaries are originally formed in the loins.

On the anterior surface of the broad ligament, you see, on either side between its layers, the *round ligament* of the uterus. This cord proceeds from the fundus of the uterus, anterior to the Fallopian tube, through the inguinal canal, like the spermatic cord in the male, and terminates in the 'mons Veneris.' Besides one or two small blood vessels, it contains muscular fibres analogous to those of the uterus: these increase very much in pregnancy, so that, about the full term, the cord becomes nearly as thick as the end of the little finger.

Side view of the female pelvis.

After the removal of the innominate bone, as described at p. 376, the vagina, rectum, and bladder should be moderately distended, and a catheter passed

Fig. 89.

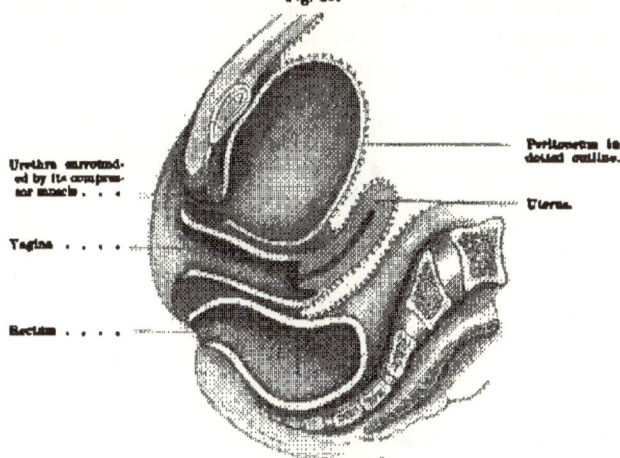

Urethra surrounded by its compressor muscle . . .

Peritoneum in dotted outline.

Uterus.

Vagina . . . .

Rectum . . . .

VERTICAL SECTION THROUGH THE FEMALE PELVIS.

into the urethra. This done, the reflections of the peritoneum must be traced.

Reflections of the peritoneum.

From the front of the rectum the peritoneum is reflected on to a small part of the vagina, thus forming what is called the 'recto-vaginal pouch.' From the vagina we trace the peritoneum over all the *back*, but only about half way down the *front* of the uterus; thence it is at once reflected over the posterior surface of the bladder, on to the wall of the abdomen. Laterally it is reflected from the uterus to the sides of the pelvis, forming the broad ligaments (p. 419).

In cases of ascites the fluid might distend the recto-vaginal pouch, and bulge into the vagina, so that it would be practicable, in some cases, to draw it off through this channel.*

Pelvic fascia.   To the description of the fascia already given in the dissection of the male pelvis (p. 378), nothing need be added except that from the side of the pelvis it is reflected over the side of the vagina and the uterus as well as the bladder.

It is this fascia which in great measure supports and braces up the uterus in its proper level in the pelvis. When, from any cause, the fascia becomes relaxed, there is a liability to 'prolapsus uteri.'

Levator ani.   For the description of this muscle see p. 386.

Bladder.   The female bladder is broader transversely, and, upon the whole, more capacious than the male. The vesical plexus of veins is not so large, and there are no vasa deferentia or prostate gland. The short urethra has a constrictor muscle, as in the male, and is supported in a similar manner by the pelvic fascia.

Venous plexus about the vagina.   Though the veins round the neck of the bladder are comparatively small in the female, attention should be directed to the plexus of large veins which surround the vagina and the rectum. They communicate in front with the vesical plexus, and behind with the hæmorrhoidal. Their congestion in pregnancy sufficiently accounts for the dark colour of the vagina and the external organs, and the frequent occurrence of hæmorrhoidal tumours.† These veins must be removed, with

---

* In the Medical Communications, vol. i., a case is related in which four gallons of fluid were drawn off by tapping through the vagina. The woman immediately afterwards passed urine, which she could not do before. See also a case in Med. and Phys. Journal, vol. vii. p. 412.

† During pregnancy, varicose tumours may form even in the vagina. In the Berlin Med. Zeitung, 1840, No. 11, a case is related of a woman who, at the sixth month, bled to death from the bursting of a large vein in the vagina. Other cases of the kind are related by Siebold.

the cellular tissue in which they are imbedded, before a clear view
of the parts can be obtained.

Urethra.   The urethra has already been described (p. 406). But
in the side view of the parts, we have the opportunity of
observing how closely the bladder and urethra are connected to the
upper wall of the vagina; and we can understand how, in cases of
protracted delivery, it sometimes happens that the contiguous coats
of the bladder and the vagina give way, and that there remains
a fistulous communication between them, which continues to be
a depending drain for the urine.

Vagina.   It is necessary to slit open the whole of the vagina
along the side, to obtain a clear idea of the manner in
which it embraces the lower end of the uterus, and of the extent to
which the neck of the uterus projects into it.

The length of the vagina, in the unimpregnated adult, is, on an
average, about 4½ inches. It may be more, or less; the difference
in each case depending upon the depth of the pelvis, the stature
and age of the individual. Owing to the curved direction of the
vagina, the anterior wall is about an inch shorter than the posterior.
The vagina, however, is never so long, that we cannot, during life,
feel the neck of the uterus projecting at the top of it; higher up,
or lower down, according to circumstances. For instance, it is a
little lower down in the erect than in the recumbent position; again,
in the early months of utero-gestation, the uterus descends a little
into the vagina, so that this canal becomes shorter: the reverse
holds good when the uterus begins to rise out of the pelvis.

The axis of the vagina is slightly curved with the concavity upwards; it corresponds with the axis of the outlet of the pelvis;
whereas, the axis of the uterus corresponds with that of the cavity
of the pelvis.

The width of the vagina is not uniform throughout. The narrowest part is at the orifice; it is also a little constricted round the
neck of the uterus. The widest part is about the middle: here a
transverse section through it presents the appearance of a broad
horizontal fissure. If therefore you would insert the bivalve speculum with the least amount of pain, the blades of the speculum

should be vertical when introduced into the orifice of the vagina, and afterwards turned horizontally.

Uterus.　　　The uterus is the receptacle which receives the ovum, retains it for nine months to bring it to maturity, and then expels it by virtue of its muscular walls. Its situation and peritoneal connections have been described (p. 409). We have now to notice that its axis slants forwards, so that, upon the whole, the axis of the vagina and uterus describes a curve nearly parallel to the axis of the pelvis. The uterus, then, is so placed that it is ready to rise out of the pelvis into the abdomen after the embryo has attained a certain size.

The uterus in the unimpregnated state is pyriform, or rather triangular with the angles rounded, and is somewhat flattened antero-posteriorly. Its average size is about three inches long, two inches broad, and one inch thick, at the upper part : but there is variety in this respect, arising from age, the effect of pregnancies, and other causes.

For convenience of description, the organ is divided into the fundus, the body, and the cervix. The term fundus is applied to that part which lies above the level of the Fallopian tubes, and is the broadest part of the viscus (p. 419). The body is the central part, while the cervix is the narrow part which projects into the vagina. The vagina is very closely attached round the neck of the uterus : observe that it is attached higher up behind than in front. The mouth of the uterus is at the apex of the neck. This is called the ' os uteri,' and by the old anatomists the ' os tincæ,' from its fancied resemblance to the mouth of a tench.

Postponing for the present the examination of the interior of the vagina and uterus, let us pass on to the vessels and nerves of these organs.

Uterine and vaginal arteries.　　In addition to the ovarian arteries (which correspond to the spermatic arteries in the male) given off from the abdominal aorta (p. 335), each internal iliac artery furnishes a branch to the uterus and another to the vagina.

The uterine artery proceeds from the anterior division of the internal iliac, towards the neck of the uterus, between the layers of the broad ligament, and then ascends tortuously by the side of the uterus, giving off numerous branches to it, which anastomose freely with each other. The fundus of the uterus is mainly supplied with branches from the ovarian arteries.

The *vaginal* artery ramifies along the side of the vagina, and sends branches to the lower part of the bladder and the rectum.

The veins, corresponding with the arteries, form the uterine and vaginal plexuses, which empty themselves into the internal iliac.

Nerves of the uterus.   The nerves of the uterus are derived from the third and fourth sacral nerves, and from the hypogastric plexus (p. 356). They accompany the blood vessels in the broad ligament to the neck of the uterus, and ascend with them along the sides of the organ.

Some very small filaments continue with the vessels, and form around them plexuses, upon which, according to the dissections of Mr. Beck,[*] minute ganglia are found. But most of the nerves soon leave the vessels, and, subdividing, sink into the substance of the uterus, chiefly about its neck and the lower part of its body. A branch may be traced passing up to the fundus of the uterus, and another to the Fallopian tube.

Whether the nerves of the uterus enlarge during pregnancy, like the arteries, is a question still undecided. Surgically speaking, the os uteri may be said to have no nerves; for it is insensible to the cautery and to the knife.

The *absorbent* vessels of the uterus are small in its unimpregnated state, but greatly increase in size when it is gravid. Those from the fundus and the ovaries proceed with the ovarian vessels to the lumbar glands; thus explaining the affection of these glands in ovarian disease. Those from the body and the lower part of the uterus accompany the uterine artery, and join the glands in the pelvis; some, however, run with the round ligament to the groin ; hence, in certain conditions of the uterus, the inguinal glands may be affected.

[*] Philosophical Transactions for 1816.

Structure of the vagina, uterus, ovaries, and Fallopian tubes.

The uterus, vagina, ovaries, and Fallopian tubes should now be collectively removed from the pelvis for the purpose of examining their internal structure.

The vagina having already been laid open (p. 412), we observe that it is lined by a mucous membrane of a pale rose colour; and that it is rough and furrowed, especially near the orifice. A more or less prominent ridge runs along its anterior; another, along its posterior wall. From either side of these, called *columnæ rugarum,* proceed a series of transverse ridges with rough, jagged margins directed forwards. They are well marked in virgins, but repeated parturition and increasing age gradually smooth them down. The use of the vaginal rugæ is to excite the sensibility of the glans in coition. They themselves also possess keen sensibility, being richly endowed with papillæ.

The mucous membrane has a thick lining of squamous epithelium, and in the submucous tissue is an abundant supply of muciparous glands, which increase in number and size towards the uterus.

The chief strength of the vagina depends upon a fibro-cellular coat, about one-twelth of an inch in thickness. If this coat be minutely injected, we find that it is composed mainly of the inosculations of blood vessels, so much so, that by some it is regarded as erectile tissue. In this coat, muscular fibres, longitudinal and circular, have been demonstrated. The orifice of the vagina is surrounded by a circular muscle, called '*sphincter vaginæ*' (p. 407).

Uterus.

Before the uterus is laid open, examine the shape of that portion of the neck which projects into the vagina. The back part of the cervix appears to project into the vagina more than the front; but this arises from the vagina being attached higher up behind it. If the vagina were cut away from the cervix, the anterior lip of the uterus would appear to project a trifle more than the posterior. For this reason, as well as on account of the natural slope forwards of the uterus, the front lip is always felt first in an examination per vaginam.* The length,

* This is the only way to reconcile the discrepancies one meets with in anatomical works, respecting the comparative length of the lips of the uterus. Kraus, Weber,

however, and the general appearance of the vaginal part of the
cervix vary according to the age of the individual; it is also considerably altered by parturition. In the adult virgin it is smooth
and round, and projects about half an inch: its mouth is a small
transverse fissure. But after parturition, it loses its plumpness,
the lips become flaccid and fissured, and the mouth larger than it
was before.[*]

The uterus must now be laid open by a longitudinal incision, to
examine its interior. In doing so, observe the thickness of its
walls, which is greatest towards the fundus. Before coming into
the proper cavity in the body of the uterus, you must slit up a
long narrow canal which leads up into it through the neck. This
canal is not of the same dimensions throughout: it is dilated in the
middle, and gradually narrows towards each end. The upper end,
which leads into the body of the uterus, is called ' os internum,'
the lower end, which leads into the vagina, ' os externum.' The
passage is called the ' canal of the cervix.' It remains unchanged
in pregnancy for some time after the cavity in the body has expanded, but gradually disappears with the increasing size of the
embryo.

The shape of the cavity in the body of the uterus is triangular,
with the apex towards the cervix. In a virgin uterus the cavity is
very small, and its sides are convex; but in a uterus which has
borne many children, the cavity has lost the convexity of its sides,
and has increased in capacity. Each angle at the base is somewhat prolonged, and leads to the minute opening of the Fallopian
tube. This prolongation of the angles is noticed more or less in

---

Hasch, and others, say the anterior is the longer; Mayer, Meckel, Quain, and others,
the posterior.

[*] Instances are recorded in which the neck of the uterus is preternaturally long. It
has been known to project even as much as an inch and a half into the vagina. In
such cases it gradually tapers, and terminates in a very narrow mouth. This is said
to be one cause of sterility, and it is recommended either to dilate the mouth, or to
cut off a portion of the neck. In support of this opinion, it is stated that Dupuytren
was once consulted by a lady on account of barrenness; finding the neck of the uterus
unnaturally elongated, he removed a portion of it, and in due time the lady became
pregnant. (Hyrtl, Handbuch der top. Anatom.)

different females, and is the last indication of the two horns of the uterus in some orders of mammalia.

The interior of the uterus is smooth at the fundus ; but the reverse at the cervix. Here there is a central longitudinal ridge, both in front and behind (as in the vagina) ; from these, other closely set oblique ridges curve off laterally, like the branches of a palm-tree. The old anatomists called it ' *arbor vitæ.*' The roughness produced by these ridges, occasions an impression as though we were touching cartilage when a metallic sound is introduced into the uterus.

The neck of the uterus is provided with small muciparous glands, of which the minute ducts open in the furrows between the ridges referred to. The secretion of these glands is glairy, albuminous, and slightly alkaline. Soon after conception, the secretion dries up so as to plug the mouth of the uterus, but shortly before and during parturition it is poured out in great quantity, to facilitate the passage of the child. It happens, occasionally that one or more of the ducts of these glands become obstructed, and then dilate into small transparent vesicles, which gradually rise to the surface and burst. These were first described by Naboth,[*] and supposed to be true ova : hence their name ' *ovula Nabothi.*'

The mucous membrane of the uterus is much more delicate than that of the vagina, with which it is continuous, and is closely united to the subjacent tissue. The greater part of it is lined by a columnar ciliated epithelium, but that which lines the cervix is squamous, like that of the vagina. Examined with a lens, the mucous membrane lining the body of the uterus is seen to be covered with minute follicles or tubes arranged at right angles to its surface. These follicles consist of simple tubes which pass outwards in a spirally coiled manner, some of them appearing branched and dilated at their extremities. These tubes become greatly developed shortly after impregnation, and are presumed to take an important part in the formation of the ' *membrana decidua.*'

The greater portion of the walls of the uterus consists of muscular fibres of the unstriped or involuntary kind, which are chiefly

* De sterilitate mulierum. Lips., 1707.

E E

aggregated at the fundus, and less so at the junction of the Fallopian tubes. The texture of these fibres is so close that in the unimpregnated uterus it is useless to attempt to make them out satisfactorily. The muscular fibres are arranged in three layers, external, middle, and internal. The *external* layer, placed immediately beneath the peritoneum, is thin, and its fibres run transversely round the uterus, some of them being continued into the round and broad ligaments. A band of longitudinal fibres passes from the anterior surface of the uterus round the fundus to its posterior aspect. The *middle* layer runs in all directions, and chiefly surrounds the blood vessels. The *internal* layer is composed mainly of concentric circles which surround the orifices of the Fallopian tubes; at the cervix its fibres are arranged transversely round it, forming a kind of sphincter. Upon the whole their collective disposition is such as to exert equal pressure on all sides, when called into operation.

At the same time that they expel the fœtus, the muscular fibres perform another very important function: they close the large venous sinuses developed for its nutrition. Therefore, little hæmorrhage accompanies the expulsion of the placenta, provided it have been attached to the fundus or the side of the uterus. But every one knows the danger of what is called '*placenta prævia.*' Here, the placenta, placed over the orifice of the uterus, is attached to a part of the organ which must of necessity expand during labour; and every uterine contraction increases, instead of checking, the bleeding. For the same reason, paralysis of the muscular fibres in immediate connection with the placenta, be it where it may, is likely to be a source of serious hæmorrhage in parturition.

Fallopian tubes.   The Fallopian tubes or oviducts are situated, one on each side, along the upper border of the broad ligament of the uterus, and convey the ovum from the ovary to the uterus (fig. 90). They are about four or five inches in length. One end opens into the uterus; the other terminates in a wide funnel-shaped mouth, surrounded by fringe-like processes called the '*fimbriated extremity.*' This termination of the Fal-

lopian tube extends about an inch beyond the ovary; and, by
floating it in water, one or two of the fimbriæ may be seen connected with the outer end of the ovary. If the Fallopian tube be
opened from the expanded end, and a probe introduced into it,
you will find that the tube runs very tortuously at first, then
straight into the uterus, gradually contracting in size, so that the
uterine orifice scarcely admits a bristle. Its mucous lining is
gathered into longitudinal wavy folds, especially at the ovarian
end, and is provided with a columnar ciliated epithelium. The
free end of the tube communicates with the cavity of the peritoneum. This is the only instance where a mucous membrane is

Fig. 90.

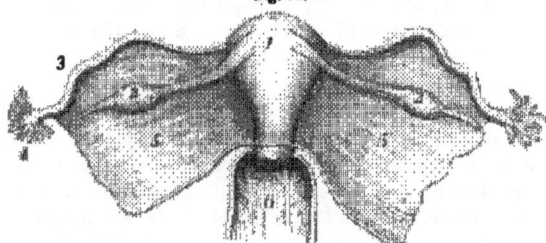

DIAGRAM OF THE UTERUS, ITS BROAD LIGAMENTS, THE OVARIES, AND FALLOPIAN TUBES.

1. Uterus.	4. Fimbriated extremity of Fallopian tube.
2. Ovary.	5. A. Broad ligament.
3. Fallopian tube.	6. Vagina.

directly continuous with a serous one. It explains how the embryo may escape into the peritoneal cavity; though this is an
extremely rare occurrence. It also explains what is said to have
occurred; namely, the escape of the fluid in dropsy through the
Fallopian tubes. In a well-injected subject, the Fallopian tubes are
seen to be well supplied with blood from the ovarian arteries.
They are provided with unstriped muscular fibres; the outer
layer being arranged longitudinally, the inner, in circles.

Ovaries.   The ovaries (called by Galen, '*testes muliebres* ')
                are suspended to the back of the broad ligament of the

uterus by a short peritoneal fold, which transmits their proper vessels and nerves: besides this, they are connected on their inner side to the uterus by a thin cord, called the *ligament* of the ovary. They are of an oblong form, with the long axis transverse, and a little smaller than the testicles. In females who have not often menstruated, their surface is smooth and even ; in after-life, they become puckered and scarred by the repeated escape of the ova.

The ovary is about an inch and a half long, and weighs about a drachm and a half. It has nearly the same coverings as the testicle ; viz. a serous coat, and beneath it a proper fibrous coat, the '*tunica albuginea.*' If a section be made through the ovary, you find that it contains transparent vesicles, embedded in a soft fibrous-looking tissue, remarkably vascular when well injected, called the '*stroma*' of the ovary. The outer part of the ovary is chiefly occupied by these vesicles; the central part, in which there are very few, is composed almost entirely of the stroma.

The transparent vesicles just alluded to are the *ovisacs* or '*Graafian*' [*] vesicles. They vary in number from eight to thirty, and in size from that of a pin's head to a pea. The smallest are near the centre ; but as they advance towards maturity, they gradually approach the surface, increasing at the same time in size. They contain a transparent albuminous fluid. On examining the contents of one of the larger vesicles under the microscope, you find in it the *ovum* or germ,[†] surrounded by a layer of granular cells called the '*discus proligerus.*' It is this ovum which, escaping from the Graafian vesicle on the surface of the ovary, is grasped by the Fallopian tube and conveyed into the uterus. The ruptured vesicle is converted soon afterwards into a yellowish-looking mass called '*corpus luteum,*' which persists for a while, and degenerates afterwards into a small fibrous cicatrix.

The ramifications of the ovarian artery through the ovary are remarkable for their convolutions : they run in parallel lines, as in the testicle. Its nerves are derived from the ovarian plexus.

---

[*] So called after De Graaf, a Dutch anatomist, who discovered them in 1672, and believed they were the true ova.

[†] This was first distinctly pointed out by Von Baer in 1827.

The ovarian veins terminate, like the spermatic in the male; the right in the vena cava, the left in the renal.

DISSECTION OF THE ABDOMINAL VISCERA.

The liver.   The liver is the largest gland in the body, and in the adult weighs from three to four pounds. Its surface is entirely covered by peritoneum, except a small part behind, which is connected to the diaphragm by cellular tissue, and in the hollow for the gall-bladder: behind, the liver is thick and round, but towards the front it gradually slopes to a thin border. The upper surface of the liver is smooth and convex, in adaptation to the diaphragm, and is marked by a white line which indicates its division into a right and left lobe, the right being the larger. The under surface is irregular and marked by five fissures and five lobes :—1. The *longitudinal fissure*, which divides the *Fissures.*   right from the left lobe, contains the round ligament (the remains of the umbilical vein). 2. The continuation of the longitudinal fissure to the posterior border of the liver, contains the remains of what was, in the foetus, the ductus venosus, and is therefore called the '*fissure of the ductus venosus.*' 3. The hollow or '*fissure for the gall-bladder.*' In the same line with this is, 4, the '*fissure of the inferior vena cava,*' which passes obliquely inwards towards the posterior border of the liver. 5. The '*transverse fissure*' unites the other fissures, and transmits the great vessels which enter the liver in the following order: in front is the hepatic duct, behind is the vena porta, and between them the hepatic artery. The relative position of these fissures may be best impressed on the memory by comparing them collectively to the letter H. The transverse fissure represents the cross-bar of the letter; the longitudinal fissure and the fissure of the ductus venosus represent the left bar; the fissures of the gall-bladder and vena cava make the right bar.

Lobes.   The lobes of the liver, five in number, are also seen on its under surface. The *right* lobe, much larger than the *left*, is separated from it by the longitudinal fissure. On the under surface of the right lobe are two shallow depressions; the anterior is for the colon, the posterior for the kidney. The remaining lobes may be considered as forming parts of the right lobe, and are, the *lobulus Spigelii*, the *lobulus caudatus*, and the *lobulus quadratus*. The lobulus Spigelii is placed between the fissures of the ductus venosus and vena cava; and behind the transverse fissure it is connected to the right lobe by a ridge—the lobulus caudatus. The lobulus quadratus is situated between the

Fig. 91.

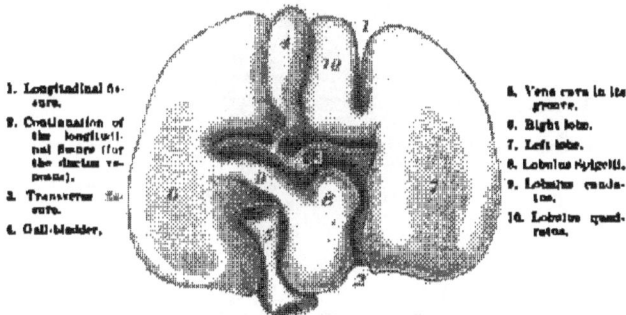

1. Longitudinal fissure.

2. Continuation of the longitudinal fissure (for the ductus venosus).

3. Transverse fissure.

4. Gall-bladder.

5. Vena cava in its groove.

6. Right lobe.

7. Left lobe.

8. Lobulus Spigelii.

9. Lobulus caudatus.

10. Lobulus quadratus.

DIAGRAM OF THE UNDER SURFACE OF THE LIVER.

gall-bladder and the longitudinal fissure. This lobe is occasionally connected with the left lobe by a bridge of hepatic substance (*pons hepatis*) which arches over the longitudinal fissure.

The liver has a thin areolar coat or capsule, best seen on those parts of it not covered by peritoneum. This coat is connected to the fine areolar tissue which surrounds the lobules, but does not send down partitions to form a framework for the interior of the gland. It is continuous, at the transverse fissure, with the sheath of loose areolar tissue called '*Glisson's capsule*,' which surrounds the vessels as they enter that fissure, and incloses them in a common sheath in their ramifications through the liver.

The interlobular areolar tissue is exceedingly delicate: hence, the great liability of the liver to be lacerated by external violence, or by the action of the abdominal muscles.

Lobules.   The liver consists of an aggregation of '*lobules*,' which range from $\frac{1}{12}$th to $\frac{1}{10}$th of an inch in diameter. These lobules vary in shape according to the direction in which they are cut; in a transverse section, they have the appearance of mosaic pavement (fig. 92); but in a perpendicular section they somewhat resemble an oak leaf (fig. 93). Each lobule consists of a

Fig. 92.

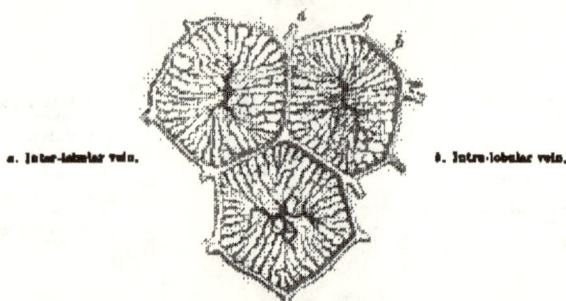

a. Inter-lobular vein.   b. Intra-lobular vein.

TRANSVERSE SECTIONS OF THREE LOBULES OF THE LIVER, MAGNIFIED TO SHOW THE PORTAL VENOUS PLEXUS.

(After Kiernan.)

minute plexus of blood vessels, ducts, and cells—*hepatic cells*—which latter fill up the spaces between the ramifications of the vessels. It will facilitate the understanding of the branchings of the different hepatic vessels, if it be borne in mind, 1, that the portal vein, hepatic artery, and hepatic duct, ramify together from first to last—they are inclosed in a sheath of areolar tissue called ' Glisson's capsule;' 2, that the hepatic veins run from first to last by themselves, and terminate in the inferior vena cava as it passes through the liver.

The *portal vein* on entering the substance of the liver gives off numerous small branches which pass between the lobules and form the '*inter-lobular veins*' (fig. 92). Some inter-lobular veins are also derived from branches (*vaginal veins*) of the portal vein, which before passing between the lobules ramify in Glisson's capsule. A minute capillary network arises from the inter-lobular veins, and penetrates into the interior of the lobules, in the centre of which it collects into a single trunk called the '*intra-lobular vein.*' This central vein opens into a *sub-lobular* vein, larger or smaller as the case may be, upon which the lobule is sessile (fig. 93). The sub-lobular veins empty themselves into the smaller hepatic veins; these unite to form the main hepatic trunks which open into the inferior vena cava.

Fig. 93.

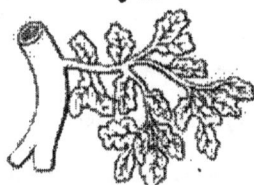

LONGITUDINAL SECTIONS OF THE LOBULES OF THE LIVER. INTRA-LOBULAR VEINS SEEN JOINING THE SUB-LOBULAR.

The *hepatic artery*, entering the liver at the transverse fissure, divides and subdivides with the portal vein, and ramifies with it between the lobules. The artery distributes branches which supply the coats of the hepatic vessels, Glisson's capsule, and the capsule of the liver; other branches run between the lobules, pass into their substance, and terminate in the capillary network.

The *hepatic ducts* form a close network round the circumference of each lobule. From this network, branches proceed on all sides, and accompany the portal vein. Doubt still exists as to the commencement of the ducts. The prevalent opinion is that they begin within the lobules by a minute plexus, surrounded by hepatic cells. The interior of each lobule, that is, the space left between the several vessels, is filled by the hepatic cells. They are nucleated, and have a diameter varying from $\frac{1}{3\,5\,8}$th to $\frac{1}{10\,0\,0}$th of an inch. They contain more or less granular matter, and in some cases fat globules: when these accumulate in large quantities, they constitute what is called a 'fatty liver.' The office of these cells is to separate the bile from the blood, and when filled with bile, discharge their contents into the hepatic ducts.[*]

[*] For further information on this subject see the original observations of Kiernan in the Philosoph. Trans. for 1833.

The *functions* of the liver may be thus briefly expressed:—1. It renders the albuminous matter (albuminose) brought to it by the portal vein capable of being assimilated by the blood. 2. It forms a substance closely allied to sugar, which passes into the hepatic veins, and being consumed in the process of respiration, helps to maintain animal heat. 3. It secretes the bile, which assists in converting the chyme into chyle, and reducing it into a state fit to be absorbed by the lacteals. 4. The bile acts as a natural aperient. 5. The bile is an antiseptic, and probably prevents the food becoming decomposed during its passage through the intestines.

Gall-bladder. The gall-bladder, a reservoir for the bile, is confined by the peritoneum in a slight depression on the under surface of the right lobe of the liver (p. 422). It is pyriform in shape, and varies in size in different subjects; generally speaking, it is about four inches long, and capable of holding about 1½ oz. of fluid. Its narrow end, or neck, makes a bend downwards, and terminates in a duct, called the '*cystic*,' which, after a course of about an inch and a half, joins the hepatic duct at an acute angle (fig. 67, p. 338). The common duct, '*ductus communis choledochus*,' formed by their union, is about three or four inches long, and opens into the back of the descending part of the duodenum, after running very obliquely through the coats of the bowel.

Exclusive of its partial peritoneal covering, the gall-bladder has two coats—the outer, consisting of fibro-cellular tissue, contains involuntary muscular fibres, which run mainly in the long axis of the gall-bladder; the inner is the mucous coat.

The gall-bladder should now be laid open. Its mucous membrane is generally tinged yellow by bile, and gathered into ridges which give it a honey-comb appearance. This appearance is most marked in the middle of the gall-bladder: in the depressions between the ridges may be seen with a magnifying glass numerous openings leading down to mucous follicles. It is covered by columnar epithelium, which secretes an abundance of viscid mucus. At the bend of the neck of the gall-bladder, both its coats project very much into the interior, making the opening considerably narrower than it appears to be outside. In the cystic duct, the mucous membrane presents a series of folds, so arranged, one after the other, as to form a complete spiral valve. The probable use of this is to prevent the too rapid flow of the bile. The gall-bladder appears to serve mainly as a reservoir for the bile, during the cessation of digestion. The bile becomes during its sojourn in the gall-bladder very viscid and intensely bitter.

Spleen. The spleen is a very vascular spongy organ, and belongs to the class of ductless glands. It varies in size according to the amount of blood in it, fluctuating in weight, consistently with health, between five and ten ounces. Usually it is of a reddish-blue colour, owing to the large amount of blood contained in it. It is more or less elliptical in shape, and in its natural position is placed with its long axis nearly vertical. Its outer surface, adapted to the diaphragm and ribs, is smooth and convex; its inner, adapted to the great end of the stomach, is concave, and divided into an anterior and a posterior portion by a vertical fissure—the *hilus*—at the bottom of which are large openings through which the vessels enter and emerge from the spleen.

The spleen is invested with two coats, a peritoneal and a fibrous. The peritoneal coat entirely covers the organ, except at the hilus, from which it is reflected to the stomach, forming the gastro-splenic omentum. Its fibrous capsule covers the spleen, and is elastic, to accommodate itself to the varying size of the viscus. This coat is intimately connected with the splenic substance, and in it are said to be some involuntary muscular fibres. It sends down into the interior numerous bands—*trabeculæ*—which cross each other in various directions, and form a network, dividing the spleen into many chambers. Besides constituting the general framework of the organ, the capsule at the hilus forms sheaths for the vessels, and supports them throughout their ramifications in the interior.

The splenic chambers are filled with a soft, reddish-brown substance, called the '*pulp*' of the spleen. Under the microscope it is found to consist mainly of cells, of a pale red colour, somewhat smaller than the red corpuscles of the blood. Interspersed among these are numerous other cells, some caudate, others nucleated, and others altered blood-cells either free or contained within larger cells. In the pulp are found numerous white spherical bodies, '*Malpighian corpuscles*,' of about the $\frac{1}{70}$th of an inch in diameter.[*] These corpuscles are not free like the smaller cells, but are attached by slender pedicles to the walls of small arteries, from whose sheaths the capsules of these bodies are derived. The artery ramifies over the surface of the corpuscles, and then terminates in a brush of capillaries, which spread out into the pulp. The interior of each corpuscle is filled with a whitish fluid, containing numerous small granular cells.

The splenic artery enters the spleen by several branches, which ramify throughout the organ, supported by sheaths derived from the capsule.[†] These branches subdivide in the trabecular tissue, and the small ramifications spread out in a brush-like manner through the pulp, and terminate in capillaries which open into the veins (and also, according to Gray, into lacunar spaces from which the veins originate). The main branches of the artery do not communicate with one another, for if injection be thrown separately into one branch, it fills only that part of the spleen to which the artery is distributed.

Thus it appears that the spleen is essentially a great blood gland; and that it consists of chambers filled with secreting gland cells of various size, between which ramify minute arteries and veins. It is presumed that the gland elaborates the albuminous materials of food, and stores them up for a time before they pass into the blood. It is considered to be a nursery for the production of the white corpuscles of the blood; and a grave-yard too, where many of the worn-out red ones undergo disintegration.

Kidneys. The kidneys are situated in the lumbar region, imbedded in a large quantity of fat. Their colour is

[*] In the human spleen they vary from $\frac{1}{70}$th to $\frac{1}{80}$th of an inch in diameter. It is useless to look for them unless the subject be exceedingly fresh, for they soon soften and melt in the pulp. It is better, therefore, to examine them in the spleen of a sheep or bullock, in which animals they are about $\frac{1}{40}$th of an inch in diameter.

[†] The ramifications of the splenic artery may be well seen by washing away the pulp, and floating the flocculent-looking spleen in water.

reddish-brown. Each weighs about five ounces in the male, rather
less in the female. The left is usually longer and somewhat
heavier than the right. The anterior surface of each is smooth
and convex; the posterior rather flattened. The outer border is
rounded; the inner presents a deep notch—the *hilus*—for the
entrance and exit of the renal vessels and duct. These have the
following relations to one another: in front lies the renal vein;
behind is the ureter; between them the renal artery.

Fig. 94.

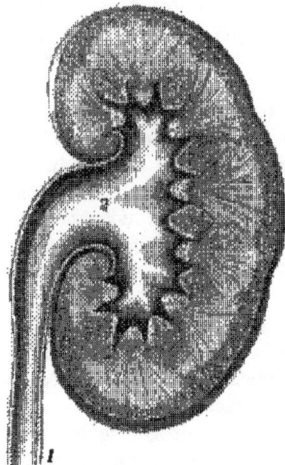

SECTION OF THE KIDNEY.

1. Ureter.
2. Pelvis of the kidney.
3, 3, 3. Papillæ.

The kidney is surrounded by a
thin fibrous capsule, to which it is
loosely connected by areolar tissue
and minute vessels. The capsule
does not penetrate into the interior
of the kidney, and can, for this
reason, when healthy, be readily
stripped off, leaving the surface
perfectly smooth.

A longitudinal section should be
made through the kidney to examine its interior. This section
displays two distinct substances, an
outer or cortical, and an inner or
medullary.

The *medullary* structure is collected into from ten to sixteen
pyramidal bundles (pyramids of
Malpighi,* fig. 94); the apices
of these, termed '*papillæ*,' project into one of the terminal divisions of the excretory tube.

These pyramids are composed of minute straight tubes, which
proceed from the cortical portion to end on the papillæ. †

* So named after Malpighi, a celebrated Italian anatomist who lived during the
middle and latter part of the seventeenth century.

† Each pyramid represents what was, in the early stage of the kidney's growth, a
distinct and independent lobe. In the human subject the lobes gradually coalesce.

The *cortical* structure, deeper in colour than the medullary, forms the outer part of the kidney, and dips down between the pyramids. It consists of convoluted tubes, and of small red bodies, called *Malpighian corpuscles.*

At the 'hilus' is the dilated commencement of the ureter, called the *pelvis of the kidney.* It is funnel-shaped, and its broad part divides into two principal channels, which again branch and form from eight to twelve cup-like excavations, called the *calices.* Into each of these calices one, sometimes two, papillæ project. Between the calices the branches of the renal artery ascend to ramify in the kidney, lying imbedded in a quantity of fat. With a lens, the papillæ may be seen studded with minute apertures, which are the terminations of the uriniferous tubes. These tubes as they pass outwards run straight, bifurcate repeatedly, and enter the cortex in bundles of straight tubes, forming the 'pyramids of Ferrein.' They vary from the $\frac{1}{500}$th to $\frac{1}{700}$th of an inch in diameter, and are largest towards their termination. On entering the cortex, the tubes become convoluted, and are surrounded by minute plexuses of blood vessels. The tubuli uriniferi, the pelvis of the kidney, and the ureter, are lined by spheroidal epithelium.*

The *Malpighian corpuscles* are situated in the cortical portion, and average about $\frac{1}{120}$th of an inch in diameter. According to Bowman,† each is formed by the dilatation of the uriniferous tube. It is composed of a homogeneous membrane, and is pierced by a small artery, which enters the capsule opposite to the commencement of the urinary tube. In the capsule the artery breaks up into a coil of minute vessels (*glomerulus*), which returns its blood by a vein (efferent vessel), which emerges from the capsule

and no trace of their primordial state remains, except the pyramidal arrangement of the tubes. But in the kidneys of the lower mammalia, of birds and reptiles, the lobes are permanently separate.

* Between the straight tubes in the Malpighian pyramids, there have recently been discovered numerous smaller tubules, named the *looped tubes of Henle.* These are said to come off from the straight tubes, to descend towards the apex of the pyramid, where they form loops, and again ascend to terminate in the Malpighian corpuscles.

† Philosoph. Trans. for 1842. Part I.

close to where the artery entered.   Instead of leaving the kidney,
as in other organs, it forms a venous plexus round the convolutions
of the urinary tube.*   The special purpose of
this plexus appears to be the secretion of the
solid matter of the urine; while the Malpighian
body filters the watery part of the urine into the
capsule, and washes the more solid part down
the tube.†   The coil of vessels in the capsule is
surrounded by the epithelium lining the interior
of the capsule.

Fig. 95.

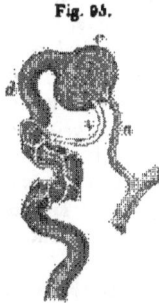

a. Artery.
v. Vein, or efferent vessel.
c. Capsule.
d. Urinary tube.

Supra-renal
capsules.

The nerves forming the renal plexus are derived from the smallest splanchnic nerves and
the solar plexus.   The lymphatics pass to the
lumbar glands.

These bodies, situated at the top of
the kidneys, belong to the class of
ductless glands.   The right resembles
a cocked hat, the left is more almond-shaped.
They measure about 1½ inch in their long diameter, and weigh
from one to two drachms.   They are surrounded by a thin fibrous
covering, which sends down partitions into the interior through
furrows upon their surface.

A perpendicular section shows that it consists of a firm exterior
or cortical part, and of an interior or medullary substance, soft and
pulpy.   The cortical portion is of a yellow colour, and forms the
principal part of the organ.   Examined under the microscope, it
appears to be composed of clusters of columns about $\frac{1}{100}$th of an
inch in diameter, arranged perpendicularly to the surface.   These
columns do not run completely through the thickness of the
cortical portion, but have a layer of cells arranged above and below

* For a summary of the opinion held by various observers, respecting these Malpighian corpuscles, consult a paper by R. Southey, M.D., St. Bartholomew's Hosp,
Reports, vol. i. 1865.

† That the vessel leaving the Malpighian body is a vein, and that a constituent
part of the urine is secreted by venous blood, is inferred from two reasons : 1. From
the analogous case of the vena porta, out of which the bile is elaborated in the liver ;
2, from the fact that in reptiles the urine is secreted from venous blood.

them.* The columns lie in the stroma of the cortex, which contains oval nucleated cells, large fat globules, and a number of minute yellowish granules. The columns are stated by some to be tubes having a distinct lining membrane; by others, to be closed vesicles; and by others to be cavities in the cortical portion. Small arteries are abundantly supplied to the cortex, and dip down between the columns. The medullary part varies in colour according to the amount of blood contained in it, being in some of a dark brown colour, in others nearly white. It consists of a plexus of minute veins, among which are numerous cells, some of whch appear branched.† The stroma is composed of areolar tissue, which forms a delicate network throughout the central part.

Of late years the minute structure and functions of the renal capsules have been much investigated, in consequence of the discovery, made by Dr. Addison, of the close relation which exists between certain diseases in these bodies and a brown discoloration of the skin. Their precise function is still unknown.

Stomach and intestines.

The alimentary canal is composed of four coats; a serous, a muscular, a submucous, and a mucous. First, is the *serous* or peritoneal coat, described at p. 332. Secondly, under the serous is a *muscular* coat, upon which the chief strength of the canal depends. It consists of two distinct strata of fibres; the outer stratum is longitudinal, the inner circular. This arrangement not only makes the bowel stronger, but regulates its peristaltic action; for the longitudinal fibres, by their contraction, tend to shorten and straighten the tube, while the circular fibres contract upon and propel its contents to greater advantage. Connecting this coat and the mucous, is a layer of areolar tissue called the *submucous coat*, in which the arteries break up before entering the mucous membrane. The *mucous* is the most complicated of all the coats, for it presents different characters

* See an article by D. Duckworth, M.D., on 'The Anatomy of the Supra-renal Capsules,' in St. Bartholomew's Hosp. Reports, vol. I. 1865.
† Consult ' A Physiological Essay on the Thymus Gland,' by Simon, London, 1845.

in different parts, according to the functions which it has to perform.

Stomach.   The stomach should be moderately distended to see its size, which varies in different subjects according to the habits of the individual. In shape it has been compared to the bag of a bag-pipe. When distended it is about twelve inches in length and about four in width. The stomach forms a large bulge to the left of the œsophagus, called the *cardiac* or *œsophageal* end : on the right side, where the food passes out, it becomes small and contracted, and is called the *pyloric* end. Just before the pylorus, the stomach bulges into a pouch, called '*antrum pylori*.' Anatomists describe the stomach as having two borders and two surfaces. The upper border is concave, and called the *lesser curve* : the lower border is convex and called the *greater curve*. The surfaces, anterior and posterior, are convex. On removing the serous investment of the stomach, the muscular coat is exposed. The fibres are of the non-striped variety and arranged in three layers, an external or longitudinal, a middle or circular, and an internal or oblique.

The *longitudinal* fibres are continuous with the longitudinal fibres of the œsophagus, and spread out over the stomach : they are most numerous along the curves of the stomach. *The circular* fibres are well marked about the middle of the stomach, but are most abundant at the pylorus, where they form a powerful sphincter muscle. The *oblique* fibres are scattered over the sides of the stomach, and are the most distinct at the entrance of the œsophagus.

When the stomach is laid open, the *mucous membrane* is seen to be of a pale colour, and gathered into longitudinal folds (*rugæ*), which disappear when the stomach is full. The mucous membrane is connected to the muscular layer by a distinct stratum of areolar tissue, called the '*submucous coat*.' Its use is to permit the muscular and mucous coats to move freely on each other, and to serve as a bed, in which the blood vessels ramify minutely before they enter the mucous membrane.

If a portion of the mucous membrane be examined under a microscope, its surface will be seen to be mapped out into small hexagonal pits or alveoli, giving it a honey-comb appearance. The pits vary from the $\frac{1}{500}$th to $\frac{1}{350}$th of an inch in diameter. At the bottom of them are a number of minute pores, the orifices of the gastric tubes. In a perpendicular section, the tubes are arranged in parallel lines at right angles to the surface, and terminate in blind sacculated ends set in the submucous tissue. The entire thickness of the mucous membrane is made up of these tubular glands. The tubules are on an average about $\frac{1}{40}$th of an inch long. In the cardiac end they are simple tubes, but at the pyloric end they are frequently branched. Their upper fourth is lined with columnar epithelium, their lower three-fourths, with spheroidal or glandular. It is presumed that these glandular cells contain the gastric juice. As fast as formed, during digestion, they pass into the stomach, discharge their contents, and disappear. Other glands—lenticular—may be found near the pyloric end of the stomach, and resemble Peyer's glands.

The mucous membrane of the stomach, and also of the upper part of the interior of the tubes, is lined by a columnar epithelium. It is exceedingly thin and delicate, and can only be seen in the stomach of an animal recently killed.

The tubes of the stomach are richly supplied with blood. The arteries form a stratum of minute inosculations in the submucous tissue, in which the closed ends of the tubes are set; from this stratum the vessels run up between the tubes to the surface of the stomach, where they again inosculate, and form the hexagonal spaces before alluded to.

The stomach is supplied with nerves from the pneumogastric and from the solar plexus.

The small intestines, consisting of the duodenum, jejunum, and ileum, form a tube from sixteen to twenty-six feet in length, according to the height of the individual. The duodenum is about twelve inches in length; the jejunum comprises two-fifths, the ileum three-fifths of the remaining part of the small intestine. As regards their external character, the duodenum and jejunum are more vascular than the ileum, and feel thicker in consequence of the peculiar arrangement of

Small intestines.

F F

their mucous membrane. Their peritoneal and muscular coats are the same throughout. The *muscular* coat consists of an outer thin longitudinal layer and an inner circular thicker layer. It is connected to the mucous membrane by the *submucous* coat.

When the small intestines are cut open from the upper end, we observe that the mucous membrane is arranged in close transverse folds or plaits, called *valvulæ conniventes.*' These differ from other folds in the alimentary canal, e.g. in the œsophagus and stomach, in that they are not obliterated when the tube is distended. Each fold extends about one-half or two-thirds round the intestine; but they are not all of equal size. They commence immediately below the openings of the biliary and pancreatic ducts, and are most largely developed in the duodenum and the upper part of the jejunum. Below this part of the tube they gradually decrease in size, and become wider apart, till they finally disappear near the middle of the ileum. The use of the valvulæ conniventes is, to increase the extent of surface for the absorption of chyle; to prevent the food passing too rapidly through the intestines, and also for secretion.

If a portion of small intestine be washed and placed in water, the surface of the mucous membrane appears like the soft fur or pile upon velvet. This appearance is produced by small processes called *villi.* These are extremely vascular projections of the mucous membrane, about a fourth of a line in length, and so close to each other that a square line contains from forty to ninety of them. Their size, however, and their number, bear a direct ratio to that of the valvulæ conniventes. Under the microscope a villus is seen to consist of an outstanding process of the mucous membrane, covered by a layer of columnar epithelium, which rests upon its proper basement membrane. Each villus is furnished with an artery which forms a network of inosculations over it, and then returns its blood by a single vein. In its interior it contains a *lacteal* or absorbing vessel, which commences in a closed end near the summit of the villus, where it is surrounded by a layer of pale unstriped muscular fibres. The cylindrical cells which cover the villi are believed to be the agents in the absorption of the chyle, and to possess the power of selection.

Intestinal glands.

There are four kinds of *glands* [*] in the small intestine, called, the glands of Lieberkühn, Brunn, Peyer, and the solitary glands. The first and last are distributed over the whole tract of the intestinal mucous membrane; the other two over particular parts.

The *glands of Lieberkühn* [†] are minute tubes with blind ends, very thickly distributed over the small and the large intestines. Under the microscope, their orifices are seen between the villi, like so many minute dots. These vary in depth from $\frac{1}{40}$th to $\frac{1}{70}$th of a line, and are lined with columnar epithelium.

The *glands of Brunn* [‡] are found only in the duodenum. They are just visible to the naked eye, and may be seen by removing the muscular coat. Their structure exactly resembles the pancreas on a diminutive scale.

The *glands of Peyer* [§] (glandulæ agminatæ) abound most in the ileum, and are seen most distinctly in children. They are arranged in groups, from twenty to forty in number, on that part of the intestine most distant from the attachment of the mesentery. These groups are from half an inch to three inches long, of an oval form, and increase in size and number towards the lower part of the ileum. If a group be examined by dissecting away the muscular coat, you find that it is composed of a number of small oval vesicles, like Florence flasks, imbedded in the submucous tissue. They are about three-fourths of a line in diameter, and contain an opaque greyish fluid. No excretory ducts have been traced from these vesicles, but they are supposed to discharge their contents by rupture of their capsules. Between the vesicles are found Lieberkühn's follicles; and the surface of the patches is covered with villi. These glands are liable to be ulcerated in typhoid fever.

[*] A satisfactory examination of the intestinal glands can be made only in specimens quite recent, taken from young persons who have died suddenly, or from a rapidly fatal disease.

[†] J. N. Lieberkühn, Diss. de fabric. et actione villorum intestin. tenuium, 1782.

[‡] J. C. Brunn. Gland. duoden. seu pancreas secundarium, 1715.

[§] Peyer, De glandulis intestinorum, 1682. These glands were first described by Nehemia Grew, in 1681.

The *solitary glands* are scattered in all parts of the small and large intestines. They resemble the glands of Peyer in structure, and only differ from them in being solitary instead of being aggregated into groups.

Large intestine. The principal external characters of the large intestine are, that it is pouched or sacculated, and that it has, attached to it, little pendulous portions of fat covered by peritoneum, called '*appendices epiploicæ.*' The pouches (sacculi) are produced by a shortening of the longitudinal muscular fibres, and by their being collected into three bands, about half an inch wide, nearly equidistant from each other. One of these bands corresponds with the attached part of the circumference of the bowel; another with the front part; a third with its concavity. If at any given part the three bands be divided, the pouches immediately disappear.

In a colon moderately distended and dried, we observe that the mucous membrane forms numerous ridges or incomplete septa (see fig. 96): they correspond to the grooves on the external surface of the bowel, and disappear, like the sacculi, when the longitudinal bands are divided.

The rectum differs from the rest of the large intestine in that its longitudinal muscular fibres are not collected into bands, but distributed equally over its whole circumference. Moreover, both the longitudinal and circular fibres are of considerable strength, like those of the œsophagus, as one might expect from the particular functions which these parts of the alimentary canal have to perform. For an inch and a half, or thereabouts, above the anus, the circular fibres are remarkably developed, and constitute the internal '*sphincter ani.*'

The mucous membrane of the large intestine differs considerably from that of the small. There are no valvulæ conniventes or villi; but the glands of Lieberkühn and the solitary glands may be seen studding the mucous membrane. The solitary glands are more abundant in the cæcum and in the appendix vermiformis than in any other part of the alimentary canal. The blood vessels present the same hexagonal arrangement on the surface as

that of the stomach. That the mucous membrane of the large
intestine may be temporarily used as a substitute for the stomach,
is proved by the fact of persons having been nourished for many
weeks, solely by injections.   The mucous membrane is lined
throughout with columnar epithelium.

At the junction of the small with the large intestine
Ilio-cæcal the mucous membrane is folded so as to form a valve :
valve. but it is not a perfect one, as is proved by pouring water
into the large intestine, or by the occasional vomiting of injections.

Fig. 96.

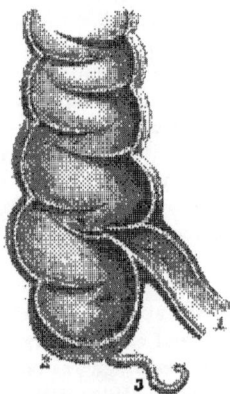

1. Ileum.
2. Cæcum or caput coli.
3. Appendix vermiformis.

SECTION THROUGH THE JUNCTION OF THE LARGE AND SMALL INTESTINE TO SHOW THE
ILIO-CÆCAL VALVE.

The arrangement of the valve is best examined in a dried preparation. The opening is a transverse fissure like a button-hole; and
the two flaps are arranged like an upper and a lower eyelid. The
flaps of the valve consist of mucous membrane and the circular
fibres of the ileum. The longitudinal fibres of the ileum are continued directly on to the cæcum: if these be divided, the ileum
can be drawn out, and the valve disappears.

In many subjects we observe that transverse or
oblique folds of the mucous membrane project into
the rectum. These cannot be seen to advantage unless
the bowel be hardened by alcohol in its natural position. Three,
more prominent than the rest, and half an inch, or thereabouts,
in width, were first pointed out by Mr. Houston.* One projects
from the upper part of the rectum, opposite the prostate
gland; another is situated higher up, on the side of the bowel;
while the third is still higher. When thickened or ulcerated,
these folds are apt to occasion great pain and obstruction in
defæcation.

Folds in the rectum.

THE DISSECTION OF THE THIGH.

An incision should be made along the groin, from the anterior
superior spine of the ileum to the spine of the pubes; another,
from the middle of the first, down the thigh for about six inches.
The skin being reflected, the superficial fascia and vessels will be
exposed.

This fascia varies in thickness according to the condition of the body. Like other superficial fascia it is
divisible into two layers, between which are situated
the inguinal glands, and the cutaneous vessels. The upper layer
is continuous with that of the abdomen; the deeper layer is best
marked in the upper part of the thigh, especially where it
stretches across the saphenous opening to form the *cribriform
fascia*.

Superficial fascia.

The cutaneous vessels come from the femoral artery and are
three in number, the *superficial epigastric*, the *superficial pudic*,
and the *superficial circumflexa ilii* arteries: the first ascends over
Poupart's ligament to the abdomen; the second crosses inwards
towards the pubes; and the third passes outwards to the ileum.
Each artery is accompanied by one, sometimes by two veins,
which empty themselves, either directly into the femoral, or into
the great cutaneous vein of the thigh, called the ' saphena.'

* Dublin Hospital Reports, vol. v.

Superficial inguinal glands.　　These are easily recognised, by their oval form and reddish-brown colour. They are divided into two sets: one, which runs parallel to Poupart's ligament, and receives the lymphatics from the penis, scrotum, and perineum; the other, which lies along the saphena vein, and transmits

Fig. 97.

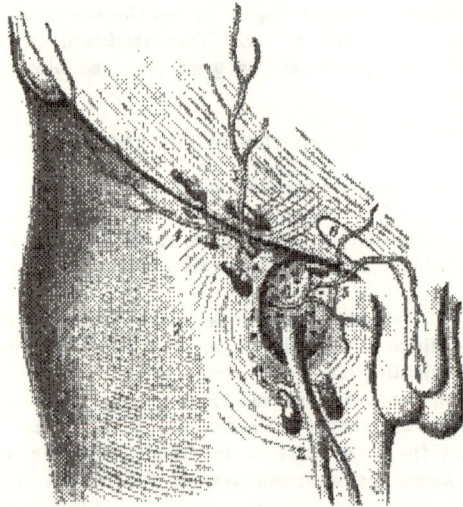

SUPERFICIAL VESSELS AND GLANDS OF THE GROIN.　SAPHENOUS OPENING WITH THE
CRIBRIFORM FASCIA.

1. Saphenous opening of the fascia lata.
2. Saphena vein.
3. Superficial epigastric a.
4. Superficial circumflexa ilii a.

5. Superficial pudic a.
6. External abdominal ring.
7. Fascia lata of the thigh.

the lymphatics from the foot and leg. This explains why, in cancer of the scrotum and syphilitic disease of the penis, the first set becomes enlarged; and the second in diseases of the lower extremity. The absorbent vessels which pass to and from the glands are small, and easily escape observation, unless specially sought.

They all pass through the femoral ring into the abdomen, and eventually empty themselves into the thoracic duct.

The glands mentioned in the preceding paragraph are all superficial. There are others, more deeply seated, close to the great vessels of the thigh: these are much smaller, and sometimes cannot be found.

The *superficial epigastric* artery comes out through the fascia lata, half an inch below Poupart's ligament, and supplies the inguinal glands. Its further course is described at p. 309.

The *superficial circumflexa ilii* runs parallel to Poupart's ligament towards the crest of the ileum, and ends in the skin and subcutaneous tissue.

The *superficial external pudic* comes out through the saphenous opening, crosses over the spermatic cord, and supplies the penis and scrotum in the male, and the labium in the female. This artery is liable to be divided in the operation for femoral hernia; also in that for phimosis, since it runs along the penis to supply the prepuce. Arising, as they all do, directly from so large an artery as the femoral, they sometimes bleed profusely; for it is an admitted fact, that when even a small branch, coming directly from a principal artery, is divided near its origin, it will sometimes pour out as much blood as if an opening were punched out of the trunk as large as the area of the divided branches.[*] There is another pudic artery, called the *deep or inferior external pudic:* this runs between the fascia lata and the pectineus, supplying that muscle, the scrotum in the male, and the labium in the female.

The incision should be prolonged down the thigh, over the knee to the tubercle of the tibia. The skin must then be reflected, to expose the subcutaneous tissue over the whole of the front of the thigh. In it will be found the cutaneous vessels and nerves, which must be carefully dissected.

[*] Mr. Liston had occasion to tie the external iliac artery for a supposed injury (by a pistol-ball) to the femoral. It was discovered, after the death of the patient, that the ball had injured only one of the superficial branches of the femoral, about an inch from its origin. See his paper in the Med.-Chir. Trans. vol. xxix. 1846.

This is the chief subcutaneous vein of the lower

Saphena vein. limb. Its roots, arising on the inner side of the foot, unite into a single trunk, which ascends *over* the inner ankle, along the inner side of the leg behind the knee, along the inner and front part of the thigh, where it passes through an opening—the ' saphenous opening '—in the fascia lata, to join the femoral vein, immediately below the crural arch (fig. 97). In this long course it receives several tributary veins, some of which are often large; and, just before its termination, it is joined by the superficial veins of the groin already alluded to. Like all subcutaneous veins, it is provided at intervals with valves to support the column of the blood.

The distribution of the cutaneous nerves of the thigh

Cutaneous nerves. varies considerably; so that a general description of their usual arrangement is sufficient. The cutaneous nerves are divided, according to their situation, into *external, middle,* and *internal.* All directly or indirectly proceed from the lumbar plexus, and are seen coming through the fascia, and dividing in the subcutaneous tissue.

a. The *external cutaneous nerve* is a branch of the second lumbar nerve. It enters the thigh beneath Poupart's ligament close to the anterior superior spine of the ileum. Here it divides into two branches, an anterior and a posterior. The anterior division runs down at first in a sheath of the fascia lata: it then comes through it, and can be traced down the outer side of the thigh as far as the knee, giving off numerous cutaneous branches. The posterior branch, after coming through the fascia, divides into branches, which are distributed to the skin over the nates and the posterior part of the thigh.

b. The *middle cutaneous nerves,* two or more in number, are derived from the anterior crural, which itself is a branch of the lumbar plexus. They pierce the sartorius four or five inches below the crural arch, and descend along the front of the thigh to the knee, distributing branches on either side (see diag., p. 453).

b. The *internal cutaneous nerves,* two or more, also branches of the anterior crural, perforate the fascia lata, one about the middle,* another about the lower third of the thigh, and supply the skin on the inner side. The last-named branch communicates with branches from the obturator, and sometimes with the saphenous, about the middle of the thigh, and again with the latter a little above the knee.

d. The *crural branch* of the *genito-crural nerve* must be sought for carefully below Poupart's ligament: it perforates the fascia external to the femoral artery, and supplies the skin in front of the thigh. About two or three inches below the crural arch it usually communicates with the middle cutaneous nerve.

e. The *ilio-inguinal nerve*, after emerging from the external abdominal ring, supplies the skin on the inner aspect of the thigh.

Fascia lata or muscular fascia.
    Remove the subcutaneous structure to examine the muscular fascia, or 'fascia lata' of the thigh. The purpose of this fascia is to cover the muscles of the thigh collectively, and to form separate sheaths for each ; so that it not only packs them together, but maintains each in its proper position. A knowledge of these sheaths is important, because they interfere with the progress of deep-seated matter towards the surface, and cause it to burrow in this or that direction according to the part in which it forms.

The fascia is not of equal strength all round the thigh. It is comparatively thin and transparent on the inner side ; exceedingly thick and strong down the outer side : here, indeed, it has the appearance of a dense expanded tendon, strapping down the vastus externus muscle ; and it certainly performs the office of a tendon, for it gives insertion to two powerful muscles—namely, the tensor fasciæ femoris, and the glutæus maximus (fig. 98).

The fascia lata is attached to the margin of the bones which constitute the framework of the lower extremity. Beginning from above, its attachment can be traced along the crest of the ileum, thence along the crural arch to the body of the pubis, and down

---

* It is important to note that one, or sometimes two, of these internal cutaneous nerves cross the sheath of the femoral artery just where the sartorius begins to overlap it ; and therefore at the spot where it is usually tied. See diag., p. 453.

the rami of the pubes and ischium. Proceeding down the thigh, it penetrates, on either side of the limb, to the linea aspera, forming what are called the 'intermuscular septa,' which separate the extensor from the flexor muscles. Below, it can be traced all round the knee-joint, and is particularly strong, especially on the outer side, where it is attached to the head of the tibia and fibula.

There are numerous small apertures in the fascia, through which the cutaneous nerves and vessels are transmitted; and one large opening —the 'saphenous opening'—through which the saphena vein passes to join the femoral. That part of the fascia lata situated external to the saphenous opening is termed the iliac portion of the fascia lata; that internal to it, the pubic portion.

Saphenous opening in the fascia lata.

The saphenous opening is an oval aperture in the fascia lata, situated immediately below the crural arch, on the inner side of the front aspect of the thigh. There is no definite edge to the saphenous opening until the fascia, which covers the opening and blends with its margin, has been removed.* The term 'cribriform' has been given to this fascia, because it is riddled with holes for the passage of the superficial vessels and absorbents. It is a thin covering over the saphenous opening, and is prolonged from the outer edge of the opening over the sheath of the femoral vessels, and

Cribriform fascia

adheres on the inner side to the fascia lata, over the pectineus muscle. Some anatomists describe this fascia as a portion of the 'superficial fascia;' others consider it as a

Fig. 98.

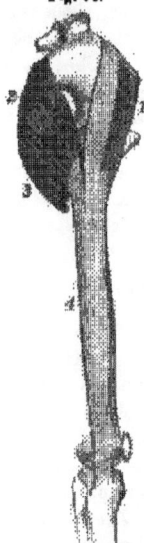

FASCIA ON THE OUTSIDE OF THE THIGH.

1. Tensor fasciæ femoris.
2. Glutæus maximus.
3. Lower fibres of ditto.
4. Fascia lata.

* According to Mr. Callender, a natural saphenous opening does sometimes exist, in consequence of the cribriform fascia becoming atrophied.—On the Anatomy of the parts concerned in Femoral Rupture, 1862.

thin prolongation of the fascia lata itself across the opening. Its chief surgical importance is derived from the fact that it forms one of the coverings of a femoral hernia.

The cribriform fascia must now be removed so as to display the saphenous opening, which will appear as represented in fig. 99.

Reverting to the saphenous opening, we observe that it is situated just below the crural arch, not far from the pubes; that it is

Fig. 99.

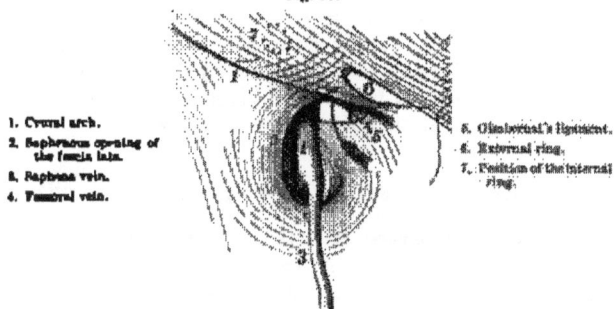

1. Crural arch.
2. Saphenous opening of the fascia lata.
3. Saphena vein.
4. Femoral vein.

5. Gimbernat's ligament.
6. External ring.
7. Position of the internal ring.

DIAGRAM OF THE FEMORAL RING.

(The arrow is introduced into the femoral ring.)

oval with the long axis vertical, and about one and a half or two inches long. Its border on the inner or pubic side is not defined; for here the fascia lata ascends under the femoral vessels, and is continuous with the iliac fascia of the pelvis.* But the outer or iliac border is defined clearly enough. This lies in front of the femoral vessels, is crescent-shaped, with the concavity towards the pubes, and called the falciform process of 'Burns.' The lower horn of the crescent curves under the saphena vein, and is lost in the fascia on the inner side of the opening. The upper horn

* On the inner side of the femoral vessels the pubic portion of the fascia is attached to the linea ilio-pectinea.

(Hey's ligament)* arches over the femoral vein, and is continued
uninterruptedly into 'Gimbernat's ligament' or into that part of
the crural arch which is inserted into the linea ilio-pectinea. The
upper horn deserves especial attention, because it forms the upper
boundary of the aperture through which a femoral hernia takes
place; and, being chiefly concerned in the constriction of the
rupture, must be divided for its relief. This may be easily
ascertained by introducing the little finger under the crural arch,
on the inner side of the femoral vein—in other words into the
femoral ring (see the arrow in the diagram). Feel how much
the upper horn of the crescent would girt the neck of a hernia,
and that its tension is greatly influenced by the position of the
limb; for if the thigh be bent and brought over to the other
side, the tension of all the parts is materially lessened.†

ANATOMY OF THE PARTS CONCERNED IN FEMORAL HERNIA.

The anatomy of the parts concerned in femoral hernia cannot be
thoroughly understood without the assistance of special dissections. The following demonstration, therefore, takes for granted
that the student has the opportunity of seeing the parts, not only
on their femoral, but also on their abdominal side.

We propose to treat the different parts of the subject in the
following order:—

　　a. The formation of the crural arch.

　　b. The arrangement of the parts which pass under the arch.

　　c. The sheath of the femoral vessels.

　　d. The crural canal and ring.

　　e. The practical application of the subject.

* This upper horn is sometimes called 'Hey's ligament,' after the surgeon who
first drew attention to it: Observations in Surgery, by W. Hey, F.R.S. London,
1810.

† We must always bear in mind, that though the crural arch and the fascia attached
to it have received particular names, they are not, on that account, distinct and separate; but all are intimately connected, and portions merely of one continuous expansion. Thus all the parts are kept in a condition of mutual tension, which depends
very much on the position of the thigh.

Crural arch or Poupart's ligament.   The lower border of the aponeurosis of the external oblique muscle extends from the anterior superior spine of the ileum to the spine of the pubes, and forms, over the bony excavation beneath, what is called the 'crural arch' or 'Poupart's ligament.' (It is marked by the dark line in fig. 100.) The direction of the arch is at first somewhat oblique, but towards its inner half, becomes nearly horizontal. In consequence of its intimate connection with the muscular fascia of the thigh, the line of the arch describes a gentle curve with the convexity downwards. The arch is attached to the spine of the pubes, and also for some distance along the linea ilio-pectinea (fig. 100). This additional attachment, called, after its discoverer, *Gimbernat's ligament*,* is of importance, for it is most frequently the seat of stricture in femoral hernia.

Gimbernat's ligament.   The best view of Gimbernat's ligament is obtained from within the abdomen, it being only necessary to remove the peritoneum. It is placed nearly horizontally, in the erect posture, and is triangular with its apex at the pubes and its base directed outwards. In front, it is continuous with the crural arch; behind, it is inserted into the linea ilio-pectinea; externally, it is continuous with the fascia lata (fig. 99). Its length is from ⅜ths of an inch to 1 inch; but it varies in different subjects, and is usually longer in the male than the female: this is one among many reasons why femoral hernia is less frequent in the male.

On putting your finger into the femoral ring, you feel the sharp and wiry edge of this ligament: observe, too, that as the body lies on the table, the plane of the ligament is perpendicular, and therefore that it *recedes from the surface.*

Arrangement of the parts which pass under the arch.   The crural arch transmits from the abdomen into the thigh (proceeding in order from the outer side) the following objects, shown in fig. 100: 1. The external cutaneous nerve; 2. The iliacus and psoas muscles, with the anterior crural nerve between them; 3. The femoral artery and vein with the crural branch of the

* Don Antonio de Gimbernat was a Spanish surgeon, who published, in 1793, A new Method of Operating for the Femoral Hernia. Madrid.

genito-crural nerve. These muscles and vessels fill up the space
beneath the crural arch, except on the inner side of the femoral
vein, where a comparatively vacant space is left for the passage of
the absorbents: this is called the *crural canal*. The muscles are
separated from the vessels by a strong vertical fibrous partition
passing from the arch to the bone, which is nothing more than a
continuation of the sheath of the psoas. The artery, too, is separated from the vein by a similar, although a much weaker parti-

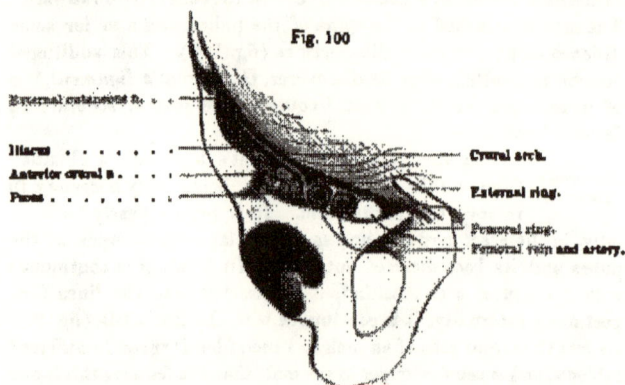

Fig. 100

External cutaneous n.

Iliacus
Anterior crural n.
Psoas

Crural arch.
External ring.
Femoral ring.
Femoral vein and artery.

POSITION OF PARTS UNDER THE CRURAL ARCH (VERTICAL SECTION).

tion, and there is a third close to the inner side of the vein. These
three partitions not only keep all the parts in their right place, but
confine the arch down to the bone, and prevent its being uplifted
by any protrusion between it and the muscles and vessels. This,
coupled with the close attachment of the iliac fascia to the crural
arch, explains why a femoral hernia rarely takes place in any other
situation than on the inner side of the femoral vein.*

* If the partitions from any cause yield, or become slack, then a rupture may descend in front of the vessels, or even (though this is rare) on the outer side of the
artery.

Sheath of the femoral vessels. The femoral vessels do not descend uncovered beneath the crural arch, but come down inclosed in a membranous sheath. This sheath appears to be derived immediately from the arch itself, but it is really formed, in front, by a prolongation from the fascia transversalis of the abdomen. This prolongation, uniting with the continuation from the iliac fascia to join the fascia lata behind the femoral vessels, forms a funnel, with the wide part uppermost, into which the femoral vessels enter.

Fig. 101.

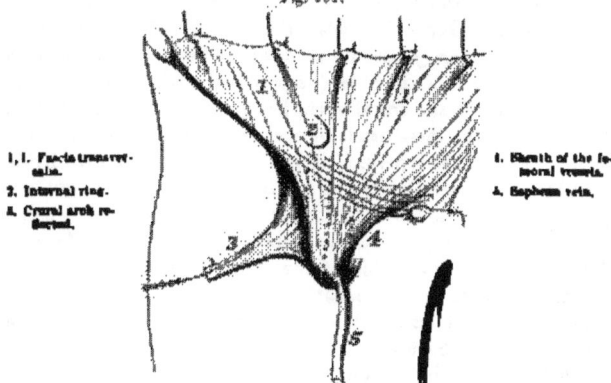

1, 1. Fascia transversalis.
2. Internal ring.
3. Crural arch reflected.

1. Sheath of the femoral vessels.
4. Saphena vein.

DIAGRAM OF THE SHEATH OF THE FEMORAL VESSELS.

This is what is described as the funnel-shaped sheath of the femoral vessels.

To examine this sheath satisfactorily, it is necessary to reflect, from its attachment to the crural arch, the upper horn of the saphenous opening, as shown in fig. 101. By this proceeding, you expose the fascia transversalis coming down over the femoral vessels, and forming the front part of their sheath. The hind part of the sheath is formed by the fascia iliaca, which runs down behind the vessels to join the pubic portion of the fascia lata. The sheath descends about as low as the lower horn of the saphenous opening, where it is gradually lost upon the proper investment of the femoral vessels. The outer part of the sheath is perforated by the crural branch of the genito-crural nerve, and the superficial arteries of the groin; the inner part by the saphena vein and some absorbent vessels.

Within the sheath of the femoral vessels, are three compartments separated from each other by partitions: the outer one is occupied by the femoral artery; the middle, by the femoral vein; the inner is the crural canal, into which the femoral hernia descends.

Practically, the sheath is important for many reasons :—

1. A femoral hernia descends inside it. 2. It forms, therefore, one of the coverings (*fascia propria*) of the hernia. 3. It contains in its substance bands of fibres (*deep crural arch*) running in the same direction as the crural arch, but quite independent of it, as shown in fig. 101; these bands lie over the neck of the sac, and are often the seat of the stricture; it is therefore necessary to divide them before the intestine can be returned.

Crural canal and femoral ring.   The hollow under the crural arch is completely occupied except for a small space, called the *crural canal*, on the inner side of the vein. This canal is from a quarter to half an inch in length. It commences, above, in the femoral ring; and ends, below, at the saphenous opening. The *femoral ring* is the upper opening of the crural canal, and is bounded, in front, by the crural arch; behind, by the bone; on the outer side, by the femoral vein; on the inner side, by the thin, wiry edge of Gimbernat's ligament. In the undisturbed condition of the parts there is no gap; it is only a weak place, which, when a hernia escapes through it, feels like a ring: hence the name of 'femoral ring.'*

The femoral ring is surrounded on all sides by unyielding structures. This accounts for the little benefit afforded by the warm bath in cases of strangulation. Mr. Lawrence was in the habit of

---

* The femoral ring is naturally occupied by a little fat and cellular membrane, by absorbent vessels, and often by a small absorbent gland. But we have never met with anything deserving the name of a 'diaphragm' or membranous septum, such as is described by Cloquet as the 'septum crurale.'

saying that he never saw a strangulated femoral hernia where the warm bath was of any avail.

Practical application of the subject. From what has been said, the student ought now to understand—1, at what point a femoral hernia escapes from the abdomen; 2, the course which it takes, and its relations to the surrounding parts; 3, the proper mode of attempting the reduction; 4, the structure and arrangement of its coverings; and, lastly, the probable seat of stricture.

The hernia escapes from the abdomen through the femoral ring —that is, under the weak part of the crural arch, between the femoral vein and Gimbernat's ligament. Here is the mouth of the hernial sac, or that part of it which communicates with the abdomen. It descends for a short distance nearly perpendicularly, and projects as a small tumour in front of the pectineus muscle. Its progress downwards, however, is soon arrested, partly by the very close adhesion of the subcutaneous structures to the lower margin of the saphenous opening; partly by flexion of the thigh. Consequently, if the hernia increase in size, it must rise over the crural arch, where the subcutaneous tissue offers less resistance; and the bulk of the hernia extends outwards towards the ilium, assuming more or less of an oblong form, with the long axis parallel to the crural arch. Since, then, the body of the hernia forms a very acute angle with the neck, the right mode of attempting its reduction is, to draw it first down from the groin, and then to make pressure on it backwards in the direction of the femoral ring.

Coverings of a femoral hernia. The *coverings* of a femoral hernia are as follow :— It first protrudes before it the peritoneum, technically called the hernial sac.* The sac is covered by more or less fat, according to the condition of the patient, called the subperitoneal fat. It next pushes before it the sheath of the femoral vessels, which forms an investment called the '*fascia propria.*' In front of this is the *cribriform fascia.* Lastly, there is the subcutaneous tissue and skin.

The *seat of stricture* is usually at the femoral ring, and the

---

* In some cases the fascia propria so much resembles the hernial sac, that it is not easy to distinguish between them. Generally speaking they are separated by a small quantity of fat.

position of the neighbouring blood vessels indicates that the proper direction in which to divide the stricture is, either directly inwards, through Gimbernat's ligament, as recommended by Mr. Lawrence, or upwards through Hey's ligament, as recommended by Sir A. Cooper.* There is no risk of wounding an artery, supposing the vessels to take their ordinary course. But it occasionally happens (as observed p. 388), that the obturator artery runs *above* (in the recumbent position) the femoral ring ; in such a case, the neck of the sac would be encircled by a large blood vessel.† From the examination of two hundred bodies, the chances are about seventy to one against this unfavourable distribution. But the possibility of it has given rise to *this rule* in practice—not to cut deeply in any one place through the stricture, but rather to notch it in several. By this proceeding we are much less likely to wound the abnormal artery, because it does not run at the base of Gimbernat's ligament, but about a line and a half from the margin of it.‡

Such is an outline of the anatomy of the parts concerned in a femoral hernia. The normal anatomy in each case being nearly the same, it might be supposed that all operations for the relief of this kind of hernia would be straightforward and pretty much alike ; but this is very far from being the case : indeed, surgeons agree that they never take the knife in hand without the expectation of meeting some peculiarity.

The fascia must now be removed from the front of the thigh, without disturbing the subjacent muscles from their relative positions. The mass of muscles, on the inner side of the thigh,

* The operation recommended by Sir A. Cooper is that usually performed now ; because, if Gimbernat's ligament be divided, its cut edges often retract to such an extent, that no truss can possibly retain the hernia when the patient assumes the erect posture.

† The museum of St. Bartholomew's Hospital contains two examples of double femoral hernia in the male, with the obturator arising on each side from the epigastric. In three out of the four hernia the obturator runs on the inner side of the mouth of the sac. See Prep. 55, 69, Series 17.

‡ During the session of 1857–58 more than half a dozen instances occurred where the obturator artery was given off by a common origin with the epigastric artery. In all these cases, however, the artery passed close by the bone, so that it would not have been injured in the operation for relief of strangulation.

consists of the adductors; that in the middle, of the extensors: the long thin muscle crossing obliquely in front from the outer to the inner side, is the sartorius. In the middle are seen the femoral vessels, and the anterior crural nerve emerging beneath the crural arch.

Sartorius. This muscle *arises* from the anterior superior spine of the ileum, and from the ridge below to the extent of an inch. It passes obliquely like a strap over the front of the thigh towards the inner side; and then descends almost perpendicularly on the inner side of the thigh as far as the knee, where it terminates in a flat tendon which expands, and is *inserted* into the inner and front part of the tibia just below its tubercle. The tendon appears all the wider on account of its broad connection with the fascia of the leg. A large bursa * is interposed between the tendon and the internal lateral ligament. The chief *action* of the muscle is to fix the pelvis steadily on the thigh. It also crosses one leg over the other, as tailors sit when at work.† Its nerve comes from the middle cutaneous branch of the anterior crural.

Scarpa's triangle. In consequence of the oblique direction of the sartorius, a triangle is formed, which has this muscle and the adductor longus for its two sides, and the crural arch for its base: the triangle is called 'Scarpa's.'‡ The contents of this important space should be carefully displayed, and their relative positions well studied. This triangle contains all the parts which pass under the crural arch; namely, from without inwards; the external cutaneous nerve, close to the anterior spine of the ileum; the iliacus internus and psoas; the anterior crural nerve and its divisions, especially the long saphenous nerve; the femoral artery with its great branch 'the profunda,' which runs

---

* In persons, females especially, who are in the habit of riding, this bursa sometimes becomes enlarged.

† Hence the name given to it by Spigelius (De corporis hum. fabric.), 'Quem ego sartorium musculum vocare soleo, quod sartores eo maxime utuntur, dum crus cruri inter consuendum imponunt.'

‡ So called in compliment to the Italian anatomist who first tied the femoral in it for popliteal aneurism.

down behind it and gives off the 'internal' and 'external circumflex;' the femoral vein, joined by the profunda vein and the
internal saphena; and, lastly, the pectineus muscle.

The triangle is important in a surgical point of view, since it is
in this space that the femoral artery is usually ligatured for popliteal aneurism. The guide to the artery is the inner border of the
sartorius. The situation at which this muscle crosses over the

Fig. 192.

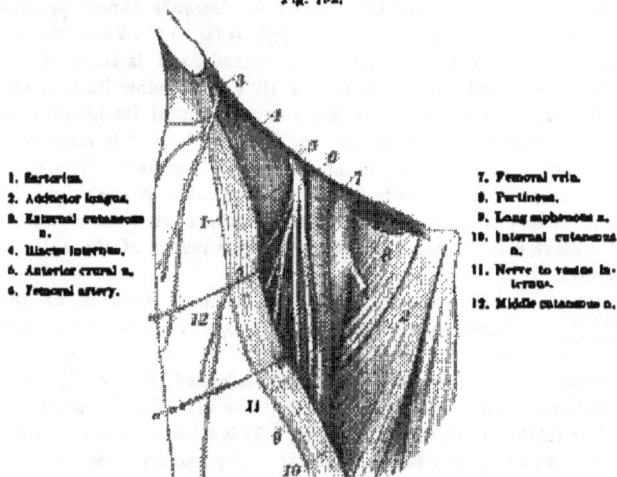

1. Sartorius.	7. Femoral vein.
2. Adductor longus.	8. Pectineus.
3. External cutaneous n.	9. Long saphenous n.
4. Iliacus internus.	10. Internal cutaneous n.
5. Anterior crural n.	11. Nerve to vastus internus.
6. Femoral artery.	12. Middle cutaneous n.

DIAGRAM OF SCARPA'S TRIANGLE.

femoral artery, varies from one and a half to four and a half inches
below Poupart's ligament; so that no rule can be laid down as to
the exact situation where the artery disappears under the sartorius.
The best way to find the inner border of the muscle during life, is
to make the patient put it into action.

Adductor muscles.   A strong group of muscles, called the 'adductors,'
extends along the inner side of the thigh, from the
pelvis to the femur. Their two most important actions

are to co-operate in balancing the pelvis steadily on the thigh, as in standing on one leg ; and (if the fixed point be reversed) to draw together or adduct the thighs. They are five in number, and are supplied, with one exception—the pectineus—by the same nerve—namely, the obturator. They are termed, respectively, the gracilis, adductor longus, pectineus, adductor brevis, and adductor magnus. The innermost is the gracilis; to clean it properly, it should be stretched by separating one thigh from the other.

Gracilis.   This long, flat muscle *arises* by a broad, ribbon-like tendon from the pubes close to the symphysis, and from the border of the pubic arch nearly as low as the tuber ischii. It descends almost perpendicularly on the inner side of the thigh, and terminates in a tendon which subsequently spreads out, and is inserted into the inner side of the tibia below the tubercle, immediately behind the sartorius. Both tendons play over the internal lateral ligament of the knee-joint, and there is a bursa common to both. This muscle assists in fixing the pelvis, and in adducting the thigh ; it also helps to bend the knee. Its nerve comes from the anterior division of the obturator.

Adductor longus.   This muscle lies external to the gracilis, and arises by a round tendon from the front of the pubes below the crest. As it descends, it becomes broader, and is inserted into the middle third of the linea aspera of the femur. It forms with the sartorius a triangular space called Scarpa's triangle (p. 452). It is supplied by the anterior division of the obturator nerve.

Pectineus.   This muscle lies on the same plane, but external to the adductor longus. It arises from the triangular surface of the pubes in front of the linea ilio-pectinea, and is inserted into the ridge leading from the lesser trochanter to the linea aspera. Its nerve comes from the anterior crural, sometimes also from the obturator (p. 358).

By separating the contiguous borders of the pectineus and the adductor longus, the adductor brevis is exposed with the anterior division of the obturator nerve lying upon it. To obtain a complete view of them, the pectineus and adductor longus must be reflected from their origin. The obturator nerve supplies all the adductors. It leaves the pelvis. through the upper part of the obturator foramen, and soon divides into an anterior and posterior branch: the anterior runs in front of the adductor brevis, and supplies the hip-joint, the adductor longus, the gracilis, and sometimes the adductor brevis; the posterior runs behind the adductor brevis, and supplies it as well as the obturator externus, the adductor magnus, and the knee-joint.

Adductor brevis.

This muscle *arises* from the front surface of the pubes near the symphysis, and from its ascending ramus; it widens as it descends, and is *inserted* into the upper third of the linea aspera. Its nerve is derived from the obturator. By reflecting it from its origin, the following muscle is exposed.*

Adductor magnus.

This muscle *arises* from the lower two-thirds of the pubic arch and from the tuberosity of the ischium. Its fibres spread out, and are *inserted*, behind the other adductors, into the whole length of the linea aspera; also into the ridge leading from it to the inner condyle. Its nerve comes from the posterior division of the obturator. Observe that all the adductor muscles are inserted into the femur by flat tendons which are more or less connected with each other.

About the junction of the upper two-thirds with the lower third of the thigh, the femoral artery passes through an oval opening in the tendon of the adductor magnus.

Psoas magnus and iliacus internus.

These muscles have been fully described in the dissection of the abdomen (p. 348).

Tensor fasciæ femoris.

This muscle is situated at the upper and outer part of the thigh. It *arises* from the external lip of the crest of the ileum, close to the anterior spine, descends with a slight inclination backwards, and is *inserted*, at the junction of the upper with the middle third, between two layers of the strong aponeurosis, generally described as part of the fascia lata (p. 443).

---

* Beneath the adductor brevis, and running parallel with the upper border of the adductor magnus, is seen the obturator externus. But the description of this muscle is deferred till the dissection of the external rotators of the thigh.

Its chief use is to fix the pelvis steadily on the thigh, and also to rotate the thigh inwards; in this last action it co-operates with the anterior fibres of the glutæus medius, with which it is almost inseparably connected. Any one may convince himself of this by placing the hand on the hip, and rotating the thigh inwards. Both these muscles are supplied by the same nerve—the superior glutæal.

To form an adequate idea of the strength, extent, and connections of the aponeurosis on the outer side of the thigh, it should be separated from the vastus externus muscle upon which it lies. There is no difficulty in doing so, for it is united to the muscle by an abundance of loose cellular tissue.* With a little perseverance the aponeurosis can be traced to the linea aspera, the head of the tibia, and the fibula. See how completely it protects the outer side of the knee-joint.

Extensor muscles. The powerful muscles situated between the tensor fasciæ on the outer and the adductors on the inner side, are extensors of the leg. One of them—the 'rectus'—arises from the pelvis; the other—the 'triceps'—arises from the shaft of the thigh bone by three portions, called, respectively, the cruræus, the vastus internus and externus. All are supplied by the anterior crural nerve.

To see the origins of the rectus femoris, dissect between the origin of the sartorius and the tensor fasciæ; in doing so, avoid injuring the branches of the external circumflex artery.

Rectus. This muscle arises from the pelvis by two strong tendons, which soon unite at an acute angle : one from the anterior inferior spine of the ileum, the other from the rough surface of the ileum, just above the acetabulum. The muscle descends perpendicularly down the front of the thigh, and is inserted into the common extensor tendon. The structure of this muscle is remarkable. A tendon runs down the centre, and the muscular fibres are implanted on either side of it, like the vane on the shaft of a feather. Its nerve comes from the anterior crural.

* When this tissue becomes the seat of suppuration, the matter is apt to extend all down the outside of the thigh, not being able to make its way to the surface by reason of the dense fascia.

This mass of muscle surrounds the greater part of *Triceps ex-* the shaft of the femur; therefore the whole extent of it *tensor.* cannot be seen without completely dissecting the thigh. It consists of an outer, middle, and inner portion, called, respectively, the vastus externus, the cruræus, and the vastus internus. The *vastus externus* arises by a very strong aponeurosis from the outer side of the base of the great trochanter, and from the outer lip of the linea aspera nearly down to the external condyle. The *cruræus* arises from the upper three-fourths of the front surface of the shaft. The *vastus internus* arises from the upper two-thirds of the inner surface of the shaft, and also from the inner lip of the linea aspera. They are all supplied by branches from the anterior crural nerve.

Common extensor tend. The tendon of the rectus, gradually expanding, becomes connected on its under surface with the tendon of the cruræus,* and on either side with that of the vasti, and is firmly fixed into the upper part and sides of the patella. From this bone the common extensor tendon, the '*ligamentum patellæ*,' descends over the front of the knee-joint, and is inserted into the tubercle of the tibia. Besides this, the lower fibres of the vasti terminate on a sheet-like tendon, which runs wide of the patella on either side, and is directly inserted into the sides of the head of the tibia and fibula, so that the knee is completely protected all round. The patella is a great sesamoid bone, interposed to facilitate the play of the tendon over the condyles of the femur: it not only materially protects the joint, but adds to the power of the extensor muscles, by increasing the angle at which the tendon is inserted into the tibia.

To facilitate the play of the extensor tendon there are two bursæ. One is placed between the ligamentum patellæ and the tubercle of

---

* A few of the deeper fibres of the cruræus are inserted into the fold of the synovial membrane of the knee-joint which rises above the patella. These are described as a distinct muscle, under the name of the '*sub-cruræus*.' Their use is to raise the synovial membrane, so that it may not be injured by the play of the patella. Since the triceps is connected to the lower part of the shaft of the femur only by loose cellular tissue, there is nothing to prevent the distention of the synovial membrane, in cases of inflammation, to the extent of several inches above the patella.

the tibia, the other between the crureus and the lower part of the femur. This last is of considerable size. In early life it is, as a rule, distinct from the synovial membrane of the knee-joint; but after a few years of friction a wide communication frequently exists between them.

Action of the extensor muscles. The extensor muscles of the thigh are among the most powerful in the body. Great power of extending the knee is one of the essential conditions of the erect attitude. Without it, how could we rise from the sitting position? When erect, how could we walk, run, or spring? The rectus, by taking origin from the pelvis, gains a double advantage; it acts upon two joints simultaneously, bending the thigh while it extends the knee, as when we advance the leg in walking: it also contributes to balance the pelvis on the head of the thigh bone, and thus prevents the body from falling backwards. We cannot have a better proof of the collective power of the extensor muscles than when the patella is broken by their contraction; an injury which sometimes happens when a man, slipping backwards, makes a violent effort to recover his balance.

Bursa over the patella. The skin over the patella is exceedingly loose, and in the subcutaneous tissue is a bursa of considerable size. Since this bursa is apt to enlarge and inflame in females who are in the habit of kneeling at their work, it is generally called 'the housemaid's bursa.' The bursa is not seated exactly over the patella, but extends some way down the ligamentum patellæ; indeed, in some cases it is entirely confined to this ligament. This corresponds with the position of the tumour which the bursa occasions when enlarged. Generally speaking, in subjects brought for dissection, the wall of the bursa is more or less thickened, and its interior intersected by numerous fibrous cords, remnants of the original cellular structure altered by long-continued friction. Again, the wall of the bursa does not always form a complete sac; sometimes there is a wide opening in it; this explains the rapidity with which inflammation, in some cases, extends from the bursa into the surrounding cellular tissue.

Below the bursa is a layer of fascia lata, and under this is a network of arteries. The immediate covering of the bone, or what may be called its periosteum, is a strong expansion derived from the extensor tendon. This is interesting for the following reason: in ordinary fractures of the patella from muscular action the tendinous expansion over it is torn also; the ends of the bone gape widely, and never unite except by ligament. But in fractures from direct mechanical violence, the tendinous expansion, being entire, maintains the fragments in apposition, so that there is commonly a bony union.

The femoral artery is a continuation of the external iliac. Passing beneath the crural arch at a point about midway between the spine of the ileum and the symphysis pubis, it descends nearly perpendicularly along the front and inner side of the thigh. At the junction of the upper two-thirds with the lower third of the thigh, it passes through an opening in the tendon of the adductor magnus, and entering the ham, takes the name of 'popliteal.' A line drawn from the point specified of the crural arch to the tubercle of the internal condyle would pretty nearly indicate the course of the artery. Its distance from the surface increases as it descends. Immediately under, and for a short distance below the crural arch, it is supported by the inner border of the psoas; lower down it runs in front of the pectineus, but separated from it by the profunda vessels; still lower down it lies upon the adductor longus, and adductor magnus.

In the upper third of the thigh, the artery is situated in Scarpa's triangle, and is comparatively superficial, being covered only by the muscular fascia. About the middle third it is more deeply seated, and is covered by the sartorius: here, being placed among powerful muscles, it is protected from pressure by a tendinous canal, which will be presently examined.

At the crural arch the anterior crural nerve is placed on the outer side of the artery, and the femoral vein on the inner side: as the vein descends, it gradually passes behind the artery. Both lie close together, and are inclosed in a common sheath.

Hunter's
canal.

In the middle third of the thigh, the femoral artery is contained in a tendinous canal * under the sartorius, called ' Hunter's canal.' This canal at its upper part is rather indistinct; but it gradually becomes stronger towards the opening in the tendon of the adductor magnus. Its boundaries are formed by the tendons of the muscles between which the artery runs. On the inner side are the tendons of the adductor longus and magnus; on the outer side is the tendon of the vastus internus; in front the canal is completed by an aponeurotic expansion thrown obliquely across from the adductors to the vastus internus, as shown in fig. 103. In a horizontal section the canal appears triangular. The adaptation of this shape to the exigencies of the case is manifest when we reflect that the muscles keep the side of the triangle always tight, and thereby prevent any compression of the vessels.

Hunter's canal contains not only the femoral artery and vein, but also the internal saphenous nerve. The vein lies behind and to the outer side; the nerve to the inner side of the artery.

It is plain that a ligature can be placed around the artery, in the upper third of the thigh, with comparative facility; not so easily in the middle third. The artery is tied for an aneurism of the popliteal, just where the sartorius begins to overlap it, for three reasons:—1, it is more accessible; 2, the coats of the artery at this distance are less likely to be diseased; 3, the origin of the profunda is sufficiently far off to admit of the formation of a coagulum. An incision, beginning about three inches below the crural arch, should be made about three inches over the line of the artery. The muscular fascia should be divided over a director to the same extent. Then, by gently

Fig. 103.

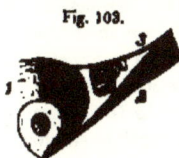

SECTION THROUGH
HUNTER'S CANAL.

1. Vastus internus.
2. Adductor longus.
3. Aponeurosis thrown across.

---

* Called 'Hunter's canal,' because it was in this part of its course that John Hunter first tied the femoral artery for aneurism of the popliteal, in St. George's Hospital, A.D. 1785. The particulars of this interesting case are published in the Trans. for the Improvement of Med. and Chir. Knowledge.

drawing aside the inner border of the sartorius, we discover the artery inclosed in its sheath with the vein. An opening should be made into the sheath sufficient to admit the passage of the aneurismal needle, which should be turned round the artery from within outwards. The nerves to be avoided are—the long saphenous, which runs along the outer side of the artery, and the cutaneous nerves which cross obliquely over it.

Having already traced the superficial branches of the femoral artery in the groin, namely, the superficial epigastric, pudic, and circumflexa ilii (p. 438), we pass on now to the profunda.

Profunda artery and branches. The profunda is the chief branch of the femoral, and is the proper nutrient artery of the thigh. It arises from the outer and back part of the femoral, about one and a half or two inches below the crural arch, and runs down behind the femoral till it reaches the tendon of the adductor longus; here the profunda passes behind the adductor, and is finally lost in the hamstring muscles. In most subjects, the profunda, for a short distance after its origin, lies rather on the outer side of the femoral and on a deeper plane, over the iliacus muscle: in this situation it might be mistaken for the femoral itself—indeed, such an error has actually occurred in practice. It soon, however, gets behind the femoral, and lies upon the adductor brevis and magnus; it is separated from the femoral artery at first, by their corresponding veins; lower down, by the adductor longus.[*]

The branches of the profunda generally arise in the following order:—1, the internal circumflex; 2, the external circumflex; 3, the perforating.

The *internal circumflex* is given off from the inner part of the profunda, and then sinks deeply into the thigh, between the psoas and pectineus. At the lower border of the obturator externus it terminates in two divisions: one, which supplies the muscles in its neighbourhood, namely, the pectineus, psoas, adductors, gracilis,

---

[*] The point at which the profunda is given off below the crural arch varies very much even in the two limbs of the same body. We have measured it in 19 bodies, or 38 femoral arteries. It varied from ½ to 3 inches. In 22 cases the profunda came off between 1½ and 2 inches; in 9 this distance was exceeded; in 7 this distance was less.

and obturator externus; the other will be seen in the dissection of
the back of the thigh, between the adductor magnus and the quadratus femoris. This division gives off a small articular branch to
the hip-joint, which runs through the notch in the acetabulum to
the ligamentum teres : it afterwards inosculates with the ischiatic
and superior perforating arteries.

The *external circumflex* artery comes off from the outer side of
the profunda, runs transversely outwards beneath the sartorius and

Fig. 104.

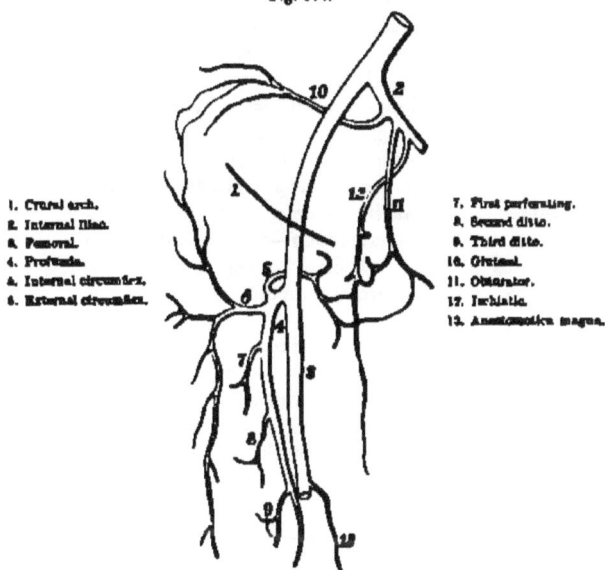

1. Crural arch.	7. First perforating.
2. Internal Iliac.	8. Second ditto.
3. Femoral.	9. Third ditto.
4. Profunda.	10. Gluteal.
5. Internal circumflex.	11. Obturator.
6. External circumflex.	12. Ischiatic.
	13. Anastomotica magna.

PLAN OF THE INOSCULATIONS OF THE CIRCUMFLEX ARTERIES.

rectus, between the branches of the anterior crural nerve, and then
subdivides into three sets of branches, 'ascending,' 'transverse,'
and 'descending.' The *ascending* run up to the outer side of

the ileum, beneath the tensor fasciæ and gluteus medius, supply these muscles, and inosculate with the terminal branches of the gluteal artery. The *transverse* are chiefly lost in the vastus externus, and inosculate posteriorly with the ischiatic artery. The *descending*, one or more in number, of considerable size, run down between the rectus and cruræus, and supply both these muscles: one branch, larger than the rest, runs down in the substance of the vastus externus, along with the nerve to that muscle, and inosculates with the articular branches of the popliteal.

The *perforating* branches of the profunda are so named because they pass through the adductors to supply the hamstring muscles. There are generally three, but they vary both in number and size. The first is the largest. It passes between the pectineus and adductor brevis, then through the tendon of the adductor magnus. The second passes through the tendon of the adductor brevis and magnus, and usually furnishes the nutrient artery of the femur. The third, through the tendon of the adductor magnus. They not only supply the hamstring muscles—namely, the biceps, semitendinosus, and semimembranosus—but, also, the vastus externus and gluteus maximus. The perforating arteries inosculate with one another, with the internal circumflex, and with the ischiatic arteries.

Arterial in-osculations. To test your knowledge of the arterial inosculations about the upper part of the thigh, reflect on the answer to the following questions. If the femoral were tied *above* the origin of the profunda, how would the circulation be carried on ? The ascending branch of the external circumflex communicates with the gluteal ; the internal circumflex communicates with the obturator and ischiatic (see fig. 104). Again—how is the circulation maintained when the femoral is tied *below* the profunda ? The descending branch of the external circumflex and the perforating branches of the profunda communicate with the articular branches of the popliteal and the tibial recurrent.[*]

* Read the account of the dissection of an aneurismal limb by Sir A. Cooper, Med. Chir. Trans. vol. ii.

The continuation of the profunda (sometimes called the fourth perforating), much reduced in size, passes through the tendon of the adductor magnus, and is distributed to the short head of the biceps, finally inosculating with the articular arteries.

The *anastomotica magna* arises from the femoral artery just before it leaves its tendinous canal. It runs in front of the tendon of the adductor magnus, in company with the long saphenous nerve to the inner side of the knee. Here it divides into two branches: one accompanies the saphenous nerve, and is subsequently distributed to the skin; the other ramifies over the capsule and communicates with the other articular arteries.*

Anterior crural nerve. The anterior crural nerve is the largest branch of the lumbar plexus (p. 358). It comes from the third and fourth lumbar nerves. It passes beneath the crural arch, lying in the groove between the iliacus and psoas, about a quarter of an inch to the outer side of the artery, and soon divides into branches, some of which are cutaneous, but the greater number supply the exterior muscles of the thigh. The cutaneous branches, already described (p. 441), and the long saphenous nerve, are given off from the superficial part of the trunk; the muscular from the deep part.

The *long saphenous nerve* descends close to the outer side of the femoral artery, and enters the tendinous canal with it in the middle third of the thigh. In the canal it crosses over the artery to its inner side. The nerve leaves the artery just before it becomes popliteal, and then runs in company with the anastomotica magna to the inner side of the knee, where it becomes superficial, between the gracilis and the sartorius. In the middle third of the thigh it gives off a small branch which communicates with the internal cutaneous and obturator nerves; and lower down another branch is distributed to the skin over the patella. Its further relations will be seen in the dissection of the leg and foot.

* In its course down the thigh the femoral artery gives off several small branches to the sartorius, and one of considerable size for the supply of the vastus internus. We may trace this branch through the substance of the vastus down to the patella, where it joins the beautiful network of vessels on the surface of that bone.

Its *muscular branches* are to be traced to the sartorius, rectus, cruraeus, and subcruraeus; the branch to the vastus externus accompanies the descending branch of the external circumflex artery, and that to the vastus internus runs parallel with, but external to, the long saphenous nerve: these two last-named branches supply articular filaments to the knee-joint. One or more branches pass under the femoral artery and vein to supply the pectineus.

The *obturator nerve*, also a branch of the lumbar plexus (p. 358), supplies the adductor muscles. It enters the thigh through the upper part of the obturator foramen with the corresponding artery, and immediately divides into two branches, of which one passes in front of, the other behind, the adductor brevis. The front branch* subdivides for the supply of the gracilis, the adductor longus, and sometimes the adductor brevis; the hind one supplies the obturator externus and the adductor brevis and magnus. In some bodies you can succeed in tracing a filament of the obturator nerve through the notch of the acetabulum into the hip-joint, and another, which runs near the popliteal artery into the back part of the knee-joint. We have frequently seen cutaneous branches from the obturator on the inner side of the thigh. This is interesting practically, since it helps to explain the pain often felt on the inner side of the knee in disease of the hip-joint.

The *obturator artery*, after passing through the foramen, divides into two branches, which form a circle round the obturator membrane. These supply the external obturator and adductors of the thigh, and inosculate with the internal circumflex artery (p. 462). It usually gives off the little artery to the ligamentum teres of the hip-joint.

* Near the lower border of the adductor longus, a filament from this branch communicates with an offset from the long saphenous nerve and with one from the internal cutaneous branch of the anterior crural nerve. This communication takes place over the femoral artery in Hunter's canal.

DISSECTION OF THE FRONT OF THE LEG.

The foot should be turned inwards, and fixed in this position. An incision must be made from the knee, down the front of the leg, over the ankle, along the top of the foot to the great toe; a second, at right angles to the first, on either side of the ankle; a third, across the basis of the toes. Reflect the skin from the front and sides of the leg and foot.

Cutaneous veins and nerves. Having traced the internal saphena vein (p. 441) to the inner side of the knee, follow it down the inner side of the leg, in front of the inner ankle * to the top of the foot. On the top of the foot notice that the principal veins form an arch, with the convexity forwards, as on the back of the hand. This arch receives the veins from the toes. From the inner side of the arch the internal saphena originates; from the outer side, the external saphena. The latter vein runs behind the external ankle, up the back of the calf of the leg to join the popliteal vein.

Long saphenous nerve. The skin on the inner side of the leg is supplied by the long saphenous nerve (p. 464). It becomes subcutaneous on the inner side of the knee, between the gracilis and sartorius. Here it meets the saphena vein, and accompanies it down the leg, distributing its branches on either side, till it is finally lost on the inner side of the foot, base of the great toe. The largest branch curves round the inner side of the knee, just below the patella, to supply the skin in this situation.

The skin on the front and outer part of the upper half of the leg is supplied by cutaneous branches from the external popliteal or peroneal nerve; the skin of the lower half, by the external cutaneous.

* The French commonly bleed from the internal saphena vein as it crosses over the inner ankle, this being a convenient and safe place for venæsection.

External cutaneous or musculo-cutaneous nerve. This is a branch of the peroneal nerve: it comes through the fascia about the lower third of the outer side of the leg; and descending over the front of the ankle, divides into two branches. Trace its subdivisions, and you will find the inner one supplies the inner side of the great toe, and the contiguous sides of the second and third toes; the outer one distributes branches to the outer side of the third toe, both sides of the fourth, and the inner side of the fifth toe.

The outside of the little toe is supplied by the external saphenous nerve, which runs behind the outer ankle with the corresponding vein.

The contiguous sides of the great and second toes are supplied by the termination of the anterior tibial nerve.[*]

Muscular fascia and annular ligaments. This is remarkably thick and strong. Besides its general purpose of forming sheaths for the muscles, and straps for the tendons, it gives origin, as in the forearm, to muscular fibres; so that it cannot be removed near the knee, without leaving the muscles ragged. The fascia is attached to the head of the tibia and the fibula: it is identified on the inner side with the expanded tendons of the sartorius, gracilis, and semi-tendinosus; on the outer side with that of the biceps: consequently, when these muscles act, it is rendered tense. Following it down the leg, you find that it is attached to the edge of the tibia, and that it becomes stronger as it approaches the ankle, to form the ligaments which confine the tendons in this situation. Of these ligaments, called 'annular,' there are three, as follow:—

a. The *anterior* extends obliquely across the front of the ankle-joint, and confines the extensor tendons of the ankle and toes. It consists of two straps, which cross each other over the front of the ankle like braces. One brace goes from the malleolus externus to the scaphoid and internal cuneiform bones; the other runs from the cuboid and os calcis upwards and inwards to the inner border

[*] Such is the most common distribution of the nerves to the upper surface of the toes. But deviations from this arrangement are frequent.

of the tibia: it is the strain of this ligament which occasions the pain in sprains of the ankle. You will see presently that it makes a beautiful pulley for the extensor longus digitorum.

b. The *external* extends from the outer malleolus to the os calcis, and confines the tendons of the peronei muscles, which draw the foot outwards.

c. The *internal* extends from the inner malleolus to the os calcis, and binds down the flexor tendons of the foot and toes.

Remove the fascia, leaving enough of the annular ligaments to retain the tendons in their places.

Muscles on the front of the leg.

The muscles on the front of the leg are:—1, the tibialis anticus; 2, the extensor communis digitorum and peroneus tertius; 3, the extensor proprius pollicis.

Tibialis anticus.

The tibialis anticus arises from the external tuberosity and the upper two-thirds of the outer side of the tibia, from the interosseous membrane, and from the fascia which covers it. About the lower third of the leg the fibres terminate on a strong flat tendon, which descends obliquely over the front of the ankle to the inner side of the foot; here it becomes a little broader, and is inserted into the internal cuneiform bone and the tarsal end of the metatarsal bone of the great toe. The synovial membrane, which lines the sheath of the tendon beneath the annular ligament, accompanies it to within an inch of its insertion; consequently it is opened when the tendon is divided for club-foot. The action of this muscle is to draw the foot upwards and inwards.* When the foot is the fixed point, it assists in balancing the body at the ankle. Its nerve comes from the peroneal.

Extensor communis digitorum.

This muscle lies along the fibular side of the preceding. It arises from the head of the tibia, from the upper three-fourths of the fibula, from the interosseous membrane, and the fascia. Its fibres terminate in a penniform manner upon a long tendon, situated on the inner side of the muscle: this tendon descends in front of the ankle and divides

* It is generally necessary to divide this tendon in distortion of the foot inwards, called 'talipes varus.'

into four slips which pass to the four outer toes. They diverge
from each other, and are inserted into the toes thus:—on the first
phalanx, each tendon (except that of the little toe) is joined on its
outer side by the corresponding tendon of the extensor brevis.
The united tendons then expand, and are inserted as on the
fingers; that is, the middle part is inserted into the base of the
second phalanx; the sides run on to the base of the third (p. 285).
Its nerve comes from the peroneal.

Immediately below the ankle the anterior annular ligament
forms a pulley through which the tendon of this muscle plays.
It is like a sling, of which the two ends are attached to the os
calcis, while the loop serves to confine the tendon. The play of
the tendon is facilitated by a synovial membrane, which is prolonged for a short distance along each of its four divisions. Besides its chief action, this muscle extends the ankle-joint.[*]

Peroneus tertius. This appears like a portion of the preceding. Its
fibres arise from the lower part of the shaft of the
fibula and the interosseous membrane, and terminate
on their tendon like barbs on a quill. The tendon passes through
the same pulley with the long extensor of the toes, and, expanding
considerably, is inserted into the tarsal end of the metatarsal bone of
the little toe. It is supplied by a branch of the anterior tibial nerve.

The peroneus tertius and the tibialis anticus are important
muscles in progression. They raise the toes and foot from the
ground. Those who have lost the use of these muscles are obliged
to drag the foot along the ground, or to swing the entire limb
outwards, in walking.

Extensor proprius pollicis. This muscle lies partly concealed between the tibialis
anticus and the extensor longus digitorum. It arises
from rather more than the middle third of the fibula,
and from the interosseous membrane. The fibres terminate in a
penniform manner on the tendon, which runs over the ankle, between the tendons of the tibialis anticus and the extensor communis

---

[*] There is often a large bursa between the tendon of the extensor longus digitorum and the outer end of the astragalus. This bursa sometimes communicates with the joint of the head of the astragalus.

digitorum, along the top of the foot, to the great toe, where it is
inserted into the base of the last phalanx. It has a special pulley
beneath the annular ligament, lined by a synovial membrane, which
accompanies it as far as the metatarsal bone of the great toe. It
is supplied by the anterior tibial, a branch of the peroneal nerve.

Now examine the course, relations, and branches of the anterior
tibial artery. Since it lies deeply between the muscles, it is
necessary to separate them from each other: this is easily done by
proceeding from the ankle towards the knee.

Course and relations of the anterior tibial artery. The anterior tibial artery is one of the two branches
into which the popliteal divides at the lower border of
the popliteus. It comes forward about 1¼ inch below
the head of the fibula, above the interosseous membrane, and then descends, lying in rather more than the first half
of its course upon the interosseous membrane, afterwards along
the front of the tibia. It runs beneath the annular ligament over
the front of the ankle, where it takes the name of the dorsal artery
of the foot. Thus, a line drawn from the head of the fibula to the
interval between the first and second metatarsal bones would nearly
coincide with its course. In the upper third of the leg it lies deep
between the tibialis anticus and the extensor communis digitorum;
in the lower two-thirds, between the tibialis anticus and the extensor proprius pollicis. But in *front of the ankle* the artery is
crossed by the extensor proprius pollicis, and lies between the
tendon of this muscle and those of the extensor communis digitorum.

The artery is accompanied by the anterior tibial nerve (a branch
of the peroneal), which runs for some distance upon its fibular
side, then in front of it, and lower down is again situated on its
outer side. It is accompanied by two veins, one on either side,
which communicate at intervals by cross branches.

The branches of the anterior tibial are as follow:—

a. The *recurrent* branch ascends close by the outer side of the
head of the tibia to the front of the knee-joint, where it inosculates with the other articular arteries derived from the popliteal.

b. Irregular *muscular* branches.

c. The *malleolar* branches, *external* and *internal*, ramify over the ankle, and supply the joint, the articular ends of the bones, and the sheaths of the tendons around them.

Extensor brevis digitorum. This muscle is situated on the top of the foot, beneath the long extensor tendons of the toes. It arises from the outer part of the os calcis, and from the ligaments uniting this bone to the astragalus. The fibres run obliquely over the foot, and terminate on four tendons, which pass forwards to the four inner toes. The innermost one is inserted by an expanded tendon into the base of the first phalanx of the great toe; the others join the fibular side of the long extensor tendons to be inserted into the ungual phalanx. The tendon to the great toe crosses over the dorsal artery of the foot. It is supplied by a branch of the anterior tibial nerve.

Dorsal artery of the foot. This artery, the continuation of the anterior tibial, runs over the instep to the interval between the first and second metatarsal bones, where it sinks into the sole and joins the deep plantar arch. On the top of the foot it runs along the outer side of the extensor proprius pollicis, and before it dips down into the sole, is crossed by the short extensor tendon of the great toe. The dorsal artery gives off the following branches:—

a. The *tarsal* branch arises near the scaphoid bone, passes beneath the extensor brevis digitorum towards the outside of the foot, supplies the bones and joints of the tarsus, and inosculates with the arteries in the sole.

b. The *metatarsal* branch generally runs towards the outside of the foot, near the bases of the metatarsal bones, and gives off the three outer interosseous arteries. These pass forwards over the corresponding interosseous muscles, supply them, and then subdivide to supply the opposite sides of the upper surface of the toes. They communicate by perforating branches with the plantar arteries.

c. The *dorsalis hallucis* is, strictly speaking, the artery of the first interosseous space. It comes from the dorsal artery just before this sinks into the sole, and runs forwards to supply both sides of the great toe and the inner side of the second toe.

Peronei muscles. These muscles are situated on the outer side of the fibula, and are named, respectively, peroneus longus and brevis.

Peroneus longus. This arises from the outer surface of the fibula along its upper two-thirds. The fibres terminate in a penniform manner upon a tendon, which runs through a groove behind the outer ankle, then along the outer side of the os calcis, and, lastly, through a groove on the under surface of the os cuboides deep into the sol It crosses the sole obliquely, and is inserted into the tarsal end of the metatarsal bone of the great toe. In its course through these several bony grooves the tendon is confined by a fibrous sheath, lined by a synovial membrane. In removing the metatarsal bone of the great toe, if possible, leave the insertion of this tendon. Its nerve comes from the peroneal.

Peroneus brevis. This muscle lies beneath the preceding. It arises from about the middle third of the outer surface of the fibula, internal to the preceding muscle. It terminates on a tendon which runs behind the outer ankle, through the same sheath with the peroneus longus, then proceeds along the outside of the foot, and is inserted into the tarsal end of the metatarsal bone of the little toe.* Its nerve is from the anterior tibial.

The *action* of the peronei is to raise the outer side of the foot.† This movement regulates the bearing of the foot in progression, so as to throw the principal part of the weight on the ball of the great toe. Its action is well exemplified in skating. Again, supposing the fixed point to be at the foot, they tend to prevent the body from falling on the opposite side, as when we balance ourselves on one leg.

Peroneal nerve. Near the inner side of the tendon of the biceps flexor of the leg, is a large nerve called the peroneal, a branch of the great ischiatic. By reflecting the upper part of

---

* On the outside of the os calcis there is a ridge which separates the tendons of the peronei. Each has a distinct sheath. The short tendon runs above, the long one below the ridge.

† In distortion of the foot outwards, called 'talipes valgus,' it is generally necessary to divide the tendons of the peronei.

the peroneus longus, you will find that this nerve runs round the
outer side of the fibula immediately below its head. Here it divides
into several branches, as follow:—1. Three articular branches to
the knee-joint, which pass in with the external articular arteries,
and the tibial recurrent artery; 2. The anterior tibial, which
accompanies the corresponding artery; 3. The external cutaneous
(p. 467), which comes through the fascia between the peroneus
longus and the extensor longus digitorum; 4. Branches which
supply all the muscles in front of the leg, namely, the extensors of
the foot and the toes and the peronei.

DISSECTION OF THE GLUTÆAL REGION.

The body having been placed on its face, rotate the thighs
inwards as much as possible, and cross them.

The incision through the skin should commence at the coccyx,
and be continued in a semicircular manner along the crest of the
ileum. Another incision should be made from the coccyx downwards and outwards for about six inches below the great trochanter.
In reflecting the skin, notice the thick cushion which the subcutaneous adipose tissue forms over the tuberosity of the ischium.

I have often seen a large bursa between the cushion and the
bone.

Cutaneous
nerves.

These are derived from several sources. The posterior divisions of the first and second lumbar nerves
descend over the crest of the ileum, near the origin of
the erector spinæ, to supply the skin over the gluteus maximus.
Internal to these, are the posterior branches of the sacral nerves,
which are distributed to the integument over the sacrum and
coccyx. Over the middle of the crest come the lateral branches
of the twelfth dorsal, and internal to it, the iliac branch of the ilio-
hypogastric. Other cutaneous nerves come up from below; they
are branches of the lesser ischiatic, and proceed from beneath the
lower border of the gluteus maximus. Lastly, some branches

from the external cutaneous nerve of the thigh are seen on the outer side of this region.

Three powerful muscles are situated on the buttock, one above the other, named, according to their relative size, the glutæus maximus, medius, and minimus.

Glutæal muscles.

This is the largest muscle of the body, and is covered by a strong fascia, which sends prolongations inwards between the muscular bundles. Its great size is characteristic of man, in reference to his erect position. Its texture is thick and coarse. It arises from the posterior fifth of the crest of the Ileum, from the lower part of the sacrum, the coccyx, and the great sacro-ischiatic ligament. The fibres descend obliquely forwards, and are inserted thus :—the anterior two-thirds terminate on a strong broad tendon which plays over the great trochanter, and joins the fascia lata on the outside of the thigh (p. 443); the remaining third is inserted into the femur, along the ridge leading from the linea aspera to the great trochanter.

Glutæus maximus.

This muscle *extends* the thigh bone upon the pelvis, and is therefore one of those most concerned in raising the body from the sitting to the erect position, and in maintaining it erect. It also propels the body—in walking, running, or leaping. It is supplied with blood by the glutæal and ischiatic arteries ; with nerves by the lesser ischiatic.

The glutæus maximus should be reflected from its origin. The best way is to begin at the front border, which overlaps the glutæus medius. The dissection is difficult, and he who undertakes it for the first time, is almost sure to damage the subjacent parts. The numerous vessels which enter its under surface must be divided before the muscle can be reflected. This having been accomplished, the following objects will be exposed :—

What is seen beneath the glutæus maximus.

The muscle covering the ileum is the glutæus medius. At the posterior border of this are the several objects which come out of the pelvis through the great ischiatic notch—namely, the pyriformis muscle, above which is the trunk of the glutæal artery and nerve, and below which are the greater and lesser ischiatic nerves, the ischiatic artery, and the pudic artery and nerve. Coming through the lesser ischiatic notch, we see the tendon of the obturator internus, and attached to it are the gemelli muscles, one above, the other below it. Extending from the tuber ischii transversely outward to the great trochanter is the quadratus femoris, and below this is seen the upper part of the adductor magnus. The origins of the semimembranosus, biceps, semitendinosus, and of the adductor magnus, from the tuber ischii, are also seen; as well as the great sacro-ischiatic ligament passing upwards to the sacrum. Lastly, the great trochanter is exposed, together with a small portion of the vastus externus; and where the tendon of the glutæus maximus plays over the trochanter major, there is a large bursa, simple or multilocular. I have seen it in some subjects sufficiently capacious to hold half a pint of fluid.

Glutæus medius. This muscle arises from the surface of the ileum, between the crest and the upper curved line; also from the strong fascia which covers it towards the front. The fibres converge to a tendon which is inserted into the upper and outer surface of the great trochanter: some of the anterior fibres —in immediate connection with the tensor fasciæ—terminate on the aponeurosis of the thigh.

Reflect the glutæus medius to see the third glutæal muscle. The line of separation between them is marked by a large branch of the glutæal artery.

Glutæus minimus. This muscle arises from the surface of the ileum below the upper curved line. Its fibres pass over the capsule of the hip-joint, and converge to a tendon which is inserted into a depression on the front part of the great trochanter. This muscle and the preceding are supplied by the glutæal nerve. Between the tendon of the last two muscles and the great trochanter are two small bursæ. The chief action of this and the preceding muscle is to assist in balancing the pelvis steadily on the thigh, as when we are standing on one leg; with the fixed point at the ileum, it is an abductor of the thigh. The anterior fibres of the glutæus medius co-operate with the tensor fasciæ in rotating the thigh inwards.

Glutæal
vessels and
nerves.

The glutæal artery is the largest branch of the internal iliac (p. 387). Emerging from the pelvis through the great ischiatic notch above the pyriformis, it divides into large branches for the supply of the glutæal muscles. Of these, some (*superficial*) proceed forwards between the glutæus maximus and medius; others (*deep*) run in curves between the glutæus medius and minimus, towards the anterior part of the ileum. Many of them inosculate with branches of the external circumflex.

The nerve which accompanies the glutæal artery is a branch of the lumbo-sacral nerve (p. 391). It subdivides to supply the glutæus medius and minimus, and the tensor fasciæ; in some subjects it sends a branch to the glutæus maximus; but this muscle is chiefly supplied by the lesser ischiatic nerve.

A practical surgeon ought to be able to cut down and tie the glutæal artery as it emerges from the pelvis. The following is the best rule for finding it:—the toes are supposed to be turned inwards. Draw a line from the posterior superior spine of the ileum to the midspace between the tuber ischii and the great trochanter. The artery emerges from the pelvis at the point where the superior third joins the two inferior thirds of this line.[*]

Now examine the series of muscles which rotate the thigh outwards—namely, the pyriformis, the obturator internus, the gemelli, the quadratus femoris, and the obturator externus.

Pyriformis.

This muscle lies immediately below and parallel to the lower fibres of the glutæus medius. It arises from the front surface of the sacrum between the holes for the sacral nerves, and from the margin of the great sacro-ischiatic notch. The fibres converge to a tendon which is inserted into the upper border of the trochanter major. Its nerve comes from the sacral plexus.

Obturator
internus.

This muscle, of which we can at present see little more than the tendon, arises within the pelvis, from the ischium between the great ischiatic notch and the obtu-

[*] The operation of tying the glutæal artery was first performed by John Bell. See his ' Principles of Surgery,' vol. i. p. 421.

rator foramen; also from the obturator membrane. The fibres
terminate on four tendons which converge towards the lesser ischiatic notch, pass round it as round a pulley, and then uniting into
one, are inserted into the top of the great trochanter. Divide the
tendon about three inches from its insertion, to see the four tendons which play over the smooth cartilaginous pulley. There is a
large synovial bursa to prevent friction. The nerve of this muscle
comes from the sacral plexus; sometimes from the pudic nerve.

Gemelli. These muscles are accessory to the obturator internus,
and are situated, one above, the other below it. The
gemellus superior arises from the spine of the ischium; the gemellus
inferior from the upper part of the tuberosity. Their fibres are
inserted into the tendon of the obturator internus. Both muscles
derive their nerves from the sacral plexus.

Quadratus This muscle arises from the ridge on the outer part of
femoris. the tuber ischii. Its fibres run horizontally outwards,
and are inserted into the back of the great trochanter, in
a line with the linea aspera. Notice that the lower border of the
quadratus femoris runs parallel with the upper edge of the adductor magnus; in fact, it lies on the same plane. Between these
muscles is generally seen a terminal branch of the internal circumflex artery. Its nerve comes from the sacral plexus.

Obturator To see this muscle reflect the quadratus femoris. It
externus. arises from the front surface of the ramus of the pubes
and ischium, and from the obturator membrane. The
fibres converge to a tendon which runs horizontally outwards over
a groove in the ischium, and is inserted into the deepest part of
the pit of the great trochanter. Its nerve is a branch of the
obturator (p. 358).

Great This large nerve is formed by the union of the sacral
ischiatic nerves (fig. 105), and is destined to supply all the flexor
nerve. muscles of the lower extremity, and the extensors of the
foot.

Emerging from the pelvis through the great ischiatic foramen
below the pyriformis, it descends over the external rotator muscles of the thigh, along the interval between the tuber ischii and

the great trochanter, but rather nearer to the former ; so that, in
the sitting position, the nerve is protected from pressure by this
bony prominence. The nerve does not descend quite perpendicularly, but rather obliquely forwards, parallel with the great sacro-

Fig. 105.

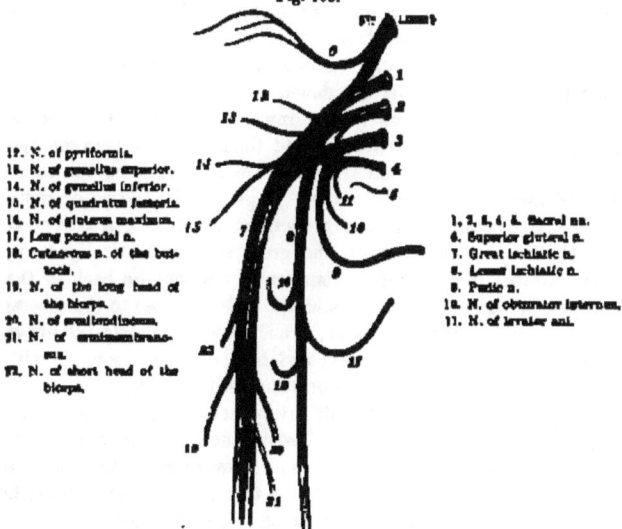

19. N. of pyriformis.
13. N. of gemellus superior.
14. N. of gemellus inferior.
15. N. of quadratus femoris.
16. N. of gluteus maximus.
17. Long pudendal n.
18. Cutaneous n. of the but-
      tock.
19. N. of the long head of
      the biceps.
20. N. of semitendinosus.
21. N. of semimembrano-
      sus.
22. N. of short head of the
      biceps.

1, 2, 3, 4, 5. Sacral nn.
6. Superior gluteal n.
7. Great ischiatic n.
8. Lesser ischiatic n.
9. Pudic n.
10. N. of obturator internus.
11. N. of levator ani.

PLAN OF THE SACRAL PLEXUS AND BRANCHES.

ischiatic ligament. It is accompanied by a branch of the ischiatic
artery, called the ' *comes nervi ischiatici.*' *

Lesser
ischiatic
nerve.

This comes from the lower part of the sacral plexus.
It leaves the pelvis with the greater ischiatic nerve,
but on the inner side of it, and in company with the

---

* The arteria comes nervi ischiatici runs generally by the side of the nerve, but
sometimes in the centre of it. This artery becomes one of the chief channels by which
the blood reaches the lower limb after ligature of the femoral. See a preparation in
the Museum of St. Bartholomew's Hospital, where the femoral was tied by John
Hunter fifty years before the man's death.

ischiatic artery. The muscular branches which it gives off are,
one or more, which enter the under surface of the glutæus maximus. All its other branches are cutaneous. One turns round the
lower border of the glutæus maximus, and supplies the skin of
the buttock. Another, the long pudendal (p. 367), turns inwards
towards the perinæum, to supply the skin of that region and the
scrotum. The continued trunk runs down the back of the thigh
beneath the muscular fascia, as low as the upper part of the calf,
supplying the skin all the way down.

Ischiatic
artery.
    This branch of the internal iliac leaves the pelvis
below the pyriformis, and then descends between the
tuber ischii and the great trochanter, along the inner
side of the great ischiatic nerve. It gives off—1, two or more
considerable branches to the glutæus maximus; 2, a coccygeal
branch, which runs through the great sacro-ischiatic ligament,
then ramifies in the glutæus maximus, and on the back of the
coccyx; 3, the comes nervi ischiatici; 4, branches to the several
external rotator muscles; lastly, branches which supply the upper
part of the hamstring muscles; and others which inosculate with
the internal circumflex and obturator arteries (p. 462).

Pudic artery
and nerve.
    The course of this artery and nerve has been fully
described (p. 374). Observe now that they pass over
the spine of the ischium, accompanied by the nerve to
the obturator internus, and that in a thin subject it is possible to
compress the artery against the spine. The rule for finding it is
this: rotate the foot inwards, and draw a line from the top of the
great trochanter to the base of the coccyx; the junction of
the inner with the outer two-thirds gives the situation of the
artery.*

Popliteal
space.
    It is advisable to examine the popliteal space at this
stage of the dissection, in order that the various parts
may be carefully made out with as little disturbance
as possible of their mutual relations.

A vertical incision must be made along the middle of the ham,

* Mr. Travers succeeded in arresting hæmorrhage from a sloughing ulcer of the
glans penis by pressing the pudic artery with a cork against the spine of the ischium.

extending from six inches above, to three inches below the knee: transverse incisions should be made at each extremity of the vertical, so that the skin may be conveniently reflected. In doing so, care must be taken to preserve the cutaneous branch of the lesser ischiatic nerve, which descends over the ham to the back of the leg.

The muscular fascia covering the space is very strong, and strengthened by numerous transverse fibres. It is traversed by the posterior saphena vein, which passes to join the popliteal vein.

The fascia having been reflected, the muscles and tendons constituting the boundaries of the popliteal space are to be cleaned. The space is formed, above, by the divergence of the hamstring muscles to reach their respective insertions; below, by the converging origins of the gastrocnemius: its shape is therefore that of a lozenge. Above it is bounded on the inner side by the semitendinosus, semimembranosus, gracilis, and sartorius; on the outer side, by the biceps; below, it is bounded on the inner side by the internal head of the gastrocnemius, on the outer, by the external head of this muscle and the plantaris.

The space is occupied by a quantity of fat, which permits the easy flexion of the knee; and in this fat are found imbedded the popliteal vessels and nerves, in the following order:—nearest to the surface are the nerves; the vessels lie close to the bone, the vein being superficial to the artery (fig. 106).

Along the outer border of the semimembranosus is the great ischiatic nerve, which, after giving off branches to the three great flexor muscles, divides, about the lower third of the thigh (higher or lower in different subjects), into two large nerves—the peroneal and the popliteal.

The *peroneal* runs close by the inner side of the tendon of the biceps* towards the head of the fibula, below which we have already traced its division into branches for the peronei, and all the extensors of the foot and toes (p. 472).

* The nerve is, therefore, very liable to be injured in the operation of dividing the outer hamstring.

The *popliteal* accompanies the popliteal artery, and is destined
to supply all the flexor muscles on the back of the leg and the
sole of the foot.

By clearing out all the fat, we observe that the popliteal vessels
enter the ham through an aperture in the adductor magnus, and

Fig. 100.

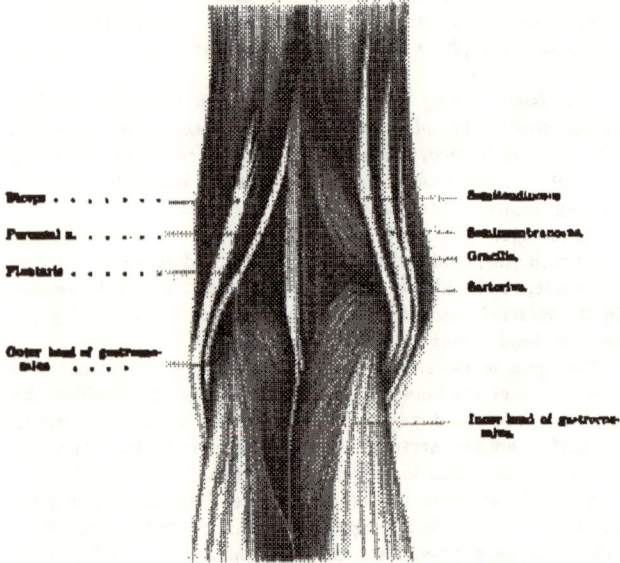

POPLITEAL SPACE.

descend close to the back part of the femur, and the back of the
knee-joint. At first they are partially overlapped (in muscular
subjects), by the semimembranosus; indeed the outer border of
this muscle is a good guide to the artery in the operation of tying
it. Arising at right angles from the popliteal artery, are the two
superior articular arteries: close to the vessel is the articular
branch of the obturator nerve which supplies the knee-joint.

I I

Absorbent glands.
Two or more absorbent glands are situated one on each side of the artery. They deserve attention, because, when enlarged, their close proximity to the artery may give them an apparent pulsation which might be mistaken for an aneurism.

DISSECTION OF THE BACK OF THE THIGH.

The incision should be continued along the back of the thigh, and the skin reflected.

Cutaneous nerves and veins.
The skin at the back of the thigh is supplied by the lesser ischiatic nerve, which runs down beneath the fascia, as low as the upper third of the calf, distributing branches on either side.

There are no subcutaneous veins of any size at the back of the thigh: here they would be liable to pressure. But near the ham we find a vein, called the 'external saphena.' It comes up the back of the calf, and joins the popliteal vein.

Muscular fascia.
Respecting this, remark that its fibres run chiefly in a transverse direction, that it becomes stronger as it passes over the popliteal space, and that here it is connected with the tendons on either side. Remove it, to examine the powerful muscles which bend the leg, called the 'hamstrings.'

Hamstring muscles.
There are three of these, and all arise by strong tendons from the tuber ischii. One, the biceps, is inserted into the head of the fibula; the other two—namely, the semitendinosus and semimembranosus—are inserted into the tibia. The divergence of these muscles towards their respective insertions occasions the space termed the 'ham,' which is occupied by soft fat, and the popliteal vessels and nerves.

Biceps.
This muscle has two origins, a long and a short. The long one takes place, by a strong tendon, from the back part of the tuber ischii; the short one, by fleshy fibres, from the linea aspera of the femur. This origin begins at the linea aspera, just below the insertion of the glutæus maximus, and con-

tinues nearly down to the external condyle. It joins the longer part of the muscle, and both terminate on a common tendon, which is inserted into the head of the fibula, by two portions separated by the external lateral ligament of the knee-joint. It also gives off a strong expansion to the fascia of the leg. The tendon covers part of the external lateral ligament of the knee-joint, and a small bursa intervenes.*

The biceps is not only a flexor of the leg, but rotates the leg, when bent, outwards. It is this muscle which dislocates the knee outwards and backwards in chronic disease of the joint. Each portion of the biceps is supplied by the great ischiatic nerve. The short head is sometimes supplied by the peroneal.

Semiten-dinosus. This arises, in common with the biceps, also by muscular fibres internal to the common origin, from the back part of the tuber ischii. The fibres terminate upon a long tendon, which spreads out below the knee-joint, and is inserted into the inner surface of the tibia, below the tendon of the gracilis, and behind that of the sartorius. Like them, it plays over the internal lateral ligament of the knee, and is provided with a bursa to prevent friction. Its nerve comes from the ischiatic.

The semitendinosus sends off from the lower border of its tendon a very strong fascia to cover the leg, which is attached along the inner edge of the tibia. The middle of the muscle is intersected by an oblique tendinous line.

Semimem-branosus. This muscle arises from the tuber ischii above and external to the two preceding, by means of a strong flat tendon, which extends nearly half way down the thigh. This tendon descends obliquely behind the biceps and semitendinosus, and terminates in a bulky muscle, which lies on a deeper plane than the others, and is inserted by a thick tendon into the posterior part of the head of the tibia. In connection with this tendon, notice three additional points:—1, that it is prolonged under the internal lateral ligament of the knee, and

* This tendon can be plainly felt as the outer hamstring in one's own person, just above the head of the fibula.

that a bursa intervenes between them ; 2, that it sends a strong prolongation upwards and outwards to the external condyle of the femur, forming the principal constituent of the '*ligamentum posticum Winslowii*,' which covers the back of the knee-joint ; 3, that a fascia proceeds from its lower border, and binds down the popliteus. Its nerve comes from the ischiatic.

A large bursa is almost invariably found between the semi-membranosus and the inner head of the gastrocnemius, where they rub one against the other. It is generally from one and a half to two inches long. The chief point of interest concerning it is, that it occasionally communicates with the synovial membrane of the knee-joint, not directly, but through the medium of another bursa beneath the inner head of the gastrocnemius. From an examination of 150 bodies, I infer that this communication exists about once in five instances; and it need scarcely be said that the proportion is large enough to make us cautious in interfering too roughly with this bursa when it becomes enlarged.[*]

Fig. 107.

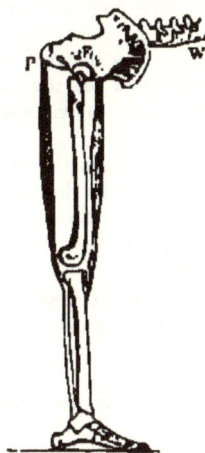

Action of the hamstring muscles.

These muscles produce two different effects, according as their fixed point is at the pelvis or the knee. With the fixed point at the pelvis, they bend the knee; with the fixed point at the knee, they form a very important part of the machinery which keeps the body erect. For instance, if, when standing, you bend the body at the hip and feel the muscles in question, you find that they are in strong action, to prevent

[*] When the bursa in question becomes enlarged, it occasions a fluctuating swelling of greater or less dimensions on the inner side of the popliteal space. The swelling bulges out, and becomes tense and elastic when the knee is extended, and vice versâ. As to its shape, it is generally oblong ; but this is subject to variety, for we know that the bursæ, when enlarged, are apt to become multilocular, and to burrow between the muscles where there is the least resistance.

the trunk from falling forwards: they, too, are the chief agents
concerned in bringing the body back again to the erect position.
In doing this, they act upon a lever of the first order, as shown in
fig. 107; the acetabulum being the fulcrum F, the trunk W, the
weight to be moved, and the power P, at the tuber ischii.

To put the action of the muscles of the thigh on the pelvis in
the clearest point of view, let us suppose we are standing upon one
leg: the bones of the lower extremity represent a pillar which supports the weight of the trunk on a ball-and-socket joint; the weight
is nicely balanced on all sides, and prevented from falling by four
groups of muscles. In front, are the rectus and sartorius; on the
inner side, the adductors; on the outer side, the glutæus medius
and minimus; behind, the hamstrings and glutæus maximus.

The semimembranosus can also rotate the knee inwards, thus
assisting the popliteus.

The hamstring muscles are supplied with blood by the perforating branches of the profunda, which come through the tendon
of the adductor magnus close to the femur. Their nerves are
derived from the great ischiatic.

Ischiatic
nerve.
This nerve descends from the buttock upon the adductor magnus, and, after being crossed by the long
head of the biceps, runs along the outer border of the
semimembranosus down the popliteal space. The further course
of this nerve has already been described (p. 480).

Deferring the course, relations, and branches of the popliteal
artery till this vessel is exposed throughout its whole course, pass
on now to the dissection of the calf.

Continue the incision down the centre of the calf to the heel,
and reflect the skin.

External or
posterior sa-
phena vein.
The large vein seen on the back of the leg is called the
'external or posterior saphena.' It commences on the
outer side of the foot, runs behind the outer ankle, and
then up the calf, receiving numerous veins in its course. It eventually passes through the muscular fascia, and joins the popliteal vein.

The chief cutaneous nerve of the calf is the external or posterior saphenous nerve; some branches, however, from the long saphenous and small ischiatic nerves, are to be traced, ramifying in the sub-cutaneous tissue of the inner and upper part of the leg.

External or posterior saphenous nerve.

The *external saphenous* nerve * is derived from the popliteal (fig. 106), and passes down between the two heads of the gastrocnemius to the middle of the calf, where it comes through the fascia. Here it is joined by a branch from the peroneal nerve (*communicans peronei*); it then descends with the saphenous vein, and is finally distributed to the outer side of the foot and the little toe.

To expose the muscles of the calf, reflect the muscular fascia by incisions corresponding to those made through the skin.

Muscles of the calf.

The great flexor muscle of the foot consists of two portions : the superficial one, called the 'gastrocnemius,' arises from the lower end of the femur; the deep one, called the 'soleus,' arises from the tibia and fibula. The force of both is concentrated on one thick tendon, called the 'tendo Achillis,' which is inserted into the heel).

Gastrocnemius.

This muscle arises by two strong tendinous heads, one from the upper and back part of each condyle of the femur (fig. 106). The inner head is the larger. The two parts of the muscle descend, distinct from each other, and form the two bellies of the calf, of which the inner is rather the lower. Both terminate, rather below the middle of the leg, on the broad com-mencement of the tendo Achillis.

The gastrocnemius should be divided transversely near its insertion, and reflected upwards from the subjacent soleus, as high as its origin. By this proceeding you observe that the contiguous surfaces of the muscles are covered by a glistening tendon, which receives the insertion of their fibres, and transmits their collected force to the tendo Achillis.

Observe also the large sural vessels and nerves (branches of the popliteal) which supply each head of the muscle. To facilitate the play of the inner tendon over the condyle, there is a bursa, which

* This nerve is sometimes called the communicans poplitei, and does not take the name of external saphenous till its junction with the communicans peronei.

generally communicates with the knee-joint; and in the substance of the outer tendon is commonly found a small piece of fibro-cartilage. Lastly, between the gastrocnemius and soleus is the tendon of the plantaris.

Plantaris. This small muscle* arises from the rough line just above the outer condyle of the femur (fig. 106). It descends close to the inner side of the outer head of the gastrocnemius, and terminates, a little below the knee, in a long tendon, which should be traced down the inner side of the tendo Achillis to the calcaneum. Its nerve comes from the popliteal.

Soleus. This muscle arises from the head and upper third of the posterior surface of the fibula, from the oblique ridge on the back of the tibia,† from about the middle third of the inner border of this bone, and from an arch thrown over the posterior tibial vessels. The fibres swell out beneath the gastrocnemius, and terminate on a broad tendon, which, gradually contracting, forms a constituent part of the tendo Achillis. The soleus is supplied with blood by several branches from the posterior tibial; also by a large branch from the peroneal. Its nerve comes from the popliteal and enters the top of the muscle. This is an important muscle in a surgical point of view, for two reasons — 1, by reflecting its tibial origin, we reach the posterior tibial artery; 2, by reflecting its fibular origin we reach the peroneal.

The *tendo Achillis* begins about the middle of the leg, and is at first of considerable breadth, but it gradually contracts and becomes thicker as it descends. The narrowest part of it is about one inch and a half above the heel; here, therefore, it can be most conveniently and safely divided for the relief of club-foot. There is no risk of injuring the deeper-seated parts, because they are separated from the tendon by a quantity of fat. Its precise inser-

---

* This is the representative of the palmaris longus of the forearm. In man it is lost on the calcaneum, but in monkeys, who have prehensile feet, it is the proper tensor muscle of the plantar fascia. It is remarkably strong in bears and plantigrade mammals.

† The tibial and fibular origins of the soleus constitute what some anatomists describe as the two heads of the muscle. Between them descend the popliteal vessels, protected by a tendinous arch.

tion is into the under and back part of the os calcis. The tendon previously expands a little : between it and the bone is a bursa of considerable size.

The *action* of the gastrocnemius and soleus is to raise the body on the toes. Since the gastrocnemius passes over two joints, it has the power (like the rectus) of extending the one while it bends the other, and it is, therefore, admirably adapted to the purpose of walking. For instance, by first extending the foot it raises the body, and then, by bending the knee, it transmits the weight from one leg to the other. Supposing the fixed point to be at the heel, the gastrocnemius is also concerned in keeping the body erect, for it keeps the tibia and fibula perpendicular on the foot, and thus counteracts the tendency of the body to fall forwards.

The tendo Achillis, in raising the body on tiptoe, acts with

Fig. 103.

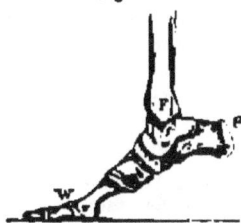

great power and under the best leverage ; for it acts upon a lever of the *first* order. The fulcrum (a movable one) is at the ankle-joint F, fig. 103 ; the weight, W, at the toes; the power at the heel, P. All the conditions are those of a lever of the first order. The power and the weight act in the same direction on *opposite* sides of the fulcrum. The pressure upon the fulcrum is equal to the sum of the pressures applied : *i. e.* $P \times F + W \times F$.[*]

COOPER AND RELATIONS OF THE POPLITEAL ARTERY.

After passing through the opening in the tendon of the adductor magnus, the femoral artery takes the name of 'popliteal.' It descends nearly perpendicularly behind the knee-joint, between the origins of the gastrocnemius, as far as the lower border of the popliteus, where it divides into the anterior and posterior tibial. In its descent it lies, first, upon the lower part of the femur, and here it is slightly overlapped by the semimembranosus ; next it lies upon the posterior ligament of the knee-joint, and, lastly, upon the popliteus.

[*] It is fair to state that some regard the foot as a lever of the second order. There is, therefore, room for two opinions on the question.

It is covered by the gastrocnemius and soleus, and is crossed by the plantaris. The vein closely accompanies the artery, and is situated superficially with regard to it, and rather to its outer side in the first part of its course. The popliteal nerve runs also in a similar direction with the vein, but is still more superficial and to the outer side (fig. 106). The vessels and the nerve are surrounded by fat, and one or two absorbent glands are generally found in the immediate neighbourhood of the artery, just above the joint.

The branches of the popliteal artery are the *articular* and the *sural.*

There are five *articular branches* for the supply of the knee-joint and the articular ends of the bone: the two *superior--external* and *internal*—run, one above each condyle, close to the bone, and are distributed partially to the vastus externus and internus, respectively; the two *inferior—external* and *internal—* run, one beneath each lateral ligament of the joint; and all four proceed towards the front of the capsule. The fifth, called the ' *azygos,*' enters the joint through the posterior ligament. These articular arteries form, over the front and sides of the joint, a beautiful network of vessels, which communicate, superiorly, with the descending branch of the external circumflex and the anastomotica magna ; inferiorly, with the anterior tibial recurrent. It is mainly through these channels that the collateral circulation is established in the leg after ligature of the femoral.

Arterial inosculations.

The *sural* arteries proceed one to each head of the gastrocnemius, and are proportionate in size to the muscle. One or two branches are distributed to the soleus. These arteries are accompanied by branches of the popliteal nerve for the supply of the muscles.

Popliteal vein.

This vein is formed by the junction of the venæ comites of the anterior and posterior tibial arteries, and is situated superficial to the artery. It crosses obliquely from the inner to the outer side of the artery, and is continued upwards under the name of femoral. It receives in the popliteal space the external saphena, the articular, and sural veins,

The insertion of the semimembranosus into the head of the tibia, alluded to p. 483, should now be more fully examined.

Popliteus. This muscle arises within the capsule of the knee-joint, from a depression on the outside of the external condyle by a thick tendon, which runs beneath the external lateral ligament. The muscular fibres gradually spread out, and are inserted into the posterior surface of the tibia above the oblique ridge on the bone. It is supplied by a branch of the popliteal nerve which enters its deep surface. Its action is to flex the leg, and then to rotate the tibia inwards. The tendon plays over the articulation between the tibia and fibula; and a bursa intervenes, which generally communicates by a wide opening with the knee-joint.

Reflect the soleus with its origin, and remove it from the deep-seated muscles, observing at the same time the numerous arteries which enter its under surface. This done, notice the fascia which binds down the deep muscles. It is attached to the margin of the bones on either side, and increases in strength towards the ankle, in order to form an annular ligament to confine the tendons and the vessels and nerves in their passage into the sole of the foot.

Deep muscles on the back of the leg. There are three:—1, the flexor longus digitorum on the tibial side; 2, the flexor longus pollicis on the fibular; 3, the tibialis posticus upon the interosseous membrane, between and beneath them both.

Flexor longus digitorum. This arises from the posterior surface of the tibia, commencing below the popliteus, and extending to within about four inches of the lower end of the bone. The fibres terminate on a tendon which runs through a groove behind the inner ankle, and entering the sole, divides into four tendons for the four outer toes. It is supplied by the posterior tibial nerve.

Flexor longus pollicis. This powerful muscle arises from the lower two-thirds of the posterior surface of the fibula. The fibres terminate on a tendon which runs through a groove on the back of the astragalus, and thence along the sole to the great toe. The action of this muscle is to raise the body on the tip of the great toe. It is essential to the propulsion of the body in walking. It is supplied by the posterior tibial nerve.

Tibialis posticus. This is so concealed between the two preceding muscles, that it cannot be properly examined without reflecting them. It arises from the interosseous membrane and from the contiguous surfaces of the tibia and fibula. In the lower part of the leg it passes between the tibia and the flexor longus digitorum. Its muscular fibres terminate on a tendon which comes into view a short distance above the inner ankle, and, running through the same groove with the tendon of the flexor longus digitorum, enters the sole, and is inserted into the scaphoid and internal cuneiform bones. Its action is to bend and turn the foot inwards. It is supplied by the posterior tibial nerve. The precise situation of the tendon of the tibialis posticus is interesting, surgically, because the tendon has to be divided for the relief of talipes varus. It lies close to, and parallel with, the inner edge of the tibia, so that this is a good guide to it. It is necessary to relax the tendon, while the knife is introduced between the tendon and the bone. Its synovial sheath commences about 1½ inch above the end of the internal malleolus, and is consequently opened in the operation.

Attention should now be directed to the *internal annular ligament*, which binds down the tendons behind the inner ankle.

It is attached to the internal malleolus and the inner border of the os calcis. It is continuous above with the deep fascia, below with the plantar fascia. Beneath it pass the tendons of the deep-seated muscles of the leg into the sole of the foot. The relative position of the structures passing under this ligament, proceeding from within outwards, are—the tendons of the tibialis posticus, and the flexor longus digitorum; the posterior tibial artery accompanied by its venæ comites; the posterior tibial nerve; and, lastly, the tendon of the flexor longus pollicis.

Course and relations of This artery is one of the branches into which the popliteal divides at the lower border of the popliteus.

the posterior It descends over the deep muscles at the back of the
tibial artery. leg to the interval between the internal malleolus and
the os calcis, and, entering the sole, divides behind the abductor
pollicis into the external and internal plantar arteries. It lies,
first, for a short distance, upon the tibialis posticus, then, on the
flexor longus digitorum; but behind the ankle it is in contact with
the tibia, so that here it can be felt beating, and effectually compressed. In the upper part of its course, it runs nearly midway
between the bones, and is covered by the gastrocnemius and soleus :
to tie it, therefore, in this situation, is very difficult. But in the
lower part of its course, it gradually approaches the inner border
of the tibia, from which, generally speaking, it is not more than
½ or ¾ths of an inch distant. Here, being comparatively superficial,
it may easily be tied. Immediately behind the internal malleolus,
it lies between the tendons of the flexor longus digitorum, on the
inner side, and the flexor longus pollicis on the outer. It has two
venæ comites, which communicate at intervals. Its branches are
as follow :—

a. Numerous branches to the soleus and the deep muscles.

b. The *peroneal* is a branch of very considerable size; often as
large as the posterior tibial. Arising about 1½ inch below the division of the popliteal, it descends close to the inner side of the fibula,
and then over the articulation between the tibia and fibula to the
outer part of the os calcis, where it inosculates with the malleolar
and plantar arteries. All down the leg it is imbedded among the
muscles: being covered, first, by the soleus, afterwards by the
flexor longus pollicis. To both these muscles, to the latter especially, it sends numerous branches, and just above the ankle it gives
off a constant one—the *anterior peroneal*—which passes through
the interosseous membrane, to the under aspect of the peroneus
tertius, then runs in front of the tibio-fibular articulation, and
inosculates with the other malleolar arteries. It supplies the
medullary artery of the fibula, and, about an inch above the os calcis,
sends off a transverse communicating branch, which inosculates
with the posterior tibial artery under the tendon of the flexor
longus pollicis.

c. The medullary artery of the tibia.

Posterior tibial nerve.   This is the continuation of the popliteal. It descends close to its corresponding artery, and, entering the sole of the foot, divides into the external and internal plantar nerve. In the first part of its course the nerve lies superficial to the artery, and rather to its inner side; but behind the ankle the nerve lies on the outer side of the artery, and on the same plane.* It supplies branches to the three deep-seated muscles, and a cutaneous branch to the sole of the foot.

DISSECTION OF THE SOLE OF THE FOOT.

Make a perpendicular incision down the middle of the sole, and reflect the skin. Notice the peculiar structure of the subcutaneous tissue. It is composed of globular masses of fat, separated by strong fibrous septa, and forms elastic pads, especially marked at the heel, and at the ball of the great and the little toe; these being the points which form the tripod supporting the arch of the foot.

In removing the subcutaneous tissue from the ball of the great and the little toe, we often meet with bursæ, simple or multilocular. They are generally placed between the skin and the sesamoid bones, and have remarkably thick walls. Very frequently we trace an artery and nerve running directly through one of these sacs, which explains the acute pain produced by their inflammation.

Cutaneous nerves.   The skin of the heel is supplied by a branch of the posterior tibial nerve; the remainder of the sole by small branches of the plantar nerves which come through the fascia, as in the palm of the hand.

Plantar fascia.   This is remarkably dense and strong. It extends from the under and back part of the os calcis to the distal ends of the metatarsal bones: it not only protects the plantar vessels and nerves, but is one of the many structures which support the arch of the foot. It acts like the string of a bow

* It sometimes happens that the nerve divides into its two plantar branches higher than usual, and then we find that one lies on either side of the artery.

(p. 508). This is exemplified in some cases of distortion, where
an unnatural contraction of the plantar fascia makes the arch of
the foot too convex; and it is necessary to divide the fascia to
relieve the deformity.

The arrangement of the fascia is like that in the palm. The
central part, where there is the greatest strain, is very strong. The
external part, which is attached to the proximal end of the fifth
metatarsal bone, is also very strong. Near the distal ends of the
metatarsal bones, the central part divides into five portions; each
of these subdivides into two slips, which embrace the corresponding
flexor tendons, and are attached to the metatarsal bones and their
connecting ligaments. Between the primary divisions of the
fascia—that is, in a line between the toes—are seen the digital
vessels and nerves.

In the interdigital folds of the skin, there are also ligamentous
fibres, which run from one side of the foot to the other, and answer
the same purpose as those in the hand (p. 257).

The plantar fascia must be partially removed to examine the
muscles. Towards the os calcis its removal is not accomplished
without some difficulty, because the muscles arise from it.

Superficial muscles. After the removal of the fascia three muscles are
exposed. All arise from the os calcis and the fascia,
and proceed forwards to the toes.[*] The central one is
the flexor brevis digitorum, the two lateral are the abductor
pollicis, and the abductor minimi digiti.

Abductor pollicis. This muscle arises from the inner and back part of
the os calcis, from the plantar fascia, and the internal
annular ligament. Its origin arches over the plantar
vessels and nerves in their passage to the sole. The fibres run
along the inner side of the sole, and terminate on a tendon which
is inserted into the inner side of the base of the first phalanx of
the great toe, through the medium of the internal sesamoid bone.
Its nerve comes from the internal plantar.

---

[*] They are separated from each other by strong perpendicular partitions—intermuscular septa—which pass in from the plantar fascia.

Abductor minimi digiti.
This muscle has a very strong origin from the under surface of the os calcis, from its external tubercle and the plantar fascia. Some of its fibres terminate on a tendon which is inserted into the proximal end of the metatarsal bone of the little toe; but the greater part runs on to a tendon which is inserted into the outer side of the first phalanx of the little toe. It is supplied by the external plantar nerve.

Flexor brevis digitorum.
This muscle arises from the under surface of the os calcis, between the two preceding, from the plantar fascia and the intermuscular septa. It passes forwards and divides into four tendons, which run superficial to those of the long flexor. Cut open the sheath which contains them; follow them on to the toes, to see that each bifurcates over the first phalanx, to allow the long tendon to pass; then the two slips, reuniting, are inserted into the sides of the second phalanx. The same arrangement prevails as in the fingers. It is supplied by the internal plantar nerve.

The three superficial muscles should now be reflected, by sawing off about half an inch of the os calcis, and then turning it downwards with the preceding muscles attached to it. This done, we bring into view the plantar vessels and nerves, the second layer of muscles, i.e. the long flexor tendon of the great toe, that of the other toes, and the flexor accessorius.

Tendon of the flexor longus digitorum.
Musculus accessorius.
Tracing this tendon into the sole, you find that an accessory muscle is attached to it. The flexor accessorius arises by muscular fibres from the inner side of the os calcis, and has often a second origin, tendinous, from the outer side. Its fibres run straight forwards, and are inserted into the fibular side of the tendon, so that their action is not only to assist in bending the toes, but to make the common tendon pull in a straight line towards the heel, which, from its oblique direction, it could not do without the accessory muscle. The common tendon then divides into four, one for each of the four outer toes. These run in the same sheath with the short tendons, and after passing through them are inserted into the bases of the ungual phalanges. Respecting the manner in which

the tendons are confined by fibrous sheaths, and lubricated by a
synovial lining, what was said of the fingers (p. 262) applies
equally to the toes. The flexor accessorius is supplied by the
external plantar nerve.

Lumbricales. These four little muscles are placed between the long
flexor tendons. Each, excepting the most internal,
arises from the adjacent sides of two tendons, proceeds forwards,
and then sinking between the toes, terminates in an aponeurosis
which passes round the inner side of the four outer toes, and joins
the extensor tendon on the dorsum of the toes. Concerning their
use, refer to p. 264. The two outer lumbricales are supplied by
the external plantar nerve, the two inner by the internal plantar.

Now trace the long flexor tendon of the great toe. From the
groove in the astragalus it runs along the groove in the lesser
tuberosity of the os calcis, above the tendon of the flexor longus
digitorum, and then straight to the base of the last phalanx.
Observe that it crosses the long flexor tendon of the toes, and that
the two tendons are connected by an oblique slip; so that we cannot bend the other toes without the great toe.

Plantar arteries. The posterior tibial artery, having entered the sole
between the origins of the abductor pollicis, divides
into the external and internal plantar arteries.

The *internal plantar* artery is very small: it passes forwards
between the abductor pollicis and the flexor brevis digitorum to
the base of the great toe, where it terminates in small inosculations with the digital arteries. Its chief use is to supply the
muscles between which it runs.

The *external plantar* is the principal artery of the sole, and
alone forms the plantar arch. It runs obliquely outwards across
the sole towards the base of the fifth metatarsal bone; then,
sinking deep from the surface, it bends inwards across the bases of
the metatarsal bones, and inosculates with the anterior tibial in the
first interosseous space. In the first part of its course, it lies
between the flexor brevis digitorum and the flexor accessorius; in
the second it lies very deep beneath the flexor tendons, and the
adductor pollicis, close to the metatarsal bones. Deeply seated as

it appears to be, a part of its curve near the fifth metatarsal bone lies immediately beneath the fascia. Here it might be more easily tied than in any other part of its course.

Fig. 109.

Its chief branches are the four digital arteries, which arise in the arched part of its course. They supply both sides of the fifth, fourth, third, and the outer side of the second toe; the great toe, and the inside of the second, being supplied by the dorsalis hallucis. Concerning the distribution of the digital arteries, refer to the account given of these arteries in the hand; they are in all respects similar (p. 259).

Besides the digital arteries, the arch gives off three small branches—the *perforating*—which ascend between the three outer metatarsal spaces, and inosculate with the dorsal interosseous arteries.

Plantar nerves.

The posterior tibial nerve divides, like the artery, into an external and internal plantar. The

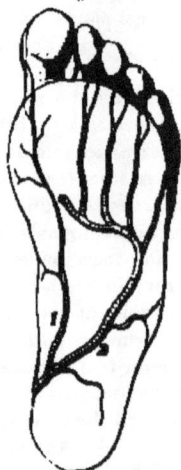

1. Internal plantar.
2. External do.

internal plantar is generally the larger, and supplies nerves to three toes and a half, like the median in the palm. It also supplies the muscles on the inner side of the sole, the abductor pollicis, the flexor brevis pollicis, the flexor brevis digitorum, the two inner lumbricales; also articular branches to the tarsus and metatarsus. The *external plantar* nerve sends branches to the flexor accessorius and the abductor minimi digiti, and then divides into a superficial and deep branch. The *superficial* branch supplies the fifth toe and the outer side of the fourth toe (like the ulnar nerve in the palm), and the flexor brevis minimi digiti. The *deep* branch furnishes nerves to the two outer lumbricales, the adductor pollicis, the transversalis pedis, and all the interossei.

Third layer of muscles. Having traced the principal vessels and nerves, divide them with the flexor tendons near the os calcis, and turn them down toward the toes, to expose the deep muscles in the sole. These are, the flexor brevis and adductor pollicis, the flexor brevis minimi digiti, and the transversalis pedis.

Flexor brevis pollicis. This muscle *arises* from the external cuneiform and cuboid bones. It proceeds along the metatarsal bone of the great toe, and divides into two portions, which run one on each side of the long flexor tendon, and are *inserted* by tendons into the sides of the first phalanx of the great toe. The inner tendon is inseparably connected with the abductor pollicis, the outer with the adductor pollicis. In each tendon there is a sesamoid bone. These bones not only increase the strength of the muscle, but both together form a pulley for the free play of the long flexor tendon ; so that in walking the tendon is not pressed upon. Its nerve comes from the internal plantar.

Adductor pollicis. This very powerful muscle *arises* from the cuboid, and the third and fourth metatarsal bones. Passing obliquely across the foot, it is *inserted* through the external sesamoid bone into the outer side of the base of the first phalanx of the great toe together with the inner head of the flexor brevis pollicis. This muscle greatly contributes to support the arch of the foot. Like the adductor of the thumb it should be considered as an interosseous muscle.

Flexor brevis minimi digiti. This little muscle *arises* from the base of the fifth metatarsal bone, proceeds forwards along it, and is *inserted* into the base of the first phalanx of the little toe.

Transversalis pedis. This slender muscle runs transversely across the distal ends of the metatarsal bones. It *arises* by little fleshy slips from the four outer toes, and is *inserted* into the first phalanx of the great toe with the adductor pollicis, of which it ought to be considered a part.

The fourth layer of muscles consists of the interossei.

Interossei.   These muscles are arranged nearly like those in the
palm. They occupy the intervals between the metatarsal bones, and are seven in number, four being on the dorsal
aspect of the foot, three on the plantar. They *arise* from the
sides of the metatarsal bones, and terminate in tendons which are
inserted, some into the inner, others into the outer side of the
first phalanges of the toes and their extensor tendons. Their use
is to draw the toes to or from each other, and they do this or that
according to the side of the phalanx on which they act. Now, if
we draw an imaginary longitudinal line through the second toe,
we find that all the dorsal muscles draw *from* that line, and
the plantar *towards* it. This is the key to the action of them all.
A more detailed account of these muscles is given in the dissection
of the palm (p. 292). Between the tendons of the interossei, that
is, between the distal ends of the metatarsal bones, there are little
bursæ to facilitate movement. These bursæ are not without
interest. They sometimes become enlarged and occasion painful
swellings between the roots of the toes. The flexor brevis minimi
digiti, the transversalis pedis, and all the interossei are supplied
by the external plantar nerve.

Now trace the tendons of the peroneus longus and tibialis
posticus. The tendon of the peroneus longus is the deepest in
the sole. It runs through a groove in the cuboid bone obliquely
across the sole towards its insertion into the outer side of the base
of the metatarsal bone of the great toe. It is confined in a strong
fibrous sheath, lined throughout by synovial membrane.

The tendon of the tibialis posticus may be traced over the
internal lateral ligament of the ankle, and thence under the
head of the astragalus to the scaphoid bone into which it is chiefly
inserted. One or two slips are sent off to the cuneiform bones.
Observe that the tendon contributes to support the head of the
astragalus, and that for this purpose it often contains a sesamoid
bone. This is one of the many provisions for the solidity of the
arch of the foot.

DISSECTION OF THE LIGAMENTS.

The sacrum is united to the last lumbar vertebra in
the same manner as one vertebra is to another. The

Ligaments of the pelvis.

same observation applies to the union between the
sacrum and the coccyx. The student should, therefore, refer to
the description of the ligaments of the spine (p. 210).

The innominate bones are connected to each other in front,
constituting the '*symphysis pubis*;' posteriorly to the sacrum,
constituting the '*sacro-iliac symphysis*.'

Fig. 110.

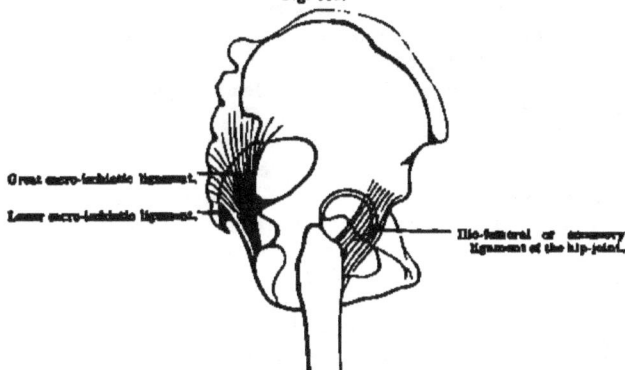

Great sacro-ischiatic ligament.

Lesser sacro-ischiatic ligament.

Ilio-femoral or accessory ligament of the hip-joint.

This is secured by, 1, an *anterior* ligament, consisting
of superficial fibres which run obliquely, and of deep

Pubic symphysis.

fibres which pass transversely; 2, a *posterior* ligament,
less distinct; 3, a *sub-pubic* ligament, or ' ligamentum arcuatum:'
it is very strong, and rounds off the point of the pubic arch; 4, a
superior ligament which passes across the upper surface of the
pubic bones; 5, an intermediate fibro-cartilage. A perpendicular
section through it shows that it consists of concentric layers, and

that its general structure resembles that between the bodies of the vertebræ. In the upper part of this fibro-cartilage is a smooth cavity lined with epithelium. The cartilage acts like a buffer, and breaks the force of shocks passing through the pelvic arch.

The ileum is connected with the fifth lumbar vertebra by the *ilio-lumbar* ligament. It is very strong, and extends from the transverse process of the last lumbar vertebra to the crest of the ileum (fig. 111).

Sacro-iliac symphysis. This is secured by, 1, an *anterior* ligament which consists of ligamentous fibres passing in front; 2, a *posterior* ligament, composed of fibres much stronger and more marked, which pass behind the articulation. The anterior part of the bones forming this articulation is crusted with articular cartilage, of which the shape is like that of the ear. Behind this is the strong *interosseous* ligament, which contributes powerfully to the security of the joint.

Sacro-ischiatic ligaments. These are two strong ligaments passing from the sacrum to the ischium. The *great sacro-ischiatic* extends from the posterior inferior spine of the ileum, and the side of the sacrum and coccyx, to the tuberosity of the ischium. The *lesser sacro-ischiatic* ligament passes from the sacrum and coccyx to the spine of the ischium. These two ligaments not only connect the bones, but also, from their great breadth, contribute to block up the lower aperture of the pelvis.

Ligaments of the hip-joint. This joint is secured by the form of the bones, and by the strength of the powerful muscles which surround it. Although a perfect ball-and-socket joint, its motion is somewhat limited: the disposition of its ligaments restricts its range of motion to those directions only which are most consistent with the maintenance of the erect attitude, and the requirements of this part of the skeleton.

Capsular ligament. The *capsular* ligament is attached above to the circumference of the acetabulum at a little distance external to the margin, and also to the transverse ligament; below to the inter-trochanteric ridge of the femur in front, and to the middle of the neck behind. The capsule is made exceedingly thick and strong in front, by a broad ligament, *ilio-femoral*, which extends from the anterior inferior iliac spine to the anterior inter-trochanteric line. This ligament is very strong, and serves as a strap to prevent the femur being extended beyond a certain limit; and to prevent the body from rolling backwards at the hip.

Open the capsule to ascertain the enormous thickness of it in front, and the strong hold it has upon the bones. This exposes the cotyloid ligament, and the ligamentum teres.

Ligamentum teres. The ligamentum teres is exposed by drawing the head of the femur out of the socket. This ligament is somewhat flat and triangular. Its base is attached, below, to the borders of the notch in the acetabulum; its apex to the fossa in the head of the femur. To prevent pressure on it, and to allow free room for its play, there is a gap at the

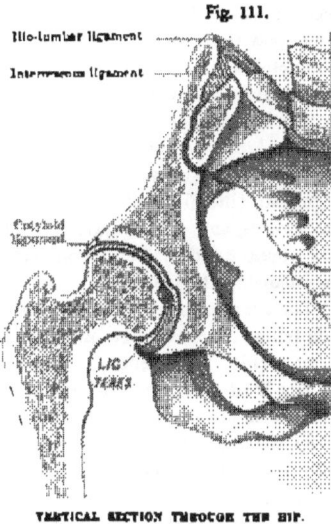

Fig. 111.

Ilio-lumbar ligament

Interosseous ligament

Cotyloid ligament

LIG TERES

VERTICAL SECTION THROUGH THE HIP.

bottom of the acetabulum. This gap is not crusted with cartilage like the rest of the socket, but is occupied by soft fat. The ligamentum teres is surrounded by the synovial membrane. A little artery runs up with it to the head of the femur. It is a branch of the obturator, and enters the acetabulum through the notch at the lower part.

The chief use of the ligamentum teres is to assist in steadying the pelvis on the thigh in the erect position. In this position, the ligament is vertical, and quite tight (fig. 111): it therefore prevents the pelvis from rolling towards the opposite side, or the thigh from being adducted beyond a certain point. Another purpose served by this ligament is to limit rotation of the thigh, both inwards and outwards.

Cotyloid ligament. The cotyloid ligament is a piece of fibro-cartilage which is attached all round the margin of the acetabulum. Its circumference is thicker than its free margin which shelves off; thus it not only deepens the cavity, but embraces the head of the femur like a sucker. It extends over the notch at the lower part of the acetabulum, and in this situation has received the name of the '*transverse*' ligament.

The ligaments of the hip are so arranged, that when we 'stand at ease,' the pelvis is spontaneously thrown into a position in which its range of motion is the most restricted; for the accessory ligament (ilio femoral) of the capsule prevents it from rolling backwards, and the ligamentum teres prevents its rolling towards the opposite side. This arrangement economises muscular force in balancing the trunk.

The synovial membrane extends down to the base of the neck of the femur in *front*, but only two-thirds down behind. It is laid upon a thick periosteum.

The head of the thigh-bone is kept in the acetabulum by atmospheric pressure; the amount of this is, of itself, sufficient to keep the limb suspended from the pelvis, supposing all muscles and ligaments to be divided. When fluid is effused into the hip-joint, the influence of the atmospheric pressure is diminished in proportion; and the bones being no longer maintained in accurate contact, it sometimes happens that the head of the femur escapes from its cavity, giving rise to what is called a spontaneous dislocation.

LIGAMENTS OF THE KNEE-JOINT. The knee-joint is a hinge-joint, and looking at the skeleton, one would suppose that it was very insecure. But nature has made up for this apparent insecurity by powerful ligaments, and by surrounding the joint on all sides with a thick capsule formed by the tendons of the muscles which move it.

First examine the tendons concerned in the con-
Capsular ligament. struction of the capsular ligament. In front is the
ligamentum patellæ; on either side are the tendons of
the vasti; at the back of the joint four tendons contribute to
form the capsule—namely, the tendons of the gastrocnemius, the
tendon of the semimembranosus, and of the popliteus. It
deserves to be noticed that the weakest part of the capsule is
near the tendon of the popliteus: here, therefore, matter formed in
the popliteal space may make its way into the joint, or *vice versâ*.

Exclusive of the capsule, the proper ligaments of the joint are
—1, the *lateral*; 2, the *crucial* in the interior.

This is a broad flat band, which extends from the
Internal lateral ligament. inner condyle of the femur to the inner side of the
tibia, a little below its head. A few of the deeper
fibres are attached to the inner semi-lunar cartilage, and serve to
keep it in place. The inferior internal articular artery, and part
of the tendon of the semimembranosus, pass underneath this
ligament. In the several motions of the joint, there is a certain
amount of friction between the liga-
ment and the head of the tibia, and consequently a small bursa is interposed.

Fig. 112.

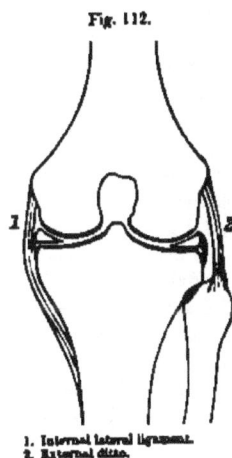

1. Internal lateral ligament.
2. External ditto.

This is a strong round
External lateral ligament. band, which extends from
the outer condyle of the
femur to the head of the fibula. This
ligament separates the two divisions
of the tendinous insertion of the biceps.
Posterior to, and running parallel with,
the external lateral ligament is a
smaller band of fibres, called the *short
external lateral* ligament.

This, which is generally
Posterior ligament. called 'ligamentum posticum Winslowii,' consists of
expansions derived from the tendons at
the back of the joint, chiefly, however,

from the semimembranosus. It not only closes and protects the joint behind, but prevents its extension beyond the perpendicular.

The joint should be opened above the patella. Observe the great extent of the fold which the synovial membrane forms above this bone.[*] The use of it is to allow the free play of the bone over the lower part of the femur. The fold extends higher above the inner than the outer condyle, which accounts for the form of the swelling produced by effusion into the joint.

Folds of synovial membrane. Below the patella a slender band of the synovial membrane proceeds backwards to the space between the condyles. It is called the '*ligamentum mucosum*;' the edges of it are called the '*ligamenta alaria*.' These are not true ligaments, but merely remnants of the partition, which, in the early stage of the joint's growth, divided it into two halves.

Immediately outside the synovial membrane there is always more or less fat; especially under the ligamentum patellæ. Its use is to fill up vacuities, and to mould itself to the several movements of the joint.

Crucial ligaments. The crucial ligaments, so named because they cross like the letter X, extend from the mesial side of each condyle to the head of the tibia. The *anterior*, a, b, the smaller, ascends from the fossa in front of the spine of the tibia, backwards and outwards to the external condyle. The *posterior*, c, d, best seen from behind, extends from the fossa behind the spine of the tibia forwards to the inner condyle.

Fig. 113.

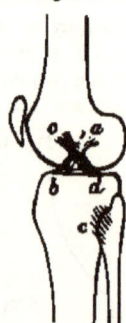

a, b. Anterior crucial ligament.
c, d. Posterior ditto.
e. Tibio-fibular.

Inter-articular or semi-lunar cartilages. Between the condyles and the articular surfaces of the tibia are two incomplete rings of fibro-cartilage, shaped like the letter C. They serve to deepen the articular surfaces of the tibia; their mobility and elasticity enable them to adapt themselves to the condyles in the

[*] In performing operations near the knee, the joint should always be bent in order to draw the synovial fold as much as possible out of the way.

several movements of the joint; they distribute pressure over a
greater surface; they equalise pressure and prevent shocks. They
are thickest at the circumference, and gradually shelve off to a
thin margin: thus they fit in between the bones, and adapt a
convex surface to a flat one, as shown in fig. 112. Their form
is suited to the condyles; the inner being oval, the outer circular.
The ends of each are firmly attached by ligaments to the pits in
front and behind the spine of the tibia; but the ends of the internal one are attached further from the spine than the external.
The cartilages are connected in front by a thin '*transverse*' ligament; and their circumference is attached round the head of the
tibia by fibrous tissue (called the '*coronary*' ligament), yet not so
closely as to restrict their range of motion.*

Action of the
ligaments.
Their respective points of attachment are such, that
when the joint is extended, all the ligaments are tight,
to prevent extension beyond the perpendicular; thus
muscular force is economised. But when the joint is bent the
ligaments are relaxed, enough to admit a slight rotatory movement
of the tibia. This movement is more free outwards than inwards;
and is effected, not by rotation of the tibia on its own
axis, but by rotation of the outer head round the inner.
Rotation outwards is produced by the biceps; rotation
inwards by the popliteus and semimembranosus.

Fig. 114.

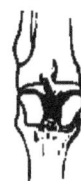

The crucial ligaments, though placed inside the joint,
answer the same purposes as the coronoid process and
the olecranon of the elbow. They make the tibia *slide*
properly forwards and backwards. The anterior especially limits extension; the posterior, flexion. They
not only prevent dislocation in front or behind, but
they prevent lateral displacement, since they cross each other like
braces, as shown in fig. 114.

---

* Of the two cartilages the external has the greater freedom of motion, because in
rotation of the knee the outer side of the tibia moves more than the inner. Consequently, it is not in any way connected to the lateral ligament; so far from this, it is
separated from it by the tendon of the popliteus, of which the play is facilitated by a
bursa communicating freely with the joint. For this reason the external cartilage is
more liable to dislocation.

There is a distinct joint between the upper ends of the tibia and fibula, although it admits of little movement. It is firmly secured by oblique ligaments in front and behind; their fibres being directed downwards and outwards (p. 505). The contiguous surfaces of the bones are crusted with cartilage. In the great majority of instances its synovial membrane is independent; but it occasionally communicates with the synovial membrane of the knee.

Ligaments connecting the tibia and fibula.

The shafts of the bones are connected by the interosseous membrane. The purpose of this is to afford additional surface for the attachment of muscles. Its fibres pass chiefly downwards and outwards from the tibia to the fibula, but some cross like the letter X. The anterior tibial artery comes forward above the interosseous membrane. It is perforated here and there for the passage of blood vessels.

Interosseous membrane.

The lower ends of the tibia and fibula are most firmly connected, for it is essential to the solidity of the ankle-joint that there be no motion between them. They are secured by an oblique ligament in front and behind, and by strong ligamentous fibres, interosseous, which connect their contiguous surfaces, and answer the purpose of rivets. Besides these, a strong fibro-cartilaginous ligament proceeds from the end of the fibula, and is attached along the posterior border of the articular surface of the tibia. The object of it is to deepen the excavation of the tibia, and enable it to adapt itself more accurately to the articular surface of the astragalus.

Inferior tibio-fibular ligaments.

From the form of the bones, it is obvious that the ankle is a hinge-joint; consequently, its security depends upon the great strength of its lateral ligaments. The hinge, however, is not so perfect but that it admits of a slight rotatory motion, of which the centre is on the fibular side, and therefore the reverse of that in the case of the knee.

Ligaments of the ankle-joint.

This ligament, sometimes called, from its shape, 'deltoid,' is exceedingly thick and strong, and compensates for the comparative shortness of the malleolus on this side (fig. 115). The great strength of it is proved by the

Internal lateral.

fact, that in dislocations of the ankle inwards, the summit of the malleolus is more likely to be broken off than the ligament to be torn. It extends from a deep excavation at the apex of the malleolus, radiates from this point, and is attached to the side of the astragalus, also to the os calcis, and the scaphoid bone. Besides this, some of its fibres are inserted into, and become

Fig. 115.

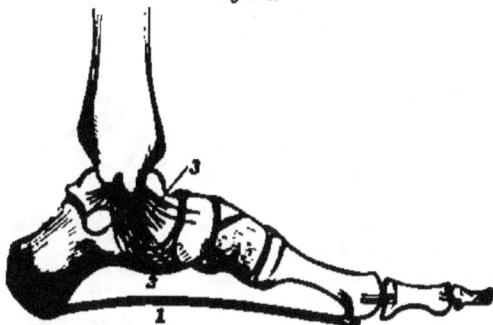

1. Plantar fascia.
2. Calcaneo-scaphoid or elastic ligament which supports the head of the astragalus.
3. Internal lateral ligament, called from its shape deltoid.

identified with, the inferior calcaneo-scaphoid ligament, so as to brace it up internally (fig. 115).

External lateral. This ligament consists of three distinct parts—an anterior, a posterior, and a middle (fig. 116). All three arise from an excavation near the summit of the external malleolus; the first two are inserted into the front and the back of the astragalus respectively; the middle into the outer surface of the os calcis.

Anterior and posterior ligament. The closure of the joint is completed, in front and behind, by an anterior and a posterior ligament attached to the bones near their articular surfaces, and sufficiently loose to permit the necessary range of motion.

Besides flexion and extension, the ankle-joint admits of a slight lateral movement, only permitted in the extended state of the joint. This is useful to us in the direction of our steps. In adaptation to this movement the internal malleolus is made shorter than the outer; it is not so tightly confined by its ligaments, and its articular surface is part of a cylinder.

Open the joint to see that the breadth of the articular surfaces of the bones is greater in front than behind. The object of this is to render the astragalus less liable to be dislocated backwards. Whenever this happens, the astragalus must of necessity become firmly locked between the malleoli.

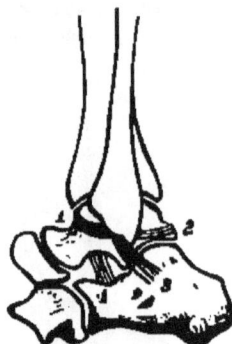

Fig. 116.

DIAGRAM OF THE EXTERNAL LATERAL LIGAMENT.

1. Anterior part.
2. Posterior part.
3. Middle part.
4. Interosseous ligament.

Ligaments connecting the bones of the foot. The astragalus is the key-stone of the arch of the foot, and supports the whole weight of the body. It articulates with the os calcis and the os scaphoides in such a manner as to permit the abduction and adduction of the foot, so useful in the direction of our steps.

The astragalus articulates with the os calcis by two distinct surfaces, respecting which remark, that the anterior is slightly convex, and the posterior slightly concave. This adaptation of itself contributes much to prevent the separation of the bones. But their principal bond of union is a strong interosseous ligament which occupies the interval between them (fig. 116).

Interosseous ligament.

In the skeleton the head of the astragalus articulates in front with the os scaphoides, but a part of it is unsupported below. In this interval it is supported by a very strong and elastic ligament, which extends from the os calcis to the os scaphoides (fig. 117). These bones, together with the

Calcaneo-scaphoid ligament.

ligament, form a complete socket for the head of the astragalus; it
is this joint, chiefly, which permits the abduction and adduction
of the foot. The chief peculiarity about the
ligament is its elasticity. It acts in all respects like a spring, and allows to the key-
stone of the arch a certain amount of play
which is of great service in preventing con-
cussion of the body. Whenever this ligament
loses its elastic property, as is often the case
with those who are in the habit of carrying
heavy burdens, the arch of the foot gradually
yields, and the individual becomes flat-footed.

The os calcis articulates with the os cuboides
nearly on a line with the articulation between
the astragalus and the os scaphoides. The
bones are most firmly connected by
means of a powerful ligament in
the sole, called the *calcaneo-cuboid*,
or 'ligamentum longum plantæ.' Some of its
fibres extend forwards as far as the second, third,
and fourth metatarsal bones.

Fig. 117.

Calcaneo-
cuboid
ligament.

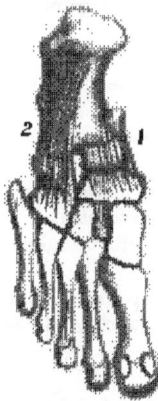

1. Calcaneo scaphoid li-
gament.
2. Calcaneo-cuboid liga-
ment.

It would be tedious to enumerate individually the several ligaments which connect the remaining bones of the tarsus and metatarsus. Let it then suffice to say, that they are firmly braced
together by very strong ligaments, both on their dorsal and their
plantar surfaces, and by interosseous ligaments which extend between their contiguous surfaces, like rivets.
Though there is very little motion between
any two bones, the collective amount is such
that the foot is enabled to adapt itself accurately to the ground; pressure is more equally
distributed, and consequently there is a firmer
basis for the support of the body. Being composed, moreover, of
several pieces, each of which possesses a certain elasticity, the
foot gains a general springiness and solidity which could not have
resulted from a single bone.

Fig. 118.

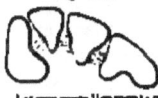

Interosseous ligaments of
the wedge bones.

Synovial membranes of the tarsus.   Exclusive of the ankle-joint and the phalanges of the toes, the bones of the foot are provided with six distinct synovial membranes; namely—

a. Between the posterior articular surface of the astragalus and os calcis.

b. Between the head of the astragalus and the scaphoid, and between the anterior articular surface of the astragalus and os calcis.

c. Between the os calcis and the os cuboides.

d. Between the inner cuneiform bone and the metatarsal bone of the great toe.

e. Between the scaphoid and the three cuneiform bones, and between these and the adjoining bones (the great toe excepted).

f. Between the os cuboides and the fourth and fifth metatarsal bones.

The phalanges of the toes are connected in all respects like those of the fingers. See the description given in the dissection of the hand (p. 306).

DISSECTION OF THE BRAIN.

Membranes of the brain.   Previous to the examination of the brain itself, we should study the structure and uses of the three membranes by which it is surrounded.

The first, the 'dura mater,' has been described (p. 5). The second is a serous membrane, termed the 'arachnoid;' the third is a very vascular one, termed the 'pia mater.'

Arachnoid membrane.   This second investment forms the smooth, polished surface of the brain, exposed after the removal of the dura mater. It is named 'arachnoid' from the delicacy of its texture, like a spider's web. It is a serous membrane, and, like all others of the kind, forms a closed sac, one part of which, the 'parietal' layer, lines the under surface of the dura mater; the other, the 'visceral,' is reflected over the brain: this reflection takes place along the nerves which leave the base of the skull.

The inner surface of this membrane is perfectly smooth, and

lubricated by a serous fluid to prevent friction; since the brain
rises and falls with a slight pulsation, caused in part by the action
of the heart, in part by respiration. The *parietal* layer is so thin
that it cannot be demonstrated as a distinct layer; it consists of
little more than a layer of squamous epithelium, lining the inner
aspect of the dura mater. But the *visceral* layer is obvious:
colourless and transparent, it is spread uniformly over the surface
of the brain, and does not dip into the furrows between the convolutions. On account of its extreme tenuity, and its close adhesion
to the pia mater, it cannot be readily separated from this membrane;
but there are parts at the base of the brain, termed 'sub-arachnoid'
spaces, where the arachnoid membrane can be seen distinct from
the subjacent tissue.

Sub-arachnoid
spaces and
fluid.   The arachnoid membrane is separated in certain
situations from the pia mater by a serous fluid (*cerebro-
spinal*) contained in the meshes of very delicate areolar
tissue. Such spaces are called '*sub-arachnoid.*' There is one in
the longitudinal fissure of the cerebrum, where the arachnoid does
not descend to the bottom, but passes across below the edge of the
falx, a little above the corpus callosum. At the base of the brain
there are two of considerable size:—one, the 'middle sub-arachnoid
space,' is situated between the pons Varolii and the commissure of
the optic nerves; the other, the 'posterior,' is situated between the
cerebellum and the medulla oblongata. In the spinal cord, also,
there is a considerable interval between the arachnoid and the pia
mater occupied by fluid. The purpose of this fluid is, not only to
fill up space, like fat in other parts, but mechanically to protect the
nervous centres from the violent shocks and vibrations to which
they would otherwise be liable.

The base of the brain may, in truth, be said to be supported by
a bed of fluid, which insinuates itself into all the inequalities of the
surface, and surrounds all the nerves down to the foramina, through
which they pass. This fluid sometimes escapes through the ear,
in cases of fracture through the base of the skull, involving the
meatus auditorius internus and the petrous portion of the temporal
bone.

Pia mater.   This, the immediate investing membrane of the brain, is extremely vascular; and composed of a network of blood vessels held together by the finest connective tissue. From its internal surface, small branches pass off at right angles into the interior of the brain. The pia mater dips into the fissures between the convolutions, and penetrates into the ventricles for the supply of their interior, forming the 'velum interpositum' and the 'choroid plexuses.'

Arteries of the brain.   The brain is supplied with blood by the two internal carotid and the two vertebral arteries.

Internal carotid.   This artery enters the skull through the carotid canal in the temporal bone, and mounts up very tortuously by the side of the body of the sphenoid, along the inner wall of the cavernous sinus. It appears on the inner side of the anterior clinoid process, and, after giving off the *ophthalmic*, divides into the anterior and middle cerebral, and the posterior communicating arteries.

a. The *anterior cerebral* artery sinks into the longitudinal fissure between the hemispheres, curves round the front part of the corpus callosum, and then runs backwards along its upper surface (under the name of artery of the corpus callosum), and terminates in branches which anastomose with the posterior cerebral. The anterior cerebral arteries of opposite sides run close together; and at the base of the brain are connected by a transverse branch, called the '*anterior communicating artery*' (fig. 119).

b. The *middle cerebral* artery, the largest branch of the internal carotid, runs deep in the fissure of Sylvius, and divides into many branches, distributed to the anterior and middle lobes. Near its origin it gives off a multitude of little arteries, which pierce the locus perforatus anticus to supply the corpus striatum.

c. The *posterior communicating* artery proceeds directly backwards to join the posterior cerebral; thus establishing at the base of the brain the free arterial inosculation called the 'circle of Willis.'

d. The *anterior choroid* artery, a small branch of the internal

L L

carotid, arises external to the posterior communicating artery. It
runs backwards, and terminates in the choroid plexus of the lateral
ventricle.

Vertebral
artery.
   This artery, a branch of the subclavian, winds backwards along the arch of the atlas, and enters the skull
through the foramen magnum, curving round the

Fig. 118.

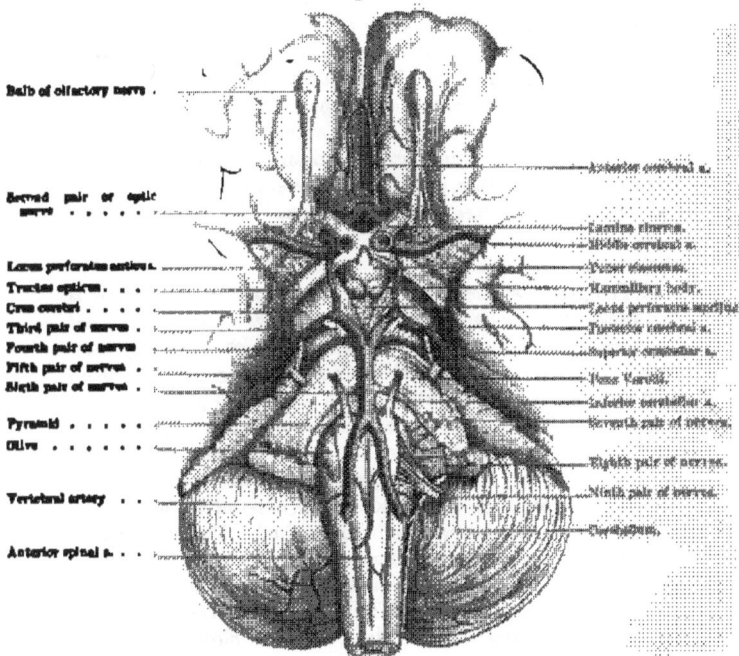

Bulb of olfactory nerve .

Second pair or optic nerve . . . . .

Locus perforatus anticus .
Tractus opticus . . .
Crus cerebri . . . .
Third pair of nerves .
Fourth pair of nerves
Fifth pair of nerves .
Sixth pair of nerves .

Pyramid . . . . .
Olive . . . .

Vertebral artery . .

Anterior spinal a. . .

Anterior cerebral a.

Lamina cinerea.
Middle cerebral a.

Tuber cinereum.
Mammillary body.
Locus perforatus anticus.
Posterior cerebral a.

Vena Varolii.
Inferior cerebellar a.
Seventh pair of nerves.

Eighth pair of nerves.
Ninth pair of nerves.

Corpus dentatum.

medulla oblongata between the hypoglossal nerve, and the anterior
root of the first cervical. At the lower border of the pons, the
two arteries unite to form the '*basilar*,' which proceeds along the

middle of the pons, and divides at its upper border into the two
posterior cerebral arteries.

Each vertebral artery before joining its fellow gives off—

a. A *posterior meningeal* branch distributed to the posterior
fossa of the skull.

b. *Anterior* and *posterior spinal arteries*, which supply the
front and back surfaces of the spinal cord.

c. The *inferior cerebellar* artery, sometimes a branch of the
basilar, but more frequently of the vertebral, passes backwards, and
supplies the lower surface of the cerebellum.

The *basilar* artery, formed by the junction of the two vertebral,
in its course along the pons gives off on each side—

a. *Transverse* branches which pass outwards on the pons: one,
the *auditory*, enters the meatus auditorius internus with the
auditory nerve; another, the *anterior cerebellar*, supplies the front
part of the lower surface of the cerebellum.

b. The *superior cerebellar*, which supplies the upper surface of
the cerebellum.

c. The *posterior cerebral*, the terminal branches, run outwards
and backwards, one on the under surface of each posterior cerebral
lobe, and divide into numerous branches, which ultimately inosculate with the outer cerebral arteries. Each gives off a small
posterior choroid artery distributed to the choroid plexus.

Circle of
Willis.

This important arterial inosculation (fig. 119) is
formed, laterally, by the two anterior cerebral, the two
internal carotid, and the two posterior communicating
arteries: in front it is completed by the anterior communicating
artery; behind, by the two posterior cerebral. The tortuosity of
the large arteries before they enter the brain is intended to miti-
gate the force of the heart's action; and the circle of Willis
provides a free supply of blood from other quarters, in case any
accidental circumstance should stop the flow of blood in any of the
more direct channels.*

* In many of the long-necked herbivorous quadrupeds a beautiful provision has
been made, in the disposition of the internal carotid arteries, for the purpose of
equalising the force of the blood supplied to the brain. The arteries, as they enter

L L 2

Peculiarities of the cerebral circulation.   Besides the 'circle of Willis,' there are other peculiarities in the circulation of the brain; namely, the tortuosity of the four great vessels as they enter the skull—their passage through bony canals—their breaking up into minute arteries in the pia mater before they enter the substance of the brain—the formation of sinuses (p. 6)—the great minuteness of the capillaries, and the extreme thinness of their walls; a fact which accounts for the slowness with which a congested brain recovers itself.

General division of the brain.   The mass of nervous matter contained within the skull, designated under the common term brain, is divided into three parts—the 'cerebrum,' or intellectual brain, which occupies the whole of the upper part of the cranial cavity; the 'cerebellum,' or little brain, which occupies the lower and back part beneath the tentorium; the 'pons Varolii,' or quadrilateral mass of white fibres, which rests upon the basilar process; and the 'medulla oblongata,' situated beneath the cerebellum. This last part passes out of the skull through the foramen magnum, and is continuous with the spinal cord.

The size of the brain varies in different subjects, but in an adult male the average weight is about 48 ounces; in an adult female, about 43 ounces.[*]

Medulla oblongata.   This term is applied to that part of the cerebro-spinal axis which is situated immediately below the pons Varolii, and is continuous below with the spinal cord. Its form is pyramidal with the broadest part above; thence it gradually tapers into the spinal cord. It is about an inch and a quarter long, and nearly an inch in its thickest part. It lies on the basilar groove of the occipital bone, and descends obliquely

the skull, divide into several branches, which again unite, so as to form a remarkable network of arteries, called by Galen, who first described it, the 'rete mirabile.' The object of this evidently is to moderate the rapidity with which the blood would otherwise enter the cranium, in the different positions of the head, and thus preserve the brain from those sudden influxions to which it would under other circumstances be continually exposed.

[*] Dr. R. Boyd, Philos. Trans., 1860.

backwards through the foramen magnum to the upper border of
the atlas, where it is continuous with the spinal cord. Its posterior
surface is received into the fossa between the hemispheres of the
cerebellum. In front and behind, the medulla is marked by a
median fissure—the *anterior* and *posterior median fissures*, which
are the continuations upwards of the median fissures of the spinal
cord. The anterior terminates below the pons Varolii in a cul-de-

Fig. 120.

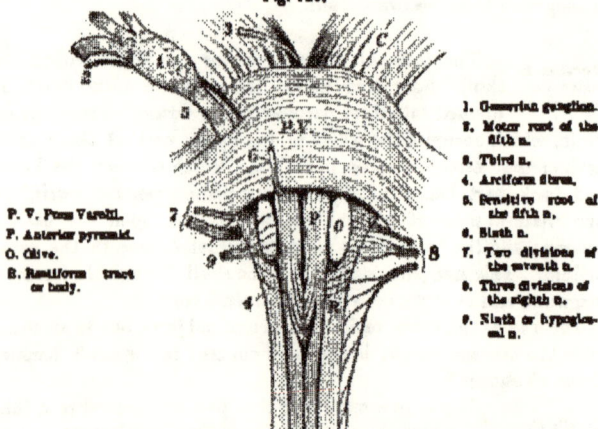

P. V. Pons Varolii.
P. Anterior pyramid.
O. Olive.
R. Restiform tract
or body.

1. Gasserian ganglion.
2. Motor root of the fifth n.
3. Third n.
4. Arciform fibres.
5. Sensitive root of the fifth n.
6. Sixth n.
7. Two divisions of the seventh n.
8. Three divisions of the eighth n.
9. Ninth or hypoglossal n.

DIAGRAM OF THE FRONT SURFACE OF THE MEDULLA OBLONGATA.

sac, named '*foramen cæcum*;' it is occupied by a fold of pia
mater. On each half of the medulla, there stand out, in relief,
four longitudinal columns. Those nearest to the anterior fissure
are called the '*anterior pyramids*.' External to these are the
'*olivary bodies*.' Still more external, and towards the posterior
part of the medulla, are the '*restiform bodies*;' lastly, on each
side of the posterior median fissure, are the '*posterior pyramids*.'

The *anterior pyramids* are narrow below, but gradually increase
in breadth as they ascend towards the pons, from which they are
separated by a transverse groove. Their component fibres are

continuous with the anterior columns of the spinal cord, and consist therefore of motor fibres. They may be traced through the pons into the lower part of the crura cerebri. By gently separating the pyramids about an inch below the pons, you observe that their fibres on each side decussate (fig. 120). This is the explanation of ' cross paralysis ; ' i. e. when one side of the brain is injured, the loss of motor power is manifested on the opposite side of the body.* The decussation, consisting of three or four bundles of fibres on each side, takes place only between the inner fibres of the pyramid ; the outer fibres run straight on without crossing over. These decussating fibres are prolongations of the deep fibres of the lateral columns of the cord, which here come forward to the surface, pushing aside the proper anterior columns.

The *olivary bodies* are two oval eminences situated on the outer side of the anterior pyramids, and separated from the pons by a deep groove. They consist, externally, of white substance ; when cut into, their interior presents a zigzag line of grey matter, called, from its shape, ' corpus dentatum.' This grey line forms a circuit, interrupted only on the upper and inner side, so that it nearly isolates the white matter in its centre. Arching round its lower part some white fibres may be observed : these constitute the *arciform fibres* of Rolando.

The *restiform bodies* are situated on the outer side of and behind the olives. They are the continuations upwards of the posterior columns of the cord, and as they ascend, diverge from each other and pass into the cerebellum, constituting its inferior crura (p. 519). In consequence of this divergence, the grey matter in the interior of the medulla oblongata is exposed ; so that the floor of the fourth ventricle (of which the restiform bodies assist in forming the lateral boundaries) is grey. The restiform bodies consist partly of longitudinal white fibres derived from the posterior and lateral columns of the cord ; partly of grey matter contained

---

* The phenomenon of 'cross paralysis' of *sensation* is explained by the fact made out by Brown Séquard, that the paths of sensory impressions cross each other in the grey matter of the cord.

in their interior, which is continuous with that in the posterior part of the spinal cord.

The *posterior pyramids* are two slender white bundles placed on each side of the posterior median fissure (fig. 121). They pass upwards and then diverge from each other, forming the apex of the fourth ventricle. They proceed with the restiform bodies for some distance, leaving which, they are lost in the cerebrum. At

Fig. 121.

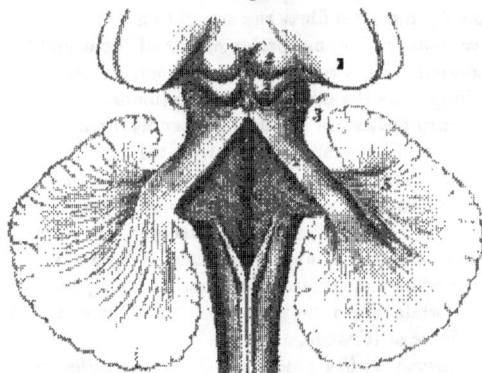

DIAGRAM OF THE FOURTH VENTRICLE AND RESTIFORM BODIES.

1. Thalamus opticum.
2. Nates and testes.
3. Origin of fourth nerve.
4. Processus a cerebello ad testes.
5. Restiform bodies diverging.
6. Origin of seventh or auditory nerve.

their point of divergence the posterior pyramids become slightly enlarged, forming what is called the '*processus clavatus.*'

When a longitudinal section is carefully made through the middle of the medulla oblongata, a number of white fibres are seen running in a horizontal direction, constituting a kind of septum between the two halves. Some of these septal fibres issue from the anterior median fissure, wind round the medulla, and constitute what are termed the *arciform fibres* of Rolando (p. 517); others, issuing from the posterior fissure, wind round in a similar manner, and form some of the transverse fibres seen on the floor of the fourth ventricle.

Pons Varolii or tuber annulare. This convex eminence (p. 517) is situated at the base of the brain, immediately above the medulla oblongata. It corresponds with the basilar groove of the occipital bone. In its antero-posterior diameter it measures rather more than an inch. Down the middle runs a slight groove which lodges the basilar artery. If the pia mater be carefully removed, we observe that its superficial fibres proceed transversely from one hemisphere of the cerebellum to the other, forming the **The great commissure of the cerebellum.** great commissure or middle peduncles of the cerebellar lobes. Throughout the mammalia its size bears a direct ratio to the degree of development of these lobes; therefore it is larger in man than in any other animal.* The superficial fibres only are transverse; if these be removed, we see that the anterior fibres of the medulla run under them at right angles into the crura cerebri, like a river under a bridge.

The pons, like the medulla oblongata, has an imperfect median septum, composed of horizontal fibres, which come from the floor of the fourth ventricle.

Besides the transverse and longitudinal fibres just described, the pons contains grey matter, which probably gives origin to fresh nerve fibres; so that the pons may be considered a source, as well as a conductor of power.

Cerebrum. The cerebrum, in man, is so much more developed than the other parts of the brain, that it completely overlays them. It is of an oval form and convex on its external aspect. It is divided in the middle line by the deep '*longitudinal fissure*' into two equal halves, termed the right and left hemispheres.† The fissure is occupied by the falx cerebri (p. 5). The

---

* Birds, reptiles, and fishes have no pons, because there are no lateral lobes to the cerebellum.

† Examples are now and then met with where the longitudinal fissure is not exactly in the middle line; the consequence of which want of symmetry is, that one hemisphere is larger than the other. Bichat (Recherches Physiologiques sur la Vie et la Mort, Paris, 1829) was of opinion that this anomaly exercised a deleterious influence on the intellect. It is remarkable that the examination of his own brain after death, went to prove the error of his own doctrine.

surface of each hemisphere is mapped out by tortuous eminences, termed 'gyri' or 'convolutions,' separated from each other by deep furrows (sulci). Many of these furrows are occupied by the large veins in their course to the sinuses; others are filled by sub-arachnoid fluid. The convolutions themselves are merely folds of the brain, for the purpose of increasing the extent of the surface upon which may be laid grey or vesicular nerve substance, now generally admitted to be the source of power. They are not precisely alike on both sides. Their number, disposition, and depth vary a little in different individuals, and, to a certain extent, may be considered as an index of the degree of intelligence.* Since this grey matter forms a sort of bark round the white brain substance, it is often called the cortical substance.† The depth of the sulci between the convolutions varies in different subjects; generally they penetrate to about an inch: hence it follows that two brains of apparently equal size may be very unequal in point of extent of surface for the grey matter, and therefore in amount of intellectual capability. Under the microscope, the cortical layer is seen to consist of four layers, two grey alternating with two of white;‡

* Those who wish to investigate the cerebral convolutions in their simplest form in the lower classes of mammalia, and to trace them through their successive complications and arrangement into groups as we ascend in the higher classes, should consult M. Leuret, Anatomie Comparée du Système Nerveux considéré dans ses Rapports avec l'Intelligence: Paris, 1839; also M. Foville, Traité de l'Anat. du Système Nerveux, &c.: Paris, 1844.

† There are two kinds of nervous matter—the grey or vesicular, and the white or fibrous. The grey is exceedingly vascular, and contains the nerve vesicles, which are generally allowed to be the source of power. The white consists of extremely delicate nerve fibres, is scantily provided with blood vessels, and is probably the mere conductor of power.

The intense vascularity of the grey matter has been demonstrated by Mr. Quekett and Mr. Smee, who have had the kindness to allow the author to inspect their beautiful preparations. Mr. Smee's injections were made by using a solution of carmine in ammonia mixed with size. The minute arteries enter the surface of the grey matter, and break up in it into a network of fine capillaries. These capillaries are peculiar in being quite naked, and not supported, as in other parts, by cellular tissue. Hence it is they are so liable to give way, and allow their contents to escape: hence it is, they are fenced round by so many provisions calculated to break the force of the current of the blood—namely, the tortuosities of the arteries at the base of the brain, their subdivisions in the pia mater, and the peculiar arrangement of the sinuses.

‡ Six layers may be demonstrated in some situations, chiefly near the corpus cal-

the external layer being always white. Some of these convolutions from their size and regularity have received special names. The most important are as follow:—

a. The *gyrus fornicatus*, or the convolution of the corpus callosum, commences close to the optic commissure, and curving along the free surface of the corpus callosum, winds round its posterior extremity, and terminates in the middle lobe forming the hippocampus major.

b. The *marginal convolution*, or the convolution of the longitudinal fissure, begins in the posterior part of the anterior lobe, courses along the margin of the fissure, and after a tortuous course is lost on the under surface of the middle lobe.

c. The *island of Reil.* This may be seen by separating the middle from the anterior lobe, deep in the fissure of Sylvius. It is composed of a number of small convolutions connected with those adjoining. It corresponds to the under surface of the corpus striatum, and might, therefore, be called the lobe of that ganglion.

The under surface of each cerebral hemisphere is not only convoluted like the upper, but presents in addition three lobes (fig. 122), an anterior, middle, and posterior, which fit into the base of the skull. The *anterior lobe,* triangular in shape, rests upon the roof of the orbit, and is separated from the middle by a cleft called the '*fissure of Sylvius,*' which receives the lesser wing of the sphenoid bone. The *middle lobe* occupies the middle fossa of the skull, formed by the sphenoid and temporal bones. The *posterior lobe* rests on the arch of the tentorium. Between this and the middle there is no definite boundary, so that some anatomists enumerate only two lobes.

Fig. 122.

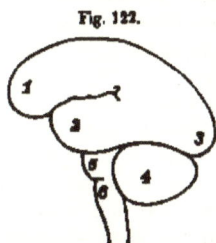

1, 2, 3. Anterior, middle, and posterior lobes of the cerebrum.
4. Cerebellum.
5. Pons Varolii.
6. Medulla oblongata.

losum. For an account of these laminæ, and the best mode of examining them, see Dalllarget, Recherches sur la Structure de la Couche Corticale des Circonvolutions du Cerveau, insérées dans les Mémoires de l'Académie de Médecine, 1840.

The several objects seen at the base of the brain in the middle line should now be examined, proceeding in order from the front (fig. 119, p. 514). In this description the cerebral nerves are omitted. These will be examined hereafter.

In the middle line dividing the anterior lobes is the longitudinal fissure. By gently separating the anterior lobes, we expose the anterior extremity of the corpus callosum, or the great transverse commissure which connects the two hemispheres of the cerebrum. Continued backwards and outwards on each side from the corpus callosum to the fissure of Sylvius, is a white band, called the *peduncle of the corpus callosum.* Extending from the corpus callosum to the optic commissure is a layer of grey matter, *lamina cinerea,* which is continued backwards to the *tuber cinereum.* Between the anterior and middle lobes is a deep fissure, ' *the fissure of Sylvius,*' at the bottom of which are situated the middle cerebral artery and the island of Reil. The *optic commissure,* formed by the union of the two optic tracts, is seen in the middle line behind the lamina cinerea. At the root of the fissure of Sylvius, and in front of the optic tract, is a space, the *locus perforatus anticus,* the surface of which is perforated by small blood vessels, which supply the corpus striatum. Immediately behind the optic commissure is a simple elevation of the surface, consisting of grey matter, called the ' *tuber cinereum.*' From this a conical tube of reddish colour, termed the ' *infundibulum,*' descends to the ' *pituitary body,*' which occupies the sella turcica of the sphenoid bone. The pituitary body consists of two lobes, the anterior and larger is of a reddish-brown colour, and concave behind to receive the posterior lobe. On section, it is composed of a soft pulpy mass of a yellowish-brown colour. Behind the tuber cinereum, are two round white bodies, the ' *corpora mammillaria or albicantia,*' which are formed by the curling round of the anterior horns of the fornix. Between the mammillary bodies and the pons is a depression of grey matter called the *locus perforatus posticus* or *pons Tarini,* the surface of which is pierced by small vessels supplying the optic thalami. From the anterior border of

the pons, two round cords of white nervous matter, about half an
inch thick, diverge from each other, one towards each hemisphere
of the cerebrum. These are the *crura cerebri.* Winding round
the outer side of each crus is a soft white band, the '*tractus
opticus*,' or root of the optic nerve.

Fig. 123.

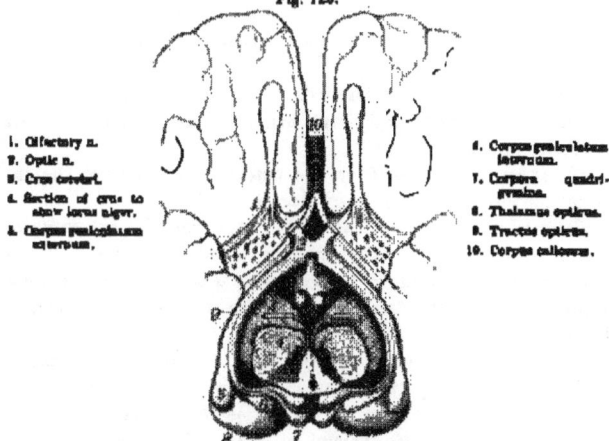

1. Olfactory n.
2. Optic n.
3. Crus cerebri.
4. Section of crus to show locus niger.
5. Corpus geniculatum externum.

6. Corpus geniculatum internum.
7. Corpora quadrigemina.
8. Thalamus opticus.
9. Tractus opticus.
10. Corpus callosum.

DIAGRAM OF THE ORIGINS OF THE OLFACTORY AND OPTIC NERVES.

ORIGIN OF THE CEREBRAL NERVES. The cerebral nerves are given off in pairs, named
the first, second, third, &c., according to the order in
which they appear, beginning from the front. There
are nine pairs. Some are nerves of special sense—as the olfactory,
the optic, the auditory; others are nerves of common sensation—
as the large root of the fifth, the glosso-pharyngeal, and the pneumogastric; others, again, are nerves of motion—as the third, the
fourth, the small root of the fifth, the sixth, the facial division of
the seventh, the spinal accessory, and the ninth.

First pair or olfactory nerve. The olfactory nerve is triangular, and fits into a
furrow between the convolutions. It proceeds straight
forwards under the anterior lobe, and terminates in

the olfactory ganglion, which lies on the cribriform plate of the ethmoid bone.

The olfactory ganglion is olive-shaped, of a reddish-grey colour and very soft consistence, due to a large amount of grey matter contained in it. It gives off from its under surface the true olfactory nerves.[*] For the description of these, see p. 109.

This nerve arises by three roots—an outer and an inner composed of white matter, and a central composed of grey (p. 524).

The *outer* root passes forwards as a thin white line from the bottom of the fissure of Sylvius, and describes a curve with the concavity outwards.

The *inner* root arises from the posterior extremity of the internal convolution of the anterior cerebral lobe.

The *middle* or grey root arises from the posterior extremity of the furrow in which the olfactory nerve is lodged; to see it, therefore, the nerve should be turned backwards. It contains white fibres in its interior which have been traced to the corpus striatum.

Second pair or optic.   These nerves proceed from the optic commissure, formed by the union of the two optic tracts. These tracts arise from the corpora quadrigemina, the corpora geniculata, and the optic thalami (p. 524). They wind round the crura cerebri, to which they are connected by their anterior borders, and join in the middle line to form the optic commissure. This commissure rests on the sphenoid bone in front of the sella turcica. From the commissure each optic nerve, invested by its

---

[*] Strictly speaking, the olfactory nerve and its ganglion are integral parts (the prosencephalic lobe) of the brain. What in human anatomy is called the origin of the nerve is, in point of fact, the crus of the olfactory lobe, and is in every way homologous to the crus cerebri or cerebelli. In proof of this, look at the enormous size and connections of the crus in animals which have very acute sense of smell. Throughout the vertebrate kingdom there is a strict ratio between the sense of smell and the development of the olfactory lobes. Again, in many animals, these lobes are actually larger than the cerebral, and contain in their interior a cavity which communicates with the lateral ventricles. According to Tiedemann, this cavity exists even in the human fœtus at an early period.

fibrous sheath, passes through the optic foramen into the orbit, and terminates in the retina.

At the commissure some of the nerve fibres cross from one side to the other. This decussation affects only the middle fibres of the nerve; the outer fibres pass from one optic tract to the optic nerve of the same side; the inner fibres pass from one optic tract round to the optic tract of the opposite side; while in front of the commissure are fibres which pass from one optic nerve to its fellow (p. 529). The purpose of this partial crossing is not thoroughly understood. It was ingeniously supposed by Dr. Wollaston * to account for single vision, since the right halves and the left halves of the eyes would derive their nerve fibres from the same optic nerve.

Third pair or motores oculorum.   The apparent origin of the third nerve is from the inner side of the crus cerebri, immediately in front of the pons. Some of its fibres, however, penetrate into the crus as far as the locus niger, and others to the corpora quadrigemina, and valve of Vieussens (p. 524). It passes through the sphenoidal fissure, and supplies all the muscles of the orbit, except the superior oblique and the rectus externus.

Fourth pair or pathetici.   The fourth nerve arises from the upper surface of the valve of Vieussens (p. 519). It runs transversely outwards, winds round the crus cerebri, enters the orbit through the sphenoidal fissure, and supplies the superior oblique muscle of the eye.

Fifth pair or trigeminal nerve.   The fifth nerve consists of two roots, both of which arise apparently from the outer side of the pons Varolii (p. 517); but their real origin is deeper. The smaller and anterior of the two roots, consisting of motor fibres only, may be traced into the pyramidal tract in the pons; the posterior and larger, consisting of purely sensitive fibres, may be traced to the floor of the fourth ventricle, between the restiform tract and the fasciculus teres. The nerve proceeds forwards over the apex of the petrous portion of the temporal bone: here is developed upon the sensitive root the great *Gasserian* ganglion. This root then divides into three branches: the *ophthalmic*, which passes through

* Philos. Trans. of the Royal Society, 1824.

the sphenoidal fissure; the *superior maxillary*, which passes through the foramen rotundum; the *inferior maxillary*, which passes through the foramen ovale. They all confer common sensibility upon the parts they supply, which comprise nearly the entire head. The small motor root passes beneath the ganglion, with which it has no connection, and accompanies the inferior maxillary division, to be distributed to the muscles of mastication.

Sixth pair or abducentes. The sixth nerve emerges from the groove between the pons and the medulla (p. 517), with both of which it is connected. Its deep origin has been traced to the floor of the fourth ventricle. It leaves the skull through the sphenoidal fissure, and supplies the rectus externus of the eye.

Seventh pair. The seventh consists of two nerves, the *portio dura*, or muscular nerve of the face, and the *portio mollis*, or proper auditory nerve. The two nerves, of which the portio dura is the more internal, arise apparently from the lower part of the pons Varolii (p. 517). The deep origin of the portio dura is stated to come from the restiform and olivary fasciculi of the medulla. The real origin of the portio mollis is from the floor of the fourth ventricle by several transverse white filaments, which emerge from the median groove. The seventh pair enters the meatus auditorius internus, where they are connected by several filaments. For the further description of the portio dura, see p. 194. The auditory nerve divides at the bottom of the meatus auditorius internus into cochlear and vestibular branches which are distributed to the internal ear.

Eighth pair. This comprises three nerves, the *glosso-pharyngeal*, the *pneumogastric*, and the *nervus accessorius* (p. 517). The first two arise by several filaments from the restiform tract of the medulla close to the olive, through which their fibres may be traced to the grey matter in the floor of the fourth ventricle. The nervus accessorius is composed of two parts, an upper or accessory portion, which arises from the side of the medulla oblongata, and a lower or spinal portion, which arises by a series of slender filaments from the lateral tract of the spinal cord as low down as the fifth or sixth cervical vertebra. The spinal portion ascends

behind the ligamentum denticulatum, into the skull through the
foramen magnum, and joins the accessory part. The nervus
accessorius then passes through the foramen jugulare, with the
pneumogastric and glosso-pharyngeal. The glosso-pharyngeal is
distributed to the mucous membrane of the pharynx and the back
of the tongue (p. 193). The pneumogastric is distributed to the
pharynx, the larynx, the heart and lungs, the œsophagus and the
stomach. The nervus accessorius supplies the sterno-mastoid and
the trapezius. For the further description of these nerves, see
pp. 21, 194.

Ninth pair or
hypoglossal.
        This nerve arises by several roots from the medulla
oblongata, along the groove between the anterior
pyramid and the olive. Its fibres may be traced to the
grey matter in the floor of the fourth ventricle. It leaves the
skull through the anterior condyloid foramen, and is distributed
to the muscles of the tongue and the depressors of the os-hyoides
and larynx.

Dissection of
the brain.
        The brain should now be laid on its base. By gently
separating the hemispheres, we expose at the bottom
of the longitudinal fissure a white band of nerve substance, which is the great transverse commissure of the cerebrum,
and termed the 'corpus callosum.'

White and
grey matter.
        Slice off the hemispheres down to the level of the
corpus callosum.* The cut surface presents a mass of
white substance surrounded by a tortuous layer of grey
matter, about one-eighth of an inch thick. This grey substance
consists of four layers—two of grey alternating with two of white,
the most external layer being white. In some places, chiefly at
the base of the brain, six layers have been demonstrated.

Corpus callo-
sum.
        This transverse portion of white substance is the chief
connecting medium between the two hemispheres, and
is called the great transverse commissure of the cere-

---

* The section of the brain at the level of the corpus callosum was called by the old
anatomists 'centrum ovale majus;' at a higher level, the section was called 'centrum
ovale minus.'

brum.* It is about four inches long, and rather nearer to the
front than to the back part of the brain. Its surface is slightly
arched from before backwards. A shallow groove, called the
' raphé,' runs along the middle of its upper surface (fig. 124); in a
fresh brain, two white streaks, named the *nerves of Lancisi*, run

Fig. 124.

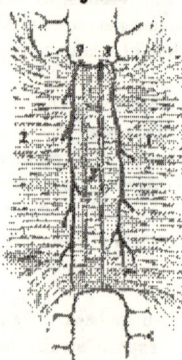

UPPER SURFACE OF COR-
PUS CALLOSUM.

1, 1. Lineæ transversæ.
2. Raphé.
3, 3. Anterior cerebral a.

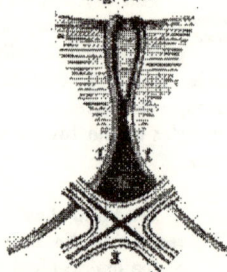

DIAGRAM OF LAMINA CINEREA.

1, 1. Peduncles of corpus callosum.
2. Lamina cinerea.
3. Commissure of optic nerves.

parallel to it. The surface of the corpus callosum is marked by
transverse lines which indicate the course of its fibres: these are
the *lineæ transversæ* of the old anatomists. The anterior cerebral
arteries proceed along the surface of the corpus callosum to the
back of the brain.

* In a brain properly hardened by spirit, the fibres may be traced congregating
towards the corpus callosum from both hemispheres: hence they were called by Gall
the *converging* fibres of the brain. This anatomist applied the above name to all
commissural fibres. Those fibres, on the other hand, which ascended from the medulla
oblongata into the hemispheres, he named the *diverging*.—Anat. et Physiol. du Système Nerv.: Paris, 1810.

M M

The anterior part of the corpus callosum turns downwards and backwards, forming a bend called its *genu*, or knee. The inferior part (rostrum) of this bend becomes gradually thinner, and terminates in two peduncles, which diverge from each other, and are lost, one in each fissure of Sylvius. Between these crura is placed the lamina cinerea (fig. 125). The posterior part of the corpus callosum terminates in a thick, round border, beneath which the

Fig. 126.

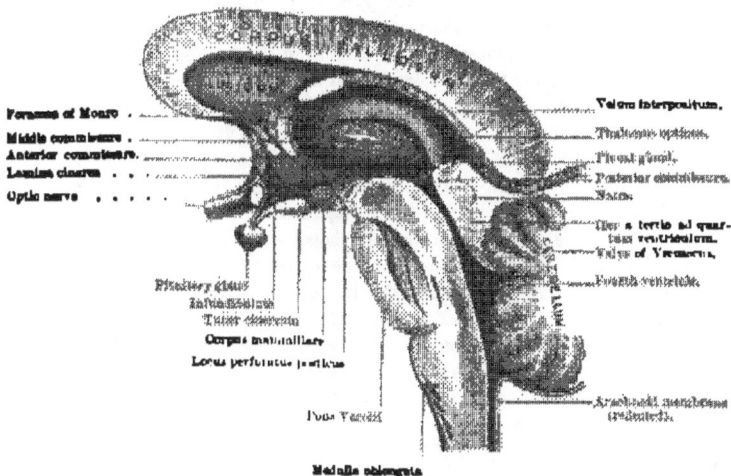

VERTICAL SECTION THROUGH THE CORPUS CALLOSUM, AND PARTS BELOW.

pia mater enters the interior of the ventricles. A satisfactory view cannot be obtained of the arch formed by the corpus callosum, of its terminations in front and behind, and of the relative thickness of its different parts, without making a perpendicular section through a fresh brain, as shown in the diagram.[*]

* The corpus callosum is more or less developed in all mammalia, but is absent in birds, reptiles, and fish. It is not absolutely essential to the exercise of the intellect.

The two cavities called the '*lateral ventricles*' are

Lateral ventricles. situated, one in each hemisphere of the brain, beneath the corpus callosum. A longitudinal incision should be made on each side, about half an inch from the raphé of the corpus callosum. Care must be taken not to cut too near the middle line, in order to preserve the delicate partition which descends from the under surface of the corpus callosum, and separates the ventricles from each other. They should be laid open throughout their whole extent. Their general form should be first examined; afterwards the several objects contained in them.

The lateral ventricles are two cavities in the general mass of the brain, occasioned by the enlargement and folding backward of the cerebral lobes over the other parts of the central nervous axis. They are lined with a ciliated spheroidal epithelium, and contain a serous fluid, which, even in a healthy brain, sometimes exists in considerable quantity: when greatly in excess, it constitutes one form of the disease termed 'hydrocephalus.'

The ventricles are crescentic in shape, with their backs towards each other. Each extends into the three lobes of the cerebral hemisphere, and consists of a central part or *body*, and three horns, or *cornua*, anterior, middle, and posterior. The body, situated in the middle of the hemisphere, is separated from its fellow by the septum lucidum. Its roof is formed by the corpus callosum; and on the floor, beginning from the front, are seen, the corpus striatum, the tænia semicircularis, the optic thalamus, the choroid plexus, and the fornix. The *anterior horn* extends into the anterior lobe, and as it passes forwards, slightly diverges from its fellow on the opposite side. The *posterior horn* may be traced into the posterior lobe, where it passes at first backwards and outwards, and then converges towards its fellow. In it take notice of an elevation of white matter, the 'hippocampus minor;' also of a triangular flat surface, called 'pes accessorius' or 'eminentia collateralis.'* The

---

for it has been found absent in the human subject without any particular intellectual deficiency. See cases recorded by Reil, Archiv. für die Phys. t. xi.; and Wenzel, de planitior Struct. Cereb. p. 802.

* The posterior horns are not always equally developed in both hemispheres, and

middle horn runs into the middle lobe, descends towards the base of the brain, making a very curious curve, like a ram's horn—that is, in a direction backwards, outwards, downwards, forwards, and inwards; the initial letters of which make the memorial word 'bodfi.' By cutting through the substance of the middle lobe, the windings of this horn can be followed; in it are the hippocampus major, the pes hippocampi, the posterior crus of the fornix, the choroid plexus, and the thalamus opticus.

Fig. 127.

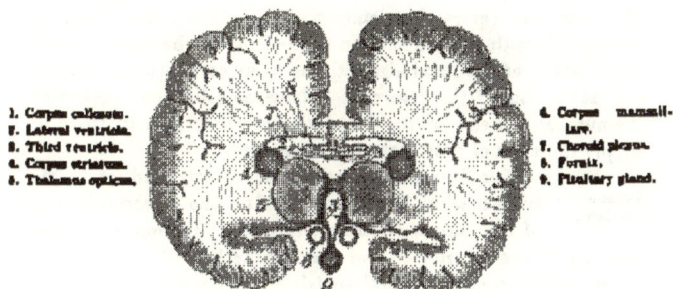

1. Corpus callosum.	4. Corpus mammillare.
2. Lateral ventricle.	6. Choroid plexus.
3. Third ventricle.	8. Fornix.
4. Corpus striatum.	9. Pituitary gland.
5. Thalamus opticus.	

TRANSVERSE PERPENDICULAR SECTION THROUGH THE BRAIN.

Appearance on perpendicular section. If a perpendicular section were made across the middle of the brain, the lateral ventricles would appear as represented in fig. 127. Together with the third or middle ventricle, their shape slightly resembles the letter T. Such a section shows well the radiating fibres of the corpus callosum, the fornix, and the velum interpositum beneath it; also the beginning of the transverse fissure at the base of the brain, between the crus cerebri and the middle lobe.

sometimes they are absent in one or in both. They are only found in the brain of man and the quadrumana.

In the carnivora, ruminantia, solipeda, pachydermata, and rodentia, the lateral ventricles are prolonged into the largely developed olfactory lobes. This is the case in the human fœtus only at an early period.

The contents of the lateral ventricles should now be examined more in detail; also the transparent septum (*septum lucidum*) by which the two lateral ventricles are separated.

Corpus striatum.

This body is so called because, when cut into, it presents alternate layers of white and grey matter.[*] It is a much larger mass of grey substance than it appears to be, for only a portion of it is seen projecting on the floor of the ventricle. The intra-ventricular portion is pear-shaped, with the large end forwards; and when traced backwards, is found to taper gradually to a point on the outside of the optic thalamus (p. 539). The under part (extra-ventricular portion) of the corpus striatum corresponds with the convolution at the base of the brain, known as the island of Reil, and also with the locus perforatus anticus—a spot at the root of the fissure of Sylvius, so called on account of the number and size of the blood vessels which pass in there to supply the mass of grey matter in question.

Tænia semicircularis.

This is a narrow semi-transparent band of longitudinal white fibres, which skirts the posterior border of the corpus striatum (fig. 129). In front it is connected with the anterior crus of the fornix; behind, it is lost in the middle horn of the lateral ventricle. A large vein from the corpus striatum passes underneath the tænia semicircularis to join the vena Galeni.

Septum lucidum.

This is a thin and almost transparent partition, which descends vertically in the middle line from the under surface of the corpus callosum, and separates the anterior part of the lateral ventricles from each other. It is attached, above, to the corpus callosum; below, to the reflected part of the corpus callosum and the fornix (p. 530). It is not of equal depth throughout. The broadest part is in front, and corresponds with the knee of the corpus callosum. It becomes narrower behind,

---

[*] The white lines in the corpus striatum are produced by the fibres of the crus cerebri, which traverse this mass of grey matter before they expand to form the hemisphere. The grey matter itself is sometimes called the anterior cerebral ganglion. It is found in all mammalia, in birds, and, to a certain extent, in reptiles. Its precise function is still unknown.

and disappears where the corpus callosum and the fornix become continuous. The septum consists of two layers, which inclose a space called the '*fifth ventricle*' (fig. 128). Each layer is made up of white substance inside, and of grey outside; the ventricle between them is closed in the adult, and lined by a delicate serous membrane, which secretes in it a minute quantity of fluid; but in fœtal life it communicates with the third ventricle between the pillars of the fornix.*

Cut transversely through the corpus callosum and the septum lucidum, and turn forwards the anterior half. In this way the

Fig. 128.

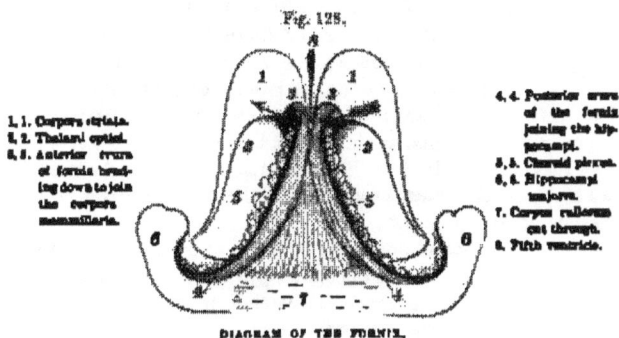

1, 1. Corpora striata.
2, 2. Thalami optici.
3, 3. Anterior crura of fornix bending down to join the corpora mammillaria.

4, 4. Posterior crura of the fornix joining the hippocampi.
5, 5. Choroid plexus.
6, 6. Hippocampi majores.
7. Corpus callosum cut through.
8. Fifth ventricle.

DIAGRAM OF THE FORNIX.

(The arrow is in the foramen of Monro.)

ventricle of the septum will appear as in fig. 128. By turning back the posterior half of the corpus callosum, a view is obtained of the fornix. This proceeding requires care, or the fornix will be reflected also, since these two arches of nervous matter are here so closely connected.

Fornix. This is a layer of white matter extending in the form of an arch from before backwards, beneath the corpus callosum. It is the 'great longitudinal commissure,' and lies

* The development of the septum lucidum commences about the fifth month of fœtal life, and proceeds from before backwards *pari passu* with the corpus callosum and fornix.

over the velum interpositum (fig. 126, p. 530). Viewed from its upper surface, it is triangular, with the base behind, as shown in diagram 128. The broad part or body is connected to the corpus callosum. From its anterior narrow part proceed two round white cords, called its *anterior crura*, one on each side of the mesial line. As they pass forwards, the crura descend towards the base of the brain, where, making a bend upon themselves, they form part of the corpora mammillaria, from which they may be traced, passing backwards to the optic thalami. Immediately behind, and below the anterior crura, is a passage through which the choroid plexuses of opposite sides are continuous with each other. This aperture is called the '*foramen of Monro*' (fig. 126).[*] Strictly speaking, it is not a foramen, but only a communication existing between the two lateral and the third ventricles. The *posterior crura* are continued downwards and outwards from the body of the fornix, as thin white bands, intimately connected with the concave side of the hippocampus major as far down as the pes hippocampi. Each band is called the *tænia hippocampi*, or the *corpus fimbriatum*.[†]

Foramen of Monro.

Hippocampus major. This is an elongated mass of grey matter covered with white, and is situated in the posterior part of the descending horn. It extends to the bottom of the horn, where it becomes somewhat expanded, and indented on the surface, so as to resemble the paw of an animal; whence its name, '*pes hippocampi*.' Attached along the front border of the hippocampus, is the posterior crus of the fornix.

Hippocampus minor. This mass, smaller than the preceding, is situated in the posterior horn. It consists of white matter externally, and corresponds to a deep convolution which projects into the ventricles. Between the hippocampus major and minor, is a triangular smooth surface, called the *pes accessorius*, or *eminentia collateralis*.

[*] Monro, 'Microscopic Enquiries into the Nerves and Brain.' Edinburgh, 1780.
[†] The fornix and septum lucidum are absent in fish; they are merely rudimentary in reptiles and birds: but all mammalia have them in greater or less perfection, according to the degree of development of the cerebral hemispheres.

The fornix should now be cut through, and its two portions reflected. On the under surface of the posterior portion is seen a number of fibres arranged transversely, constituting what is termed the *lyra.*

Between the fornix and the upper surface of the cerebellum is the '*transverse fissure,* or *fissure of Bichat,*' through which the pia mater enters the ventricles. The fissure extends downwards on each side to the base of the brain, and terminates between the crus cerebri and the middle lobe. It is of a horse-shoe shape, with the concavity directed forwards.

Velum interpositum and choroid plexus. The *velum interpositum,* which supports the fornix, should now be examined. This is a portion of the pia mater, which penetrates into the ventricles through the fissure of Bichat, beneath the posterior border of the corpus callosum, as shown at p. 530. The shape of this vascular veil is like that of the fornix, and its borders are rolled up so as to form the red fringe called the '*choroid plexus.*' These plexuses consist almost entirely of the tortuous ramifications of minute arteries.[*] In front, they communicate with each other through the foramen of Monro; behind, they descend with the middle horns of the lateral ventricles, and become continuous with the pia mater at the base of the brain, between the middle lobe of the cerebrum and the crus cerebri. From the under surface of the velum, two small vascular processes are prolonged into the third ventricle forming the choroid plexuses of that cavity.

Vena Galeni. Along the centre of the veil run two large veins, called '*venæ Galeni,*' which return the blood from the ventricles into the straight sinus.

The velum interpositum, with the choroid plexus, must now be reflected to expose the following parts shown in diagram 129:—
1. A full view of the thalamus opticus. 2. Between the thalami optici is the '*third ventricle of the brain,*' a deep vertical fissure, situated in the middle line. 3. Behind the fissure is the '*pineal*

---

[*] In preparations where the choroid plexus is well injected, we see that they are covered with beautiful vascular villi. The villi themselves are covered with epithelium.

gland,' a vascular body, about the size of a pea. From the gland
may be traced forwards two slender white cords, called its ' peduncles '—one along the inner side of each optic thalamus. 4. Passing
transversely across are *three commissures* —anterior, middle, and
posterior, connecting the opposite sides of the brain. 5. Immediately behind the pineal gland are four elevations, two on each
side, called the '*corpora quadrigemina*,' or ' *nates* and *testes*.'
6. These bodies are connected to the cerebellum by two bands,
one on each side, termed the '*processus a cerebello ad testes*.'
7. Between these bands extends a thin layer of grey substance,
called the '*valve of Vieussens*,' beneath which lies the fourth
ventricle.

Thalamus opticus.

This is the oval elevation seen on the floor of the
lateral ventricle, immediately behind the corpus striatum and tænia semicircularis. Though white on the
surface, its interior consists of alternate layers of white and grey
matter, like the corpus striatum.* The under surface of the
thalamus rests upon its corresponding crus cerebri, and forms the
roof of the descending or middle horn of the lateral ventricle.
Beneath the posterior part of the thalamus are two small eminences, termed the '*corpus geniculatum internum, and externum*. These eminences are produced by small accumulations
of grey matter beneath the surface. A narrow band of white
matter connects the external one with the nates, and a similar
band connects the internal one with the testes.†

Third ventricle.

This is the narrow fissure which exists between the
optic thalami, and reaches down to the base of the
brain. Its roof is formed by the velum interpositum;
the floor, which increases in depth in front, by certain parts at the

* The elevation called the optic thalamus is occasioned by the interposition of a
quantity of grey matter among the fibres of the crus cerebri. Gall termed it the
inferior ganglion of the cerebrum, in opposition to the corpus striatum, which he
termed the superior ganglion (Anat. et Phys. du Système Nerv.: Paris, 1810). The
epithet 'optic' applied to the thalamus might lead us to suppose that it presides over
vision; but that it exercises very little influence over sight is rendered probable by
comparative anatomy, by experimental physiology, and by pathology.

† These bands are faintly marked in man, but more apparent in the lower animals.

base of the brain—namely, the locus perforatus posticus, corpora
mamuillaria, tuber cinereum, infundibulum, and lamina cinerea:
all of which are best seen in a vertical section, as shown p. 530.   In
front it is bounded by the anterior crura of the fornix, and the
anterior commissure; behind, it communicates with the fourth
ventricle through the 'iter a tertio ad quartum ventriculum;'
a long canal beneath the corpora quadrigemina.

Commissures.   By gently separating the optic thalami in a fresh
brain, you see that they are connected by a transverse
layer of grey matter about half an inch in breadth.   This is the
Middle.   middle commissure, sometimes called the soft, on
account of its delicate consistence: in most brains it is
generally torn before it can be examined.*   The optic thalami
Posterior.   are also connected by a round white cord, called the
posterior commissure.   It is situated immediately in
front of, and rather below the pineal gland.   The corpora striata
Anterior.   are connected by a round white cord, called the anterior
commissure: it lies immediately in front of the anterior
crura of the fornix.   This commissure may be traced extending
transversely through the corpus striatum of each side; then arching backwards, its fibres are lost near the surface of the middle
cerebral lobe.

The third ventricle communicates with the lateral ventricles
through the foramen of Monro, and with the fourth ventricle
through the Iter a tertio ad quartum ventriculum.

Pineal gland.   This very vascular heart-shaped body is situated
immediately in front of the corpora quadrigemina.   It
is wrapped up in the velum.   It has two white peduncles or crura,
which extend forwards, one on the inner side of each optic thalamus, and terminate by joining the crura of the fornix.   In its
interior is some gritty matter, consisting of phosphate of lime.

* The soft commissure does not appear to be a very essential constituent part of
the brain.   It is not found before the ninth month of fœtal life; and in some instances,
according to our observation, is never developed.   The brothers Wenzel state that it
is absent about once in seven subjects (De plenitiori Struct. Cerebri Hom. et Brut.
Tubingen, 1812).

Although the pineal gland is found in all mammalia, birds, and reptiles, in the same typical position, its functions are entirely unknown.

Fig. 129.

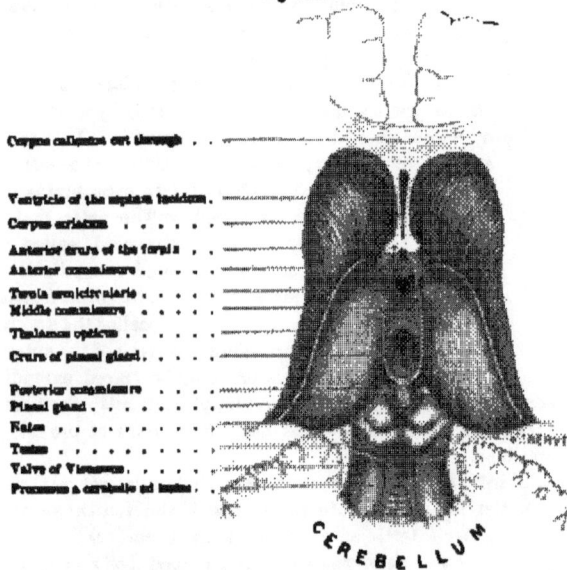

Corpus callosum cut through . .
Ventricle of the septum lucidum .
Corpus striatum . . . . . .
Anterior crura of the fornix . .
Anterior commissure . . . . .
Tænia semicircularis . . . . .
Middle commissure . . . . .
Thalamus opticus . . . . . .
Crura of pineal gland . . . . .
Posterior commissure . . . .
Pineal gland . . . .
Nates . . . .
Testes . . . .
Valve of Vieussens . . . . .
Processus a cerebello ad pontem .

CEREBELLUM

These are four eminences, situated, two on each side, behind the pineal gland. Though white on the surface, they contain grey matter in the interior: this grey matter is accumulated here for the purpose of giving origin to the optic nerve. A more appropriate term for them would be the 'optic lobes,' instead of 'nates and testes,' handed down from the old anatomists.[*]

Tubercula quadrigemina.

* Eminences homologous to the corpora quadrigemina are found in all vertebrate animals: they are the mesc-cephalic lobes; they invariably give origin to the optic

Processus a
cerebello
ad testes.
By gently drawing back the overlapping cerebellum, two broad white cords are seen, which pass backwards, diverging from each other, from the corpora quadrigemina to the cerebellum (fig. 129). These are the '*superior crura of the cerebellum.*' They connect the cerebrum and the cerebellum. The space between them is occupied by a thin layer of grey matter, which covers the fourth ventricle. This layer is called the '*valve of Vieussens.*' The fourth nerve arises from it by several filaments. Two white bands proceed on each side from the corpora quadrigemina to join the optic thalamus and the optic tract.

Iter a tertio
ad quartum
ventriculum,
or aquæduct
of Sylvius.
The third ventricle is connected with the fourth by means of a canal large enough to admit a probe, which runs backwards beneath the posterior commissure and the corpora quadrigemina (p. 530). This passage, together with the third and fourth ventricles, are persistent parts of the central canal which, in early fœtal life, extended down the middle of the spinal cord.

Fourth
ventricle.
This cavity is situated between the cerebellum and the posterior part of the medulla oblongata and pons Varolii. It is only a dilated portion of the primordial canal alluded to in the last paragraph. To obtain a perfect view of its boundaries, a vertical section should be made, as in diagram (p. 530). It appears triangular, and its boundaries are as follow:—The front or base is formed by the medulla oblongata and pons Varolii; the upper wall, by the valve of Vieussens and the aqueduct of Sylvius; the posterior wall, by the inferior vermiform process of the cerebellum; below, by the continuation of the arachnoid membrane on to the spinal cord; and, laterally, by the processus a cerebello ad testes, posterior pyramids, and restiform bodies. The pia mater is prolonged for a short distance into the lower part of the cavity, and forms the 'choroid plexus of the fourth ventricle.*

nerves, and their size bears a direct relation to the power of sight. They are relatively smaller in man than in any other animal. In birds there are only two eminences, and these are very large, especially in those far-seeing birds which fly high, as the eagle, falcon, vulture, &c., who require acute sight to discern their prey at a distance.

* Tiedemann proposes to call the fourth ventricle the first; because, in the fœtus, it

The anterior wall of the fourth ventricle is lozenge-shaped, and on it are the following objects, which should be separately examined (p. 519):—1. A median furrow, the remains of the primitive axis canal; running parallel to it on each side is a slight elevation, the *fasciculus teres*. 2. From the lower part of the furrow two white cords (the *restiform columns* or *inferior crura cerebelli*) pass off from the medulla oblongata, diverging like the branches of the letter V, and enter the lateral lobes of the cerebellum. The divergence of these cords with the median furrow was called by the old anatomists the '*calamus scriptorius*.' 3. The floor of the fourth ventricle is covered by grey matter, which is the grey substance of the medulla exposed by the divergence of its posterior or restiform columns: one mass, placed external to the fasciculus teres, has received the name of '*locus cœruleus*.' 4. On its anterior surface are seen a number of transverse white lines, emerging from the median groove, some of which form part of the origin of the auditory nerves.

Cerebellum. This portion of the brain is situated in the occipital fossa, beneath the posterior lobes of the cerebrum, from which it is separated by the tentorium. Its form is elliptical, with the broad diameter transverse. When the arachnoid membrane and the pia mater are removed, you observe that its surface is not arranged in convolutions like those of the cerebrum. It is laid out upon a plan adapted to produce a much greater superficial extent of grey matter. It consists of a multitude of thin plates, disposed in a series of concentric curves, with the concavity forwards. By a little careful dissection, it is easy to separate some of the plates from each other, and to see that the intervening fissures increase in depth from the centre towards the circumference of the cerebellum. The fissure at the circumference itself is the deepest of all, and nearly horizontal, so that it seems to divide the cerebellum into an upper and a lower segment.

is formed sooner than any of the others; because it exists in all vertebrated animals, whereas the lateral ventricles are absent in all osseous fishes; and because the ventricle of the septum lucidum is absent in all fishes, in reptiles, and in birds.

The upper surface of the cerebellum slopes on each
side, having a ridge along the middle line, called the
'*superior vermiform process*.' Comparative anatomy
proves that this is really the fundamental part of the cerebellum.
The sides, called the '*hemispheres*,' are merely offsets or wings,
superadded for special purposes, and increase in size as we ascend
in the vertebrate series, till in man they form by far the largest
part of the organ. They are separated posteriorly by a perpendicular fissure, which receives the '*falx cerebelli*.' On the upper
surface of the cerebellum are two lobes, which have received
names, i.e. the *quadrate* lobe, situated on its external and anterior
aspect, and the *posterior* lobe, placed along its posterior border.

Upper surface.

On the under surface of the cerebellum, its division
into two hemispheres is clearly perceptible. The deep
furrow between them is called '*the valley*.' The front
part of it is occupied by the medulla oblongata. To examine the
surface of the valley, the medulla must be raised, and the hemispheres separated from each other. Along the middle line of the
valley, is the '*inferior vermiform process*,' which is the under
surface of the fundamental part of the cerebellum. Traced forwards, this process terminates in the '*nodule*;' traced backwards,
it terminates in a small conical projection, called the '*pyramid*;'
between these, is a tongue-like body called the '*uvula*.'

Under surface.

Each hemisphere presents on its under surface certain secondary
lobes, to which fanciful names have been applied. That portion
which immediately overlays the side of the medulla oblongata is
called the 'tonsil' (*amygdala*): at the anterior part of each
hemisphere, near the middle line, is a little lobe called the '*floc-
culus*,' or pneumogastric lobe.

From either side of the uvula may be traced a thin valve-like
fold of white substance, which proceeds in a semicircular direction
to the flocculi. These folds form the *posterior medullary velum*.*
To see this satisfactorily, the tonsils should be carefully separated
from each other.

---

* These were first pointed out by Tarini, and are sometimes called the '*velum of
Tarini*' (Advers. Anat. prima: Paris, 1750).

In addition to the amygdala and flocculi already mentioned, other lobes have been described on the under surface of the cerebellum. Thus, there is the *digastric* lobe, situated external to the amygdala; and behind this are successively the slender and the inferior posterior lobes.

Appearance of the interior.

To examine the internal structure of the cerebellum, a longitudinal section should be made through the thickest part of one of the hemispheres. There is then seen in the centre a large nucleus of white matter, from which branches radiate into the grey substance in all directions. Each of these branches corresponds to one of the plates of the cerebellum, and from it other smaller branches proceed and again subdivide. This racemose appearance of the white matter in the substance of the grey has been likened to the branches of a tree deprived of its leaves, and is generally known as the '*arbor vitæ*;' it is a beautiful contrivance for bringing an extensive surface of the two kinds of nervous matter into connection with each other.

Corpus rhomboideum.

In the centre of the white nucleus of each hemisphere is an oval space, circumscribed by a zigzag line of grey matter. To this the name 'corpus dentatum or rhomboideum' has been given. It is displayed both by a vertical and by a horizontal section.

Peduncles of the cerebellum.

The cerebellum is connected with the cerebro-spinal axis by three *peduncles* or *crura*—superior, middle, and inferior. With the medulla oblongata it is connected by means of the restiform tracts—these are called the processus a cerebello ad medullam or its inferior crura; with the cerebrum, by means of the processus a cerebello ad testes—these are called its superior crura. The transverse fibres of the pons constitute the middle crura.

Function.

Respecting the function of the cerebellum, the arguments furnished by comparative anatomy render probable that it is a co-ordinator of muscular movements—e.g. in the action of walking, flying, swimming, &c.

DISSECTION OF THE SPINAL CORD.

To see the spinal cord covered by its membranes, the arches of the vertebræ must be removed by the saw. The first thing to be noticed is, that the cord does not occupy the whole area of the spinal canal. The dura mater does not adhere to the vertebræ, and does not form their internal periosteum, as in the skull. Between the bones and this membrane, a space intervenes, which is filled by a soft, reddish-looking fat, by watery cellular tissue, and by the ramifications of a plexus of veins.

The spine is remarkable for the number of large and tortuous veins which ramify about it, inside and outside the vertebral canal.* They are—1. The *dorsal veins*, which form a tortuous plexus outside the arches of the vertebræ. They send off branches, which pass through the ligamenta subflava, and end in the plexus inside the vertebral canal. 2. The *veins from the bodies of the vertebræ* emerge from their posterior surface, and empty themselves into, 3, the *anterior longitudinal spinal veins*: these, two in number, extend all down the spinal canal, behind the bodies of the vertebræ. 4. The *posterior longitudinal spinal veins*, like the anterior, run along the whole length of the spinal canal. They are situated inside the vertebral arches, and communicate with the anterior longitudinal veins by cross branches at frequent intervals. 5. The proper *veins of the spinal cord*, which lie within the dura mater. This complicated system of spinal veins discharges itself through the intervertebral foramina, in the several regions of the spine, as follow:—in the cervical, into the vertebral veins ; in the dorsal, into the intercostal veins; in the lumbar, into the lumbar veins. None are provided with valves, hence they are liable to become congested in diseases of the spine.

(margin note: Spinal system of veins.*)*

* An accurate description and representation of these veins has been given by Breschet, Essai sur les Veines du Rachis, 4to.; Traité Anatomique sur le Système Vineux, fol. avec planches.

Peculiari-
ties of the
membranes
of the cord. The membranes of the spinal cord, though continuous with those of the brain, differ from them in certain respects, and require separate notice.

Dura mater. The 'dura mater' of the cord is a tough fibrous membrane like that of the brain, but does not adhere to the bones, because such adhesion would impede the free movement of the vertebræ upon each other. It is attached above to the margin of the foramen magnum, and may be traced downwards as a canal as far as the first bone of the sacrum, from which it is prolonged as a cord to the coccyx, where it becomes continuous with the periosteum. It forms a complete canal, which loosely surrounds the spinal cord, and sends off prolongations over each of the spinal nerves. These prolongations accompany the nerves only as far as the intervertebral foramina, and are then blended with the periosteum.

Cut through the nerves which proceed from the spinal cord on each side, and remove the cord with the dura mater entire. Then slit up the dura mater along the middle line, to examine the arachnoid membrane.

Arachnoid
membrane. The 'arachnoid membrane' of the cord is a continuation from that of the brain, and, like it, consists of a *visceral* layer which surrounds the cord, and of a *parietal*, which lines the inner surface of the dura mater. The visceral layer is not in immediate contact with the pia mater underneath, but is separated from it by a transparent watery fluid contained in the meshes of the subarachnoid tissue (p. 548). This cerebrospinal fluid cannot be demonstrated unless the cord be

Cerebro-spi-
nal fluid. examined very soon after death, and before the removal of the brain.* The nerves proceeding from the cord

* The existence and situation of the cerebro-spinal fluid were first discovered by Haller (Element. Phys. vol. iv. p. 87), and subsequently more minutely investigated by Magendie (Récherches Phys. et Cliniques sur le Liquide Cephalo-rachidien, in 4to. avec atlas: Paris, 1842). This physiologist has shown that if, during life, the arches of the vertebræ are removed in a horse, dog, or other animal, and the dura mater of the cord punctured, there issue jets of a fluid which had previously made the sheath tense. The fluid communicates, through the fourth ventricle, with that in the general ventricular cavity. The collective amount of the fluid varies from 1 to 2 oz. or more.

N N

are loosely surrounded by a sheath of the arachnoid; but this only accompanies them as far as the dura mater, and is then reflected upon that membrane.

Pia mater. The pia mater of the cord is the protecting membrane which immediately invests it. It is quite different from that of the brain, since it does not form a bed in which the arteries break up, but serves rather to support and strengthen the cord: consequently it is much less vascular, more *fibrous* in its structure, and more adherent to the substance of the cord. The fibres of which it is composed are rendered very evident by immersion for a time in water. It sends down thin folds into the anterior and posterior fissures of the cord, and is prolonged upon the spinal nerves, and forms their investing membrane, or 'neurilemma.'

From the upper part of the second lumbar vertebra, the pia mater is continued down as a slender filament, called the '*filum terminale*,' which runs in the middle of the bundle of nerves into which the spinal cord breaks up. It is prolonged to the sacrum, where it becomes continuous with the dura mater of the cord. In its upper part may be traced some nerve matter, continued from the spinal cord, and a small artery and vein.

Ligamentum denticulatum. The pia mater sends off from each side of the cord, along its whole length, a fibrous band, '*ligamentum denticulatum*,' which gives off a series of processes to steady and support the cord. They are triangular, their bases being attached to the cord, and their points to the inside of the dura mater (fig. 130). There are from eighteen to twenty-two of them on each side, and they lie between the anterior and posterior

It can be made to flow from the brain into the cord, or *vice versâ*. This is proved by experiments on animals, and by that pathological condition of the spine in children termed 'spina bifida.' In the latter instance, coughing and crying make the tumour swell; showing that fluid is forced into it from the ventricles. Again, if pressure be made on the tumour with one hand, and the fontanelles of the child examined with the other, in proportion as the spinal swelling decreases so is the brain felt to swell up, accompanied by symptoms resulting from pressure on the nervous axis generally. See also some remarks by Dr. Barrows, On Diseases of the Cerebral Circulation, p. 50, 1846.

roots of the spinal nerves. The first process passes between the vertebral artery and the hypoglossal nerve; the last one is found at the termination of the cord.

Spinal cord.   The spinal cord is that part of the cerebro-spinal axis contained in the vertebral canal. It is the continuation of the medulla oblongata, and extends from the foramen magnum down to the upper border of the second lumbar vertebra, where it terminates in a pointed manner, after having given off the great bundle of nerves Cauda equina. termed 'cauda equina,' for the supply of the lower limbs.[*]

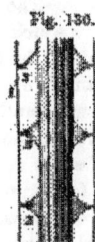

Fig. 130.

DIAGRAM OF THE LIGAMENTUM DENTICULATUM.

1. Dura mater.
2, 2, 2. Ligamentum denticulatum.

The length of the cord is about seventeen or eighteen inches, and its general form is cylindrical, slightly flattened in front and behind. It is not of uniform dimensions throughout. It presents a slight enlargement in the lower part of the cervical region; another in the lower part of the dorsal, where the great nerves of the upper and lower limbs are given off. The upper or cervical enlargement reaches from the third cervical to the first dorsal vertebra; the lower or lumbar is situated opposite to the last dorsal vertebra.

Fissures.   The cord is divided into two symmetrical halves by a fissure in front and behind (fig. 131). The *anterior fissure* is the most distinct, and penetrates about one-third of the substance of the cord; it contains a fold of pia mater full of blood vessels for the supply of the interior. At the bottom of this fissure

---

[*] Although the nerve substance of the cord itself terminates at the second lumbar vertebra, yet the pia mater is continued as a slender filament, called '*filum terminale*,' down to the base of the coccyx. The explanation of this is, that, at an early period of fœtal life, the length of the cord corresponds with that of the vertebral canal; but after the third month, the lumbar and sacral vertebræ grow away, so to speak, from the cord, in accordance with the more active development of the lower limbs. See Tiedemann, Anatomie und Bildungsgeschichte des Gehirns im Fœtus des Menschen, &c.; Nüremberg, 1816.

is a transverse layer of white substance, named the *anterior commissure*, connecting the two anterior halves of the cord. The *posterior fissure* is so much less apparent than the anterior, that some anatomists altogether deny its existence; but it can be demonstrated by careful preparation, and, indeed, penetrates to a greater depth than the anterior, so that it reaches down to the grey matter in the centre of the cord.

Besides the anterior and posterior fissures, along each half of the cord are two superficial grooves, from which the anterior and posterior roots of the spinal nerves respectively emerge. These are the *anterior* and *posterior lateral grooves*. The posterior

Fig. 131.

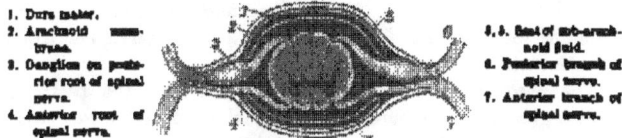

1. Dura mater.
2. Arachnoid membrane.
3. Ganglion on posterior root of spinal nerve.
4. Anterior root of spinal nerve.

5, 5. Sac of sub-arachnoid fluid.
6. Posterior branch of spinal nerve.
7. Anterior branch of spinal nerve.

DIAGRAM OF A TRANSVERSE SECTION THROUGH THE SPINAL CORD AND ITS MEMBRANES.

leads down to the posterior horn of the grey matter in the interior of the cord; the anterior is less distinct, and does not reach down to the anterior horn of grey matter. By these lateral grooves each half of the cord is divided into three longitudinal columns—an *anterior*, a *posterior*, and a *lateral*. The anterior are motor columns, the posterior sensitive, the lateral probably contain both motor and sensitive filaments.

Columns.

A transverse section through the cord (fig. 131) shows that, externally, it is composed of white nerve substance, and that its interior contains grey matter, arranged in the form of two crescents placed one in each half of it, and connected across the centre by a portion called the '*grey commissure*.'*

Interior.

* The grey matter in the interior of the cord of man and animals presents somewhat different appearances in its different parts. These have been accurately de-

The posterior horns of the crescents are long and narrow, and extend to the posterior lateral fissure, where they are connected with the posterior roots of the spinal nerves. The anterior horns are short and thick, and come forwards towards the line of attachment of the anterior roots of the nerves, but do not reach the surface.

SPINAL NERVES.

Thirty-one pair of nerves arise from the spinal cord —namely, 8 in the cervical region, 12 in the dorsal, 5 in the lumbar, 5 in the sacral, and 1 in the coccygeal. Each nerve comes off by two distinct series of roots—one from the front, the other from the back of the cord. Sir Charles Bell first noticed the fact that the anterior roots consist exclusively of motor filaments, the posterior exclusively of sensitive. All converge and unite in the corresponding intervertebral foramen to form a single nerve, composed of both motor and sensitve filaments.

Two roots, sensitive and motor.

The *posterior* or sensitive roots proceed from the posterior lateral groove of the cord, and are thicker and more numerous than the anterior.* Previous to their union with the anterior roots, they are collected together and pass through a ganglion. This ganglion is of an oval form, and lies in the intervertebral foramen, where the roots of the nerves pass through the dura mater.†

The *anterior* root arises from the groove between the anterior and lateral columns of the cord, and passes in front of the

scribed and figured by Rolando, Richerche Anatomiche sulla Struttura del Midollo Spinale, con Figure, art. tratto dal Dizionario Periodico di Medicina, Turino, 1824, 8vo. p. 55.

* The researches of Blandin, Anat. descript. t. ii., p. 548, 1838, have led him to establish the following relation between the respectivo size of the anterior and posterior roots of the nerves in the several regions of the spine:—

The posterior roots are to the anterior in the cervical region   :: 2 : 1
     „   „   „   dorsal   „   :: 1 : 1
     „   „   „   lumbar and sacral :: 1½ : 1

This relation quite accords with the greater delicacy of the sense of touch in the upper extremity.

† The ganglia of the two last sacral nerves lie within the dura mater.

ganglion on the posterior root, which it joins in the intervertebral foramen.

The compound nerve formed by the junction of the two roots divides, outside the Intervertebral foramen, into an anterior and a posterior branch. See diagram, p. 548.

Variation in length of the roots.
The direction and length of the roots of the nerves vary in the different regions of the spine, because the respective parts of the cord from which they arise are not opposite the foramina through which the nerves leave the spinal canal. In the upper part of the cervical region, the origins of the nerves and their point of exit are nearly on the same level: therefore the roots proceed transversely, and are very short. But as we descend from the neck, the obliquity and length of the roots gradually increase, so that the roots of the lower dorsal nerves are at least two vertebræ higher than the foramina through which they emerge. Again, since the cord itself terminates at the second lumbar vertebra, the lumbar and sacral nerves must of necessity pass down from it almost perpendicularly through the lower part of the spinal canal. To this bundle of nerves the old anatomists have given the name of 'cauda equina,' from its resemblance to a horse's tail.

Cauda equina.

In brief, then, it appears that the spinal cord consists of two precisely symmetrical halves, separated in front and behind by a deep median fissure; that the two halves are connected at the bottom of the anterior fissure by an anterior or white commissure —at the bottom of the posterior fissure by the posterior or grey commissure; that each half of the cord is divided into three tracts or columns of longitudinal nerve fibres— an anterior, a posterior, and a lateral—the boundaries between them being the respective lines of origin of the roots of the spinal nerves; that the interior of the cord contains grey matter disposed in the form of two crescents placed with their convexities towards each other, and connected by a transverse bar of grey matter, which is the posterior commissure.

Blood vessels of the cord.
The cord is supplied with blood by—1, the *anterior spinal* artery, which commences at the medulla ob-

longata by a branch from the vertebral of each side, and then runs down the cord, receiving, through the intervertebral foramina, numerous branches in its course from the vertebral, ascending cervical, intercostal, and lumbar arteries; 2, the *posterior spinal* arteries, which proceed also from the vertebral, intercostal, and lumbar arteries, and ramify very irregularly on the back of the cord.

On the posterior part of the bodies of the vertebræ, the spinal arteries of opposite sides communicate by numerous transverse branches along the entire length of the spine, thus resembling the arrangement of its venous plexuses.

Functions of the columns of the cord. The *anterior* columns consist exclusively of motor fibres which originate from the grey matter of the brain or that of the spinal cord, and carry the commands of the will and the power of reflex movement to the muscles.

The *posterior* columns consist exclusively of sensitive fibres, which carry sensations, not, as was formerly believed, direct to the brain, but to the grey matter of the cord, through which *alone*, according to the recent experiments of Brown Séquard,* they are transmitted to the brain. The same experimentalist has also proved another unexpected fact—that sensations do not run up on the same side, but on the opposite. They cross in the cord; for instance, if the posterior column on the *right* side were injured, the *left* leg and not the right would be deprived of sensation.

In the interior of the grey matter of the upper part of the spinal cord may be seen a *central canal*, the remains of the primordial canal of fœtal life, which extends through the whole length of the cord.

Minute structure of the medulla oblongata and pons Varolii. These are among the most complicate parts of the central nervous system. They contain white and grey matter,† intermixed. The white matter consists in part of a continuation of the longi-

* See an able article on Brown Séquard's experiments in the British and Foreign Medico-Chirurgical Review by Mr. Thomas Smith.

† The grey matter in the medulla oblongata is collected in three situations—1. In the olives; 2. In the restiform tracts; 3. On the floor of the fourth ventricle.

tudinal fibres of the cord, in part of a new system of horizontal
fibres. We will endeavour to trace the longitudinal fibres first;
then the horizontal.

Anterior columns of the cord. The anterior columns (8), (fig. 132), having reached
the lower part of the medulla oblongata, are not con-
tinued straight up through it, but diverge from each
other, so as to allow a part of the lateral columns (9) to come

Fig. 132.

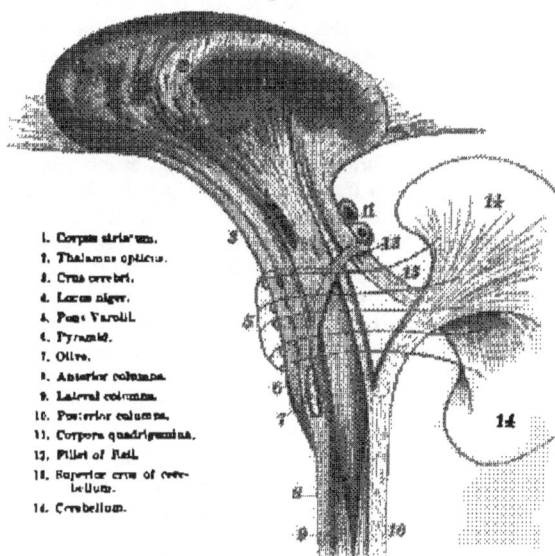

1. Corpus striatum.
2. Thalamus opticus.
3. Crus cerebri.
4. Locus niger.
5. Pons Varolii.
6. Pyramid.
7. Olive.
8. Anterior columns.
9. Lateral columns.
10. Posterior columns.
11. Corpora quadrigemina.
12. Fillet of Reil.
13. Superior crus of cere-
    bellum.
14. Cerebellum.

DIAGRAM OF THE COURSE OF THE FIBRES OF THE CORD.

forward, and after decussation to form the pyramids (6). In their
further progress the fibres of the anterior columns are disposed of
thus: a small number of them run up and contribute to form the
outer portion of their own pyramid; all the rest, after embracing
the olive, pass up through the deep strata of the pons, and then

divide into two bundles: one of these, called the fillet of Reil (12), mounts over the superior crus of the cerebellum to the corpora quadrigemina, beneath which it meets with the corresponding fillet of the opposite side; the other proceeds with the crus cerebri to the cerebrum.

Lateral columns of the cord. The lateral columns (9), on reaching the medulla oblongata, are disposed of in three ways, as follows —Some of its fibres come forward between the diverging anterior columns, decussate in the middle line, and contribute to form the pyramid of the opposite side; others ascend with the restiform tract into the cerebellum; a third set ascend along the floor of the fourth ventricle* (concealed by its superficial grey matter), and then along the upper part of the crus cerebri into the cerebrum.

Posterior columns of the spinal cord. The posterior columns (10) ascend under the name of the restiform tracts at the back of the medulla oblongata, diverge from each other, and are, for the most part, continued into the cerebellum, forming its inferior crura; but some of their fibres run on along the floor of the fourth ventricle (external to the fibres from the lateral columns), then along the upper part of the crura cerebri into the cerebrum.

Horizontal fibres. The horizontal fibres in the medulla oblongata and the pons were first accurately described and delineated by Stilling.† Some of them form a raphé, and divide the medulla oblongata and pons into symmetrical halves; others, arising apparently from the raphé, pass outwards in an arched manner through the lateral halves of the medulla; so that, when seen in a transverse section by transmitted light, they describe a series of curves, with the convexity forwards, throughout the entire thickness of the medulla. Some of these transverse fibres appear on the surface over the pyramid and the olive; these have received the name of 'arciform fibres' (p. 517). It is difficult to determine the object of this system of transverse fibres, or what parts

---

* These fibres constitute what are sometimes called the 'round cords' of the fourth ventricle.

† Ueber die Medulla Oblongata. Erlangen, 1843.

they connect. Stilling and Kölliker,[*] who have deeply studied the
subject, are both of opinion that they originate in the restiform
tracts, and thence arch forwards—some on the surface, others
through the substance of the medulla, and that they eventually
join the fibres of the raphé.

Internal struc-
ture of pons
Varolii.   The pons consists of transverse and longitudinal
white fibres, with a considerable quantity of grey
matter in its interior. The superficial layer of
fibres is obviously transverse, and connects the two wings of the
cerebellum. After removing this first layer, we come upon the
longitudinal fibres of the pyramids in their course to the crura
cerebri (p. 552): these longitudinal fibres, however, are intersected by the deep transverse fibres of the pons, which, like the
superficial, are continued into the cerebellum. The third and
deepest layer of the pons consists entirely of longitudinal fibres,
derived partly from the lateral, partly from the restiform tracts
of the medulla.

Crura cerebri.   These are composed of longitudinal fibres, derived
from the pyramids, from part of the lateral and restiform columns of the cord, and from the grey matter in the pons
Varolii. If one of the crura he divided longitudinally, we find in
the middle of it a layer of dark-coloured nervous matter, called
'locus niger;' it separates the crus into an upper and a lower
stratum of fibres. The lower stratum is tough and coarse, and
consists of the continuation of the fibres proceeding from the
pyramid and the pons. The upper stratum is much softer and
finer in texture, and has received the name of the 'tegmentum:'
it is composed of the fibres proceeding from the lateral and the
restiform columns; also from the superior commissure or crus of
the cerebellum.

Tracing the fibres of the crus cerebri into the cerebral hemisphere, we find that they diverge from each other, that its lower
fibres ascend chiefly through the corpora striata, its upper fibres
through the thalami optici. In passing through these great

<hr/>

[*] Mikroskopische Anatomie, p. 451.

ganglia, the crus receives a very large addition to its fibres: these then branch out widely towards all parts of the hemisphere, in order to reach the cortical substance on the surface.

From what has been said, it appears that the crura or roots of the cerebellum and the cerebrum contain part of the motor and part of the sensitive tracts of the spinal cord.

DISSECTION OF THE EYE.

Since the human eye cannot be obtained sufficiently fresh for anatomical purposes, the student should examine the eyes of animals, of the sheep or pig. The first thing to be done is to remove the conjunctival coat, and the loose connective tissue which unites it to the sclerotica.

The *conjunctiva* is the mucous membrane which lines
the ocular surface of the eyelids and the front part of

Membrana
conjunctiva.

the eyeball. It is attached by loose folds to the sclerotic coat, so as not to impede the motions of the globe. The *palpebral* portion of it is very vascular, and provided with fine papillæ which are abundantly supplied with nerves.* It is continued into the Meibomian glands, the puncta lachrymalia, and the ducts of the lachrymal gland. The *ocular* portion is thinner and has no papillæ. It is nearly colourless, except when inflamed; it then becomes intensely vascular and of a bright scarlet colour. An abundant supply of nerves has been bestowed upon the membrane for the purpose of giving it that degree of sensibility necessary to guard the eye.

The *corneal* portion is composed chiefly of epithelial cells, arranged in layers. This portion of the conjunctiva cannot be separated by dissection in recent eyes, but it possesses the same acute sensibility as the rest of the conjunctiva. Changes produced by inflammation of the conjunctiva are often continued over the cornea,

* These papillæ were first pointed out by Ehle, Ueber den Bau und die Krankheiten der Bindehaut des Auges.

and cause the blood vessels on its surface to become injected, and its texture thickened and opaque.* Blood vessels ramify round the margin of the cornea, forming a network arranged in loops.

The human eye is very nearly spherical, and would be quite so, but that the transparent part in front—the cornea—forms a segment of a smaller sphere than the rest. Consequently, the antero-posterior diameter of the ball—about one inch—exceeds the transverse by about one line. The convexity of the cornea, however, varies in different persons, and at different periods of life; this is one cause of the several degrees of near-sight and far-sight.

Coats and humours of the eye.   The globe is composed of three coats arranged one within the other. The external coat, consisting of the 'sclerotic and cornea,' is fibrous, thick, and strong. The second coat, consisting of the 'choroid, the iris, and ciliary processes,' is composed of blood vessels, muscular tissue, and pigment cells, and is very dark in colour. The third coat, called the 'retina,' consists of the expansion of the optic nerve for the reception of the impression of light. The bulk of the interior is filled with a transparent humour called the 'vitreous.' Imbedded in the front of this, and just behind the pupil, is the crystalline lens for the purpose of concentrating the rays of light. In front of the lens is placed a movable curtain, called the 'iris,' in order to regulate the quantity of light which shall be admitted through the pupil. The space in which the iris is suspended is filled with a fluid termed the 'aqueous' humour.

Sclerotic coat.   The sclerotic is the tough protecting coat of the eye, and consists of white glistening fibres interlacing in all directions.† It covers about ⅘ths of the globe, the re-

---

* The facts of comparative anatomy confirm this view. In the serpent tribe, which annually shed their skin, the front of the cornea comes off with the rest of the external surface of the body. In the eel the surface of the cornea is often drawn off in the process of skinning. In some species of rodents which burrow under the ground like the mole, the eye is covered with hair like other parts.

† The sclerotic coat of the eye in fishes is of extraordinary thickness and density, for obvious reasons; and in birds this coat is further strengthened by a circle of bony plates, fourteen or fifteen in number, arranged in a series round the margin of the cornea. Similar plates are found in some of the reptiles, and particularly in the fossil icthyosauri and plesiosauri.

maining ⅔th being completed by the cornea.   The thickest part of
the sclerotic coat is at the back of the globe (fig. 134), and thinnest
a short distance behind the cornea.
The back of the sclerotic is perforated by the optic nerve, which enters it a little on the nasal side of
the axis of vision. The optic nerve
at its entrance into the sclerotic is
very much constricted, and instead
of passing through a single large
aperture in this coat, enters it
through a porous network of fibrous
tissue called the *lamina cribrosa*.*
Around the optic nerve the sclerotic
is perforated by the ciliary arteries,
veins, and nerves, for the supply of
the choroid coat and the iris. Towards the front, the sclerotic
becomes much thinner, and about a quarter of an inch from the
cornea it receives the insertion of the recti muscles; here also
it is perforated by the anterior ciliary arteries, which come forward along the tendons of these muscles, and form a vascular ring
round the margin of the cornea.

The sclerotic is composed of fibro-cellular tissue arranged in
bundles which run, some longitudinally and some transversely.
The longitudinal fibres are the most external and abundant.
Under the microscope fusiform and stellate cells can be seen interspersed among the fibres, between which fine elastic fibres may
also be demonstrated. The inner surface of the sclerotic is coated
by a thin layer of areolar tissue impregnated with dark pigment
cells. It is called '*lamina fusca*.' At present it is believed that
no nerves exist in the sclerotic.

To examine the cornea, it should be removed with the sclerotic
coat. This should be done under water, by making a circular cut

Fig. 133.

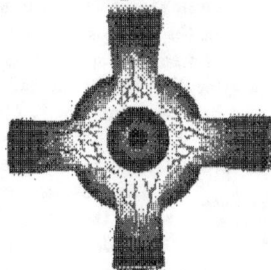

INSERTION OF THE RECTI MUSCLES WITH
ANTERIOR CILIARY ARTERIES.

---

* In the centre of the lamina cribrosa is an opening larger than the rest, which
serves for the transmission of the arteria centralis retinæ. It is sometimes called the
porus opticus.

with scissors about a quarter of an inch from the margin of the
cornea. With a little care, it is easy to remove the outer coat of
the eye without injuring the dark choroid coat, the ciliary ligament, or the iris. In the loose dark-brown cellular tissue between
the sclerotic and the choroid are seen the ciliary nerves passing

Fig. 131.

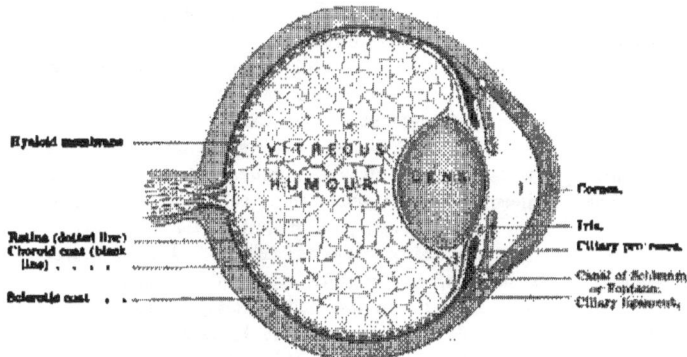

Hyaloid membrane

VITREOUS HUMOUR

LENS

Cornea.

Iris.

Retina (dotted line)
Choroid coat (black
line) . . . .

Ciliary processes.

Canal of Schlemm,
or Fontana.

Sclerotic coat . .

Ciliary ligament,

DIAGRAM OF A VERTICAL SECTION OF THE EYE.

1. Anterior chamber filled with aqueous humour.
2. Posterior chamber.   3. Canal of Petit.

forwards towards the iris; their white colour makes them very
conspicuous on the dark ground.

Cornea.   The cornea is the brilliant and transparent coat
which occupies about the anterior fifth of the globe.
Although apparently delicate, yet it is quite as tough and thick as
any part of the sclerotica. It is nearly circular in diameter and
is about the $\frac{1}{24}$th of an inch in thickness. It is firmly connected
at its margin to the sclerotic, with the fibres of which it is continuous. The margin of the sclerotic is beveled on the inside;
that of the cornea on the outside; so that the former overlaps the
latter (fig. 134).

Structure.   The cornea consists of five layers, which are not all composed of the same kind of tissue. The first layer is the conjunctival. This consists of several strata of epithelial cells, the superficial ones being flattened; the deeper ones, the more numerous, being placed vertically. The second layer is about the $\frac{1}{1700}$th of an inch thick, and consists of an extremely elastic tissue. It is perfectly structureless, and, when peeled off, has a remarkable tendency to curl up. Boiling, or the action of acids, does not render it opaque like they do the other layers of the cornea.[*] Very delicate fibres pass obliquely inwards from it, and serve to connect it to the next layer. The third layer (*cornea proper*) consists of transparent fibrous tissue, upon which the thickness and strength of the cornea mainly depend. The fibres are arranged in layers about sixty in number, between which are branched fusiform cells, communicating freely with each other. The fourth layer is again elastic, and resembles the second layer in structure, except in being somewhat thinner. The fifth layer consists of a layer of epithelial cells, resembling those which line serous membranes.[†] In its healthy state, the cornea contains no blood vessels; they run back in loops as soon as they reach its circumference. Its nerves, which are numerous, are derived from the ciliary nerves, and ramify in the transparent fibrous tissue.

Choroid coat.   After the removal of the sclerotic and cornea, we expose the *choroid coat*[‡]—a white ring, consisting of the *ciliary ligament* and *ciliary muscle*, which bounds its anterior parts; also the *iris* and *ciliary processes*, of which the outer circumference is attached to this ring (fig. 134).

The choroid is the soft and flocculent tunic of the eye, recog-

---

[*] Dr. Jacob calls it 'the elastic cornea.'—Med. Chir. Trans., vol. xii. p. 503. Its use, according to Dr. Jacob, is probably to preserve the correct curve of the cornea proper.

[†] For a detailed investigation of the structure of the cornea, see Todd and Bowman, Physiological Anatomy.

[‡] So called, because its outer flocculent surface somewhat resembles the chorion, or external investment of the ovum.

nised by its dark-brown colour and great vascularity. Posteriorly
there is a circular aperture in it for the passage of the optic nerve.
In front, the choroid is attached to the ciliary ligament, under
which it extends forwards, round the circumference of the crystalline lens, in a series of plaited folds, called the *ciliary processes.* It is connected to the sclerotic by fine cellular tissue—
the lamina fusca—through which the ciliary vessels and nerves
pass forwards.

Under the microscope the choroid is found to consist of three
layers—an external, composed of arterial and venous ramifications; a middle, composed of capillaries, and an internal, composed of pigment cells. The outer layer consists of the branches
of the blood vessels, the arteries being chiefly arranged on its
inner, the veins on its outer surface. The veins are arranged
with great regularity in drooping branches (*vasa vorticosa*), like
a weeping willow (fig. 135), and converge to four nearly equidistant trunks, which, after running backwards for a short distance, perforate the sclerotica not far from the entrance of the
optic nerve, and empty themselves into the ophthalmic vein.

The arteries which ramify on the inner side of the veins perforate the sclerotica near the optic nerve, and then divide and
subdivide into a very minute network. Between the vessels are
found a number of stellate pigment cells, which communicate
with each other. This middle layer, formed by the minute
subdivisions of the ciliary arteries, is termed, after the Dutch
anatomist Ruysch, '*tunica Ruyschiana.*' It consists of a very
delicate capillary network, which extends forwards to the ciliary
processes.

The inner layer is the pigment-matter of the choroid. It is
merely adventitious, for, if the choroid be washed in water or spirit,
the colour is entirely removed, leaving the membrane of a greyish
tint. In man this pigment is dark brown, but in most animals it
is jet black. Under the microscope, it is found to consist of
minute hexagonal nucleated cells, filled with pigment granules,
which are most numerous towards the margins of the cells. On
the choroid it exists only as a single layer, but on the iris and

ciliary processes several layers may be demonstrated.* The use of the pigment is to absorb the rays of light which pass through the retina, and prevent their being reflected. It serves the same purpose as the black paint with which the inside of optical instruments is darkened. Albinos, in whom the choroid has little or no pigment, are, consequently, dazzled by daylight, and see better in the dusk.†

Ciliary body and processes.

These structures are best seen when the globe has been divided by a vertical section into an anterior and a posterior half, the vitreous humour being left undisturbed. They should be regarded as a continuation of the choroid, and are arranged as a black circle, about three lines broad, surrounding the lens. The posterior boundary of this ring is smooth and flat, and defined by a dentated line. The anterior part presents a number of longitudinal plaits or folds, from sixty to seventy in number, alternately long and short, and arranged in a radiated manner round the circumference of the lens. One of these is seen in the diagram, p. 558. The entire ring is called the ciliary body; and the folds of it in front, the ciliary processes. The processes are kept in place by being attached to the ciliary ligament: they fit into corresponding depressions in the vitreous humour, and their free ends project for a short distance into the posterior chamber. They consist of convolutions of minute arteries, and their dark colour arises from the pigment on their surface. Their use is unknown.

Ciliary ligament.

The ciliary ligament (fig. 135) is a whitish grey ring, about the ⅛th of an inch broad, situated just beneath

* Dalrymple speaks of a very delicate membrane (membrane of Bruch) as lining the inner surface of the choroid, for the purpose of keeping the dark pigment in its place. A similar membrane may be detected on the posterior surface of the iris; otherwise the pigment there would be apt to be washed away by the aqueous humour.

† In many of the nocturnal carnivorous quadrupeds, the inner surface of the choroid at the bottom of the eye presents a brilliant colour and metallic lustre. It is called the tapetum. By reflecting the rays of light a second time through the retina, it probably causes the animal to see better in the dusk. It is the cause of the well-known glare of the eyes of cats and other animals; and the great breadth of the luminous appearance arises from the dilatation of the pupil.

the union of the sclerotica and the cornea. It serves as the connecting medium between several structures—namely, the choroid,
the iris, the ciliary processes, and the sclerotica.

Between the sclerotic, the cornea, and the ciliary ligament, is
placed a minute circular canal, termed the *sinus circularis iridis*
or *canal of Schlemm* (fig. 134). It is probably a venous sinus, for
it can always be injected from the arteries.

Fig. 135.

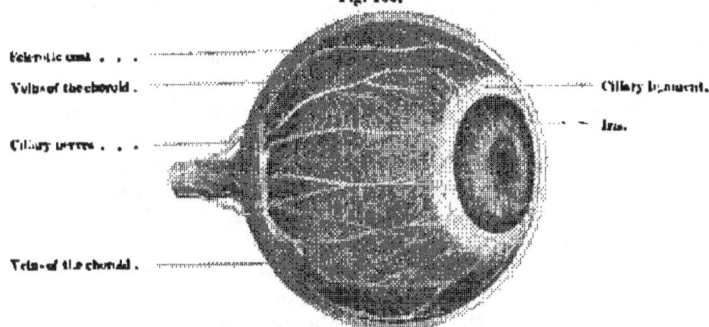

SCLEROTIC COAT REMOVED TO SHOW THE CHOROID, CILIARY LIGAMENT, AND NERVES.

Ciliary muscle.
 This muscle consists of unstriped fibres, and is
attached to the line of junction of the sclerotic and
cornea; thence its fibres radiate backwards over the
ciliary ligament, and are lost in the choroid behind the ciliary
processes.[*] Its action is probably to accommodate the eye to objects at various distances, by rendering the lens more or less
convex.

Iris.
 The iris is a movable curtain suspended in the clear
fluid, which occupies the space between the cornea and
crystalline lens. The iris divides this space into two unequal
parts, called the *anterior* and *posterior chambers* (fig. 134); these

---

[*] Sir Philip Crampton has noticed that this muscle is well developed in birds. In
them its fibres are of the striped kind, just as the circular fibres of the iris are.

communicate with each other through a circular aperture in the centre, called the *pupil*.* Its use is to regulate the amount of light which shall be admitted into the eye: for this purpose its inner circumference is capable of dilating and contracting according to circumstances, while its outer circumference is immovably connected to the ciliary ligament, the choroid, and the cornea.

The colour of the iris varies in different individuals, and gives the peculiar tint and brilliancy to the eye. The colouring matter or pigment is contained in minute cells (*pigment cells*) lining the anterior and posterior surfaces of the iris. The posterior surface of the iris, called the *uvea*,† is covered by a thick layer of black pigment.

When the iris is laid under water, and viewed with a low magnifying power, a number of fine fibres are seen converging from all sides towards the pupil; many of them unite and form arches. When the pupil is contracted, these fibres are stretched, and *vice versâ*. Whether they co-operate in producing the dilatation of the pupil is uncertain.

The contractile power of the iris depends upon muscular fibres of the non-striped kind, arranged some in a radiating, others in a circular manner. The radiating (*dilatator*) converge towards the pupil, where they blend with the circular fibres; the circular (*sphincter*) are aggregated on the posterior aspect of the pupillary margin, where they form a ring about $\frac{1}{40}$th of an inch in width.‡

A considerable amount of *fibrous tissue* is present in the iris, and consists of circular and radiating fibres; the circular are found at the circumference of the iris, the radiating converge towards the pupil.

When minutely injected, the iris appears to be composed almost

---

* The size and shape of the pupil vary in different animals. In the bullock, sheep, horse, &c., it is oblong; in carnivorous quadrupeds it is often a mere vertical slit during the day, but dilates into a large circle at night.

† Strictly speaking, the term uvea was applied by the old anatomists to the choroid and iris collectively, which they very properly considered as one coat, and called the 'χιτὼν ῥαγοειδὴς,' because its dark colour made it like the berry of the grape.

‡ The circular fibres of the iris in the bird are of the striped variety, and discernible without difficulty.

entirely of blood vessels; * so much so that some anatomists consider it to be a kind of erectile tissue, and that its power of con
tracting and expanding depends upon this property alone. Its blood

Its blood vessels.   vessels are derived from two sources—the posterior
or long, and the anterior or short ciliary arteries. The
posterior, 15 to 20 in number, perforate the sclerotica
round the optic nerve, and then run on upon the choroid to the
iris; the *anterior* proceed from the tendons of the recti (p. 182),
and perforate the sclerotica round the margin of the cornea. It
is from the enlargement of these latter vessels that the red zone
round the cornea is produced in inflammation of the iris.

Its nerves.   The nerves of the iris, twelve or more in number, proceed from the lenticular ganglion, and from
the nasal branch of the ophthalmic division of the fifth pair
(p. 178). They perforate the back of the sclerotica like the arteries, and run along the choroid to the iris.

Membrana papillaris.   Until the seventh or eighth month of fœtal life, the
pupil is closed by a delicate membrane, termed ' *mem-
brana pupillaris.*' Its vessels are arranged in loops,
which converge towards the centre of the pupil. It has been lately
discovered that this membrane, which has always been regarded
as a distinct structure, is identical with the anterior layer of the
capsule of the crystalline lens.†

Retina.   To obtain a view of the retina, the choroid coat must
be removed while the eye is under water; this should
be done with the forceps and scissors. The optic nerve, having
entered the interior of the globe through the sclerotic and the
choroid, expands into the delicate nervous tunic called the retina.
In passing through the coats of the eye, the nerve becomes suddenly constricted, and reduced to one-third of its diameter; at
this point, too, it projects slightly into the interior of the globe,

* In well-injected preparations one may see that the chief blood vessels are disposed in two circles on the front surface of the iris, one near the outer, and the other
near the inner circumference.

† See a paper by John Quekett in the Transactions of the Microscopic Society of
London, vol. iii. p. 9.

forming a little prominence to which the term 'papilla conica' has been applied.* In front the retina terminates in a thin serrated border (ora serrata), which ends a short distance behind the posterior margin of the ciliary processes.

Precisely opposite the pupil there is a bright yellow spot, macula lutea, in the retina, about ⅒th of an inch in diameter, fading off gradually at the edges, and having a black spot, fovea centralis, in the centre. This central spot was believed by its discoverer, Soemmering,† to be a perforation; but it is now ascertained to depend upon the absence of the yellow colour in the centre: so that the dark pigment of the choroid becomes conspicuous. These appearances are lost soon after death, and are replaced by a minute fold, into which the retina gathers itself, reaching from the centre of the spot to the prominence of the optic nerve. The use of this yellow spot is not understood.‡

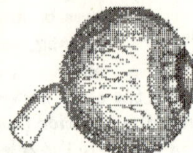

Fig. 136.

ARTERIES OF THE RETINA.
Canal of Petit (inflated).
Zone of Zinn (exaggerated).

Its elaborate organisation.   Although to the naked eye the retina appears a simple, soft, semi-transparent membrane, yet, when examined with the microscope, it is found to be most minutely and elaborately organised. It varies in thickness from the ⅒th to the ⅛th of an inch, and consists of four layers, named from without inwards, the columnar layer or membrana Jacobi, the granular layer, the nervous layer, and the vascular layer.

The columnar layer or membrana Jacobi§ is composed of minute cylindrical transparent rods arranged at right angles to the surface of the retina. Their outer extremities are imbedded to a greater or less depth in the dark pigment of the choroid, so that

* This prominence is remarkable, in that it is insensible to the rays of light.
† De foramine centrali, &c., retinæ humanæ; in Comment. Soc. Gotting. t. 13.
‡ In birds the retina has throughout the yellowish colour seen only at one part in the human eye.
§ After its discoverer, Dr. Jacob of Dublin, who described it in the Philosophical Transactions, 1819.

when viewed from without, the rods have the appearance of mosaic pavement.* Among the rods are intermingled numerous flask-shaped bodies, called *cones*: their outer extremities taper off towards the choroid, with which they are in contact, their inner broad ends join the fibres of Müller. The rods are absent in the macula lutea.

The *granular* layer consists of two horizontal collections of oval cells, separated by a variable amount of granular material.

The *nervous* layer is composed of the terminations of the optic nerve fibres, and of branched nerve cells. The fibres of the optic nerve, consisting only of the axis cylinders, run forwards as a continuous layer, and terminate in the nerve cells. The fibres are absent on the yellow spot.†

The *vascular* layer is formed by the ramifications of the arteria centralis retinæ, which form a close network of blood vessels throughout the nervous substance for its nutrition. After a short maceration in water, the nervous substance can be brushed off with a camel's hair brush, and then, in an injected eye, the network formed by the vessels can be distinctly seen. The larger branches, however, are visible without injection; one of them runs round the free margin of the retina.

The retina is separated from the vitreous humour by a perfectly transparent membrane, the *membrana limitans*. At the yellow spot the retina has no rods, and over the fovea centralis it is destitute of the granular layer and the nerve fibres.

The aqueous humour consists of a few drops of alkaline clear watery fluid, which fills up the space between the cornea and crystalline lens. The iris floats freely in it, and divides the space into two chambers of unequal size—an anterior and a posterior. The posterior is much the smaller of the two: indeed, the iris is so close to the lens that they are separated by a mere film of fluid. This accounts for the frequent

Aqueous humour.

---

* See Hannover, Recherches Microscop. sur le Système nerveux, 1844.

† H. Müller has described a number of *radiating fibres*, which are connected externally with the rods and cones, and after passing through the whole thickness of the retina, end in triangular expansions which rest on the membrana limitans.

adhesions which are apt to take place, during inflammation, between the pupil and the capsule of the crystalline. Some anatomists describe the anterior chamber as lined by a serous membrane, which they call the membrane of the aqueous humour. A delicate layer of epithelium exists on the posterior surface of the cornea, but nothing like a continuous serous membrane can be demonstrated on the iris or the capsule of the lens. The anterior chamber is remarkable for the rapidity with which it absorbs and secretes, as is proved, in the one case, by the speedy removal of extravasated blood; in the other, by the rapid re-appearance of the aqueous humour after the extraction of a cataract.

Vitreous humour and hyaloid membrane.   The vitreous humour is a transparent, gelatinous-looking substance, which fills up nearly four-fifths of the interior of the globe (p. 558). It consists of a watery fluid contained in the meshes of a cellular structure, called the 'hyaloid membrane,' from its perfect translucency: the cells communicate freely with each other; for, if any part of it be punctured, the humour gradually drains off. The membrane itself is so delicate, that it is difficult to obtain it separately; but it may be rendered slightly opaque by strong spirit or diluted acids. It is of somewhat firmer consistence on the surface, so that it answers the purpose of a capsule for the vitreous humour, and is sufficiently strong to keep it in shape after the stronger tunics of the eye have been removed.*

In the fœtus, a branch of the retinal artery runs through the centre of the vitreous humour, and ramifies on the back of the capsule of the lens. It is lodged in a tubular canal in the hyaloid membrane, termed the hyaloid canal; but this entirely disappears in the adult.

The vitreous humour presents in front a deep depression, in

---

* The cells of the vitreous humour may sometimes be demonstrated by freezing the eye and then dividing it. The figure and size of the cells are shown by the portions of ice which they contain. Again, by macerating the eye in chromic acid, it is found that the vitreous humour is intersected by 180 delicate partitions, disposed like those in the pulp of an orange—with this difference, however, that the partitions do not quite reach the centre, but leave a cylindrical space in the axis of the humour. Up this space the central artery runs in the fœtus.

Zone of Zinn. which the crystalline lens is imbedded; around this depression is the 'zone of Zinn.'[*] This zone is best exposed by removing the ciliary body. It then appears like a dark disk, and extends from the front margin of the retina nearly to the capsule of the lens: its surface is marked by prominent ridges which correspond with the intervals between the ciliary processes (fig. 136). It is supposed to form the suspensory ligament for maintaining the lens in its proper position.

Canal of Petit. If the transparent membrane between the zone of Zinn and the margin of the lens be carefully punctured, and the point of a small blow-pipe gently introduced, we may succeed in inflating a canal which encircles the lens, and, when inflated, resembles a circle of small glass beads: this is the canal of Petit, or 'canal godronné' (fig. 136, p. 565). How this canal is formed, whether by the separation of the hyaloid membrane into two layers or not, and what is its use, are questions not satisfactorily determined.

Crystalline lens. The crystalline lens (fig. 134) is a perfectly transparent solid body, situated immediately behind the pupil, and partly imbedded in the vitreous humour. It is convex on both surfaces, but more so behind. Its shape and consistence vary at different periods of life. In early life it is nearly spherical and soft, but it becomes more flattened, firmer, and amber-coloured with advancing age. In the adult, its transverse diameter is about three-eighths of an inch; its anteroposterior, one-fifth of an inch.

The lens is surrounded by a capsule equally transparent as itself. The capsule is composed of tissue exactly similar to the elastic layer of the cornea. It is four times thicker in front than behind, as might be expected, for the sake of more effective support. No vascular connection whatever exists between the lens and its capsule.[†]

* Zinn was Professor of Anatomy at Göttingen about the middle of the eighteenth century, and author of 'Descriptio Anat. Oculi Humani.'

† The vessels of the capsule of the lens are derived from the arteria centralis retinæ, and, in mammalia, can only be injected in the fœtal state. In the reptilia, however, the posterior layer of the capsule is permanently vascular. According to Quekett,

The lens protrudes directly the capsule is sufficiently opened. The lens is nourished by means of an extremely delicate layer of nucleated cells on its surface, which absorb nourishment from the capsule. Some anatomists speak of a layer of fluid (*liquor Morgagni*) as existing between the lens and its capsule; but no such fluid can be detected during life, and if there be any after death, it is, in all probability, imbibed by the capsule from the aqueous humour.

Minute structure.
The minute structure of the lens is very remarkable. It is gelatinous in consistence outside, but grows gradually denser towards the centre. After immersion in nitric acid, alcohol, or boiling water, it becomes hard and opaque. It may then be seen that it is divided into three equal parts, by three lines which radiate from the centre to within one-third of the circumference. Each of these portions is composed of hundreds of concentric layers, arranged one within the other, like the coats of an onion. If any single layer be examined with the microscope, we find that it is made up of fibres about $\frac{1}{5000}$th of an inch in thickness, and connected together by finely serrated edges. This beautiful dovetailing of the fibres of the lens was first pointed out by Sir David Brewster; and, to see it in perfection, one ought to take the lens of the common cod-fish.

The use of the lens is to bring the rays of light to a focus upon the retina.

DISSECTION OF THE ORGAN OF HEARING.

The parts constituting the organ of hearing should be examined in the following order:— 1. The outer cartilage or pinna; 2. The meatus auditorius externus; which leads to, 3. The tympanum or middle ear; and, 4. The labyrinth or internal ear, comprising the vestibule, cochlea, and semicircular canals.

the membrana pupillaris of anthors is nothing more than the anterior layer of the capsule. In taking the eye to pieces, it is quite a matter of accident whether the membrane adhere to the iris, or remain in its proper place in front of the lens. See Quekett's paper in the 'Transactions of the Microscopic Society of London,' vol. iii.

Pinna.   The pinna is irregularly oval, and has on its external aspect numerous eminences and hollows, which have received the following names:—The outer folded border is called the *helix*; the ridge within it, the *anti-helix*; between these is a curved groove called the *fossa of the helix*. The anti-helix bifurcates towards the front, and bounds the *fossa of the anti-helix*. The conical eminence in front of the meatus is termed the *tragus*, on which hair generally grows. Behind the tragus, and separated from it by a deep notch, is the *anti-tragus*. The *lobule* is the soft pendulous part, and consists of fat and fibrous tissue. The deep hollow which collects the sonorous vibrations, and directs them into the external meatus, is termed the *concha*. The pinna is formed of yellow fibro-cartilage, which is attached by an anterior ligament to the root of the zygoma, and by a posterior to the mastoid process.

Muscles of the pinna.   The muscles which move the cartilage of the ear as a whole, have been described (p. 2). Other small muscles extend from one part of the cartilage to another; but they are so indistinct, that, unless the subject be very muscular, it is difficult to make them out. The following six are usually described—four on the front of the pinna, and two behind it:—

a. The *musculus major helicis* runs vertically along the front margin of the pinna.

b. The *musculus minor helicis* lies over that part of the helix which comes up from the bottom of the concha.

c. The *musculus tragicus* lies vertically over the outer surface of the tragus.

d. The *musculus anti-tragicus* proceeds transversely from the anti-tragus to the lower part of the anti-helix.

e. The *musculus transversus* is on the back of the pinna; it passes from the back of the concha to the helix.

f. The *musculus obliquus* extends vertically from the cranial aspect of the concha to the convexity below it.

The arteries of the pinna are derived from the posterior auricular, and from the auricular branches of the temporal and occipital.

The nerves are furnished by the auriculo-parotidean branch of the cervical plexus, the temporo-auricular branch of the inferior maxillary, the posterior auricular branch of the facial, and Arnold's nerve from the pneumogastric.

Meatus auditorius externus.

This passage leads down to the membrana tympani, or drum of the ear. It is about an inch and a quarter in length; its external opening is broadest in its vertical direction; its termination is broadest in its transverse. The canal inclines at first upwards and forwards, and then curves a little downwards.*

It is not throughout of the same calibre, the narrowest part being about the middle; hence the difficulty of extracting foreign bodies which have passed to the bottom of the canal. It is formed partly by a tubular continuation of the concha, partly by an osseous canal in the temporal bone. The *cartilaginous portion* is about half an inch long, and the *osseous portion* three-fourths of an inch. The skin and the cuticle are continued down the passage, and becoming gradually thinner, form a cul-de-sac over the membrana tympani. The outer portion is furnished with hairs and ceruminous glands, of which the peculiar bitter secretion is for the purpose of keeping the passage moist, and preventing insects from lodging in it. Its arteries are derived from the posterior auricular, internal maxillary, and temporal; its nerve, from the temporo-auricular.

Tympanum.

The *tympanum*, or middle ear, is an irregular cavity in the petrous part of the temporal bone, and lined by mucous membrane. It is filled with air, which is freely admitted through the Eustachian tube; so that the atmospheric pressure is equal on both sides of the membrana tympani. It contains a chain of small bones, of which the use is to communicate the vibrations of the membrana tympani to the internal parts of the ear. For this purpose one end of the chain is attached to the membrana tympani, the other to the fenestra ovalis. The antero-posterior

---

* To obtain a correct knowledge of the length and dimensions of the meatus, sections should be made through it in different directions, or a cast of it taken in common plaster.

diameter of the tympanum is rather less than half an inch, its
vertical and transverse diameter about a quarter of an inch. The
cavity is bounded by a roof, a floor, an external, an internal, an
anterior, and a posterior wall. Its *roof* and *floor* are formed by
thin plates of bone. Its *external wall* is formed by the membrana
tympani, and partly by bone; the latter is pierced by the fissura
Glasseri, and the canal for the exit of the chorda tympani nerve.
The *internal wall* presents the following objects, beginning from
above: a *ridge* indicating the line of the aqueductus Fallopii; the
'*fenestra ovalis*,' which leads into the vestibule of the internal ear,
but is closed in the recent state by a membrane, to which is
attached the base of the stapes. Below the fenestra ovalis is a bony
prominence, the '*promontory*;' it is occasioned by the first turn
of the cochlea, and is marked by grooves, in which lie the
branches of the tympanic plexus of nerves. Still lower is the
'*fenestra rotunda*;' it leads into the scala tympani of the cochlea,
but is closed in the recent state by membrane. Immediately
behind the fenestra ovalis, is a small conical eminence, named the
'*pyramid*;' in the summit of which is a minute aperture, from
which the tendon of the stapedius emerges.

The *posterior* wall presents a large opening which leads into the
mastoid cells, and conveys air into them from the tympanum.

The *anterior wall* leads into the '*Eustachian tube*,' and the
'*canal for the tensor tympani*,' which are separated from each
other by a bony septum, the '*processus cochleariformis*.' Lastly,
a nerve called the chorda tympani (a branch of the portio dura)
runs across it.

Membrana
tympani.

The membrana tympani completely closes the bottom
of the meatus auditorius. It is nearly circular, and its
circumference is set in a bony groove, so that it is
stretched somewhat like the parchment of a drum on the outer
wall of the tympanum. Its plane is not vertical, but slants from
above downwards, forming, with the lower part of the meatus, an
angle of 45°: it is slightly conical, the apex being directed inwards
towards the tympanum, and firmly united to the handle of the
small bone called the '*malleus*.' The structure of the membrane

is essentially fibrous; some of the fibres radiate from the centre, others are circular. Its inner surface is lined by mucous membrane; its outer surface is covered by an extremely thin layer of the true skin. This accounts for the great sensibility of the membrane, and its vascularity when inflamed.

For a complete account of the Eustachian tube see p. 159. It proceeds from the anterior part of the tympanum downwards and forwards to the pharynx.

Eustachian tube.

The four small bones in the tympanum are named, after their fancied resemblance to certain implements, the malleus, incus, os orbiculare, and stapes. They are articulated to each other by perfect joints, and are so placed that the chain somewhat resembles the letter Z. Their use is to transmit the vibrations of the membrana tympani to the membrane of the fenestra ovalis, and, through it, to the fluid contained in the internal ear. But they have another use, which would be incompatible with a single bone—namely, to permit the tightening and relaxation of the membrana tympani, and thus adapt it either to resist the impulse of a very loud sound, or to favour a more gentle one.

Tympanic bones.

The handle of the malleus is nearly vertical, and attached along its whole length to the upper half of the membrana tympani. The long process (processus gracilis) projects at right angles from the body of the bone, runs into the Glasserian fissure, and receives the insertion of the laxator tympani. The short process receives the insertion of the tensor tympani.

The incus, or anvil bone, is shaped like a bicuspid molar tooth with unequal fangs. Its broad part articulates with the malleus; its long process articulates with the stapes, or stirrup bone, through the os orbiculare; its short process is directed backwards, and its point is fixed in a small hollow at the commencement of the mastoid cells.

The stapes is horizontal, and its base is attached to the membrane covering the fenestra ovalis. The stapedius muscle is inserted into its neck.

These muscles, by moving the tympanic bones, tighten or

MUSCLES OF THE TYMPANUM. relax the membrane of the tympanum. The 'tensor tympani' runs in the canal above and parallel to the Eustachian tube, from the cartilaginous part of which it arises. It passes backwards, and terminates in a round tendon, which enters the fore part of the tympanum through a special bony canal, and is inserted into the root of the handle of the malleus. Its nerve comes from the otic ganglion. Its action is to draw the membrana tympani inwards, and thus render it tense. The 'laxator tympani' arises from the spine of the sphenoid, and is inserted into the long process of the malleus. It is supplied by a branch from the facial nerve. Its action is to relax the membrana tympani. The 'stapedius' arises from a tube in the pyramid,* and its tendon is inserted into the neck of the stapes. Its nerve is derived from the facial. Its precise use is not thoroughly understood.

Chorda tympani. A branch of the portio dura (chorda tympani) enters the tympanum through a foramen at the base of the pyramid; it then crosses the tympanum between the handle of the mallens and the long process of the incus (see p. 195), and leaves the tympanum through a canal (canal of Huguier), which runs close to the Glasserian fissure.

The tympanum is supplied with blood, 1, by the tympanic branch of the internal maxillary, which runs in through the fissura Glasseri; 2, by the stylo-mastoid branch of the posterior auricular; 3, by small branches which enter with the Eustachian tube; 4, by branches from the internal carotid artery; and, 5, by the petrosal branch of the arteria meningea media.

INTERNAL EAR. This, in consequence of its complexity, is appropriately termed 'the labyrinth.' It consists of cavities excavated in the most compact part of the temporal bone. These cavities are divided into three—a middle one, called 'the vestibule,' as being a centre in which all communicate with each other; an anterior, named, from its resemblance to a

---

* There is a little sheath, lined by synovial membrane to facilitate the play of the tendon in the pyramid.

snail's shell, the *cochlea*; and a posterior, consisting of *three semi-circular canals*. These cavities are filled with a clear fluid, called the endo-lymph, and contain a membranous expansion (the *membranous labyrinth*), upon which the filaments of the auditory nerve are expanded.

Vestibule. The vestibule, or central chamber, communicates in front with the cochlea, through the scala cochleæ; behind, with the semicircular canals; on the outside with the tympanum, through the fenestra ovalis; on the inside is a shallow depression, the *fovea hemi-spherica*, through which are transmitted the branches of the auditory nerve. In the roof is an oval depression—the *fovea hemi-elliptica*. In some subjects there is the opening of a small canal, termed the '*aqueductus vestibuli*.' It leads to the posterior surface of the temporal bone, and transmits a small vein.

Semicircular canals. The semicircular canals, three in number, are situated above and rather behind the vestibule. Each canal is about the $\frac{1}{10}$th of an inch in diameter, and forms $\frac{2}{3}$rds of a circle. They open at each extremity into the vestibule: therefore, there should be six apertures for them; but there are only five, since one of the apertures is common to the extremity of two canals. The canals are not precisely of equal diameter throughout; each presents at one end a dilatation termed the '*ampulla*.' This dilatation corresponds to a similar dilatation of the membranous sac upon which the auditory nerve expands. Each canal differs in its direction: they are named, accordingly, *superior, posterior,* and *external.* The *superior s. c.* is also the most anterior of the three: its direction is vertical, and runs across the petrous bone: the ampulla is at the outer extremity. Its non-ampullated extremity opens by a common orifice with the posterior s. c. The *posterior s. c.* is also vertical, runs parallel to the posterior surface of the petrous bone, and, consequently, at right angles to the preceding: the ampulla is at the lower end. The *external s. c.* is horizontal in position with the convexity of the arch directed backwards: the ampulla is at the outer end.

Cochlea. The cochlea is the most anterior part of the internal ear: it very closely resembles a common snail's shell, and is placed so that the base of the shell corresponds to the bottom of the meatus auditorius internus, while the apex is directed forwards and outwards. It consists of the spiral convolutions of two parallel and gradually tapering tubes, which wind round a central pillar, called the '*modiolus.*' The partition by which the tubes are separated is termed the '*lamina spiralis.*' In the dry bones this partition is only partial; but, in the recent state, it is completed by a membrane. At the apex of the cochlea (*helicotrema*) the partition is altogether absent, so that here the tubes communicate with each other. These tubes are called the scales of the cochlea, and are filled with fluid. The upper one opens into the vestibule, and is therefore called the vestibular scale; the lower one leads to the membrane which closes the foramen rotundum of the tympanum, and is termed the tympanic scale. If unwound, they would be about 1½ inch long. Each makes two turns and a half round the central pillar, from left to right in the right ear, and *vice versâ* in the left.

The central pillar of the cochlea is called the '*modiolus.*' It is of considerable thickness at the base, but gradually tapers towards the apex. Its interior is traversed by numerous canals, for the purpose of transmitting the filaments of the auditory nerve. One of these canals, larger than the others, runs down the centre of the modiolus nearly to the apex, and transmits a small artery, the '*arteria centralis modioli.*'

The *lamina spiralis*—the partition between the two tubes or scales of the cochlea—is made up, on the inner half, of bone, on the outer half, of membrane. The bony part has a number of minute canals in it, which come off at right angles from the modiolus. They are for the lodgment of the filaments of the auditory nerve in their course to the membranous part, which is the most important element of the cochlea, since it receives the undulations of the fluid in the interior.[*]

* There is an extremely delicate little muscle, termed the 'cochlearis,' for the purpose of tightening or relaxing, according to circumstances, the membranous part

The osseous labyrinth is lined throughout by a delicate fibro-serous membrane, which secretes the fluid called the 'peri-lymph,' or 'liquor Cotunnii.'

Membranous labyrinth.   If the bony labyrinth just now described be properly understood, there is no difficulty in comprehending the membranous labyrinth in its interior—a structure intended to support the ultimate ramifications of the auditory nerve, and to expose them to the undulations of the fluid in the internal ear.

The membranous labyrinth is a sac, situated partly in the vestibule, partly in the semicircular canals—that situated in the vestibule is termed the *vestibular portion*; that in the bony canals, the *membranous semicircular canals*. The semicircular canals present the same dilatations or ampullæ at one end, and just at this part they nearly fill their bony cases; but in the rest of their extent the diameter of the membranous canal is not more than one-third that of the bony one.

The sac in the vestibule is constricted, so as to appear like two sacs of unequal size. The larger of the two, generally called the *utricle*, is lodged in the fovea hemi-elliptica, and communicates with the semicircular canals. The smaller, called the *saccule*, lies in the fovea hemi-spherica, and communicates with the vestibular scale of the cochlea. Both sacs are filled with the *endo-lymph*, besides which, each contains a minute quantity of calcareous matter, called by Breschet the *otoliths*. These masses of cretaceous substance seem to be suspended in the fluid contained in the sacs by the intermedium of a number of nerve filaments proceeding from the auditory nerve.[*]

The membranous labyrinth is protected, inside and out, by fluid. There is the proper fluid in the interior, termed the 'endo-lymph,'

of the lamina spiralis. It is placed along the outer circumference of the membrane, and, in fact, forms an integral part of it. Its fibres are of the non-striped kind, like the ciliary muscle of the eye. See Todd and Bowman, Phys. Anat. Part iii. p. 79.

[*] From the universal presence of these chalky bodies in the labyrinth of all mammalia, and from their much greater hardness and size in aquatic animals, there is little reason to doubt that they perform some office of great importance in the physiology of hearing.

and the thin layer of fluid, the 'peri-lymph,' between it and the bone.

Distribution of the auditory nerve.

The auditory nerve, or portio mollis of the seventh pair, passes down the meatus auditorius internus, and, at the bottom of it, divides into an anterior and a posterior branch: a branch for the cochlea, and a branch for the vestibule. These nerves then break up into numerous fasciculi, which pass through the foramina at the bottom of the meatus into the osseous labyrinth. Here the filaments are grouped into six bundles, corresponding to the parts which they supply—namely, two for the vestibular sac, one for each of the ampullæ of the semicircular canals, and one for the cochlea.

The *cochlear* nerve divides into filaments, which run through the canals of the modiolus, and then along those of the lamina spiralis, in order to terminate upon the membranous part of this lamina. The precise manner in which the filaments terminate is still dubious: according to Breschet,[*] they communicate and form a series of minute arches.

Respecting the other nerves, little more need be said than that their ultimate ramifications are lost upon the vestibular sac, and upon the ampullæ of the semicircular canals: some of them, however, pass into the sac, and come into contact with the otoconies, or ear-dust, in its interior.

Blood vessels of the labyrinth.

The internal auditory artery—a branch of the basilar —runs with the auditory nerve to the bottom of the meatus, and divides into branches corresponding with the divisions of the nerve. Its ultimate ramifications terminate, in the form of a fine network, on the membranous labyrinth, and on the spiral lamina of the cochlea. The auditory vein pours its blood into the superior petrosal sinus.

* Recherches Anat. et Phys. sur l'Organe de l'Ouïe, &c. (Mém. de l'Acad. de Med. t. v. fasc. iii. 1836.)

DISSECTION OF THE MAMMARY GLAND.

The form, size, position, and other external characters of the mammary gland, are sufficiently obvious. The longest diameter of the gland is in a direction upwards and outwards towards the axilla; its thickest part is at the centre; and the fullness and roundness of the gland depend upon the quantity of fat which is situated about it and between its lobes. Its deep surface is flattened in adaptation to the pectoral muscle, to which it is loosely connected by an abundance of areolar tissue.

It is inclosed by a fascia which not only supports it as a whole, but penetrates into its interior, so as to form a framework for its several lobes; hence it is that, in cases of mammary abscess, the matter is apt to be circumscribed, not diffused.

The *nipple* (*mammilla*) projects a little below the centre; it is surrounded by a coloured circle termed the 'areola:' this circle is of a rose-pink colour in virgins, but, in those who have borne children, of a dark brown. It begins to enlarge and grow darker about the second or third month of pregnancy, and these changes continue till parturition. The areola is also abundantly provided with papillæ, and with subcutaneous sebaceous glands, for the purpose of lubricating the surface during lactation.

Structure. The gland itself consists of distinct lobes held together by firm connective tissue, and provided with separate lactiferous ducts. Each lobe divides and subdivides into lobules, and the duct branches out accordingly.* Traced to their origin, we find that the ducts commence in clusters of minute cells, and that the blood vessels ramify upon these cells in rich profusion; altogether, then, a single lobe might be compared to a bunch of grapes, of which the stalk represents the main duct. The main ducts (*galactophorous ducts*) from the several lobes, from fifteen

---

* It is observed, in some cases, that one or more lobules run off to a considerable distance from the main body of the gland, and lie imbedded in the subcutaneous tissue. One should remember this when it is necessary to remove the entire gland.

to twenty in number, converge towards the nipple, and, just before they reach 'it, become dilated into small sacs or reservoirs two or three lines wide; after this they run up to the apex of the nipple, and terminate in separate orifices.

The arteries of the gland are derived from the long thoracic and internal mammary: the nerves come from the anter or and lateral cutaneous branches of the intercostal nerves.

DISSECTION OF THE SCROTUM AND TESTIS.

Structure of the scrotum.

The scrotum is composed of six tunics:—1. The skin; 2. The tunica dartos; 3. A layer of cellular tissue; 4. The spermatic fascia derived from the external abdominal ring; 5. The cremaster, or suspensory muscle; 6. The infundibuliform fascia derived from the internal ring.

Each of these coverings cannot be demonstrated under ordinary circumstances, because they are so blended together; but they can be shown in the case of old and large herniæ when in a state of hypertrophy.

Dartos.

The *dartos* is a thin layer consisting of muscular fibres of the non-striped kind, like those of the bladder and intestines. Its use is to corrugate the loose and extensible skin of the scrotum, and in a measure to support and brace the testicle.

Layer of cellular tissue.

Beneath the dartos is a large quantity of loose cellular tissue, remarkable for the total absence of fat. Together with the dartos, it forms a vertical partition between the testicles, termed '*septum scroti*.' It is not a complete partition, since air or fluid will pass from one side to the other. The great abundance and looseness of this tissue explains the enormous swelling of the scrotum in cases of anasarca, and in cases where the urine is effused into it in consequence of rupture or ulceration of the urethra.

The spermatic fascia, cremaster muscle, and infundibuliform fascia have been described (pp. 318, 321).

The testicle is a gland of an oval shape, with flattened
sides, suspended obliquely, so that the upper end points
forwards and outwards, the lower end in the reverse direction.
The left is generally a little the lower of the two. The ordinary
weight of each gland is about six drachms; but few organs present
greater variations in size and weight, even in men of the same

Testis.

Fig. 137.

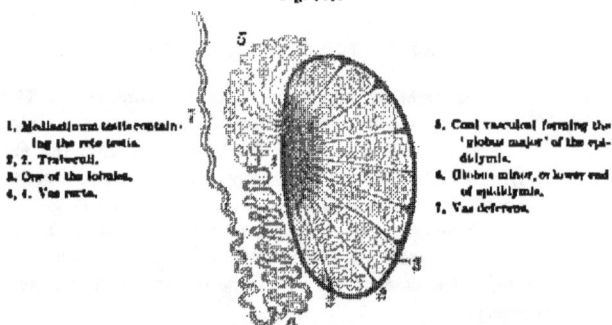

1. Mediastinum testis containing the rete testis.
2, 2. Trabeculi.
3. One of the lobules.
4, 4. Vas recta.

5. Coni vasculosi forming the
'globus major' of the epididymis.
6. Globus minor, or lower end
of epididymis.
7. Vas deferens.

DIAGRAM OF THE TESTICLE.

age; generally speaking, the left is the larger. Along the posterior part of the gland is placed a long narrow body,
termed the 'epididymis:' this is not a part of the
testicle, but an appendage to it, formed by the convolutions of its
long excretory duct. Its upper larger end is called the 'globus
major,' and is connected to the testicle by the efferent ducts; the
lower end, 'globus minor,' is only connected to the testicle by
fibrous tissue.

Epididymis.

The coverings of the testicle, are—1, a serous membrane, called the 'tunica vaginalis,' to facilitate its
movements; 2, a strong fibrous membrane, called the
'tunica albuginea,' to support and form a case for the glandular
structure within; 3, a delicate stratum of minute blood vessels,

**Proper co-
verings of
the testicle.**

which some anatomists have described as a distinct coat, under
the name of tunica vasculosa.

Tunica
vaginalis.   The *tunica vaginalis* is a serous sac, one part of
which (tunica vaginalis propria) adheres closely to the
testicle; the other (tunica vaginalis reflexa) is reflected
loosely around it. If the sac be laid open, you see that it completely covers the testicle, except behind, where the vessels and
duct are placed (fig. 138); and that it also covers part of the
outer side of the epididymis. The interior of the sac is smooth
and polished, like all other serous membranes, and lubricated by
a little fluid. An excess of this fluid gives rise to the disease
termed ' hydrocele.'

The tunica vaginalis was originally derived from the peritoneum. In some subjects it still communicates with that cavity
by a narrow neck, and is therefore liable to become the sac of a
hernia (see diagram, p. 324). Such herniæ are termed *congenital*
—a bad name, since they do not, as a matter of course, take place
at birth, but often in adult age. Sometimes the communication
continues through a very contracted canal, open to the passage of
fluid only; or the communication may be only partially obliterated,
and then one or more isolated serous sacs are left along the cord.
Such an one, when distended by fluid, gives rise to hydrocele of
the cord.

Tunica
albuginea.   This tunic is a dense, inelastic membrane, composed
of fibrous tissue, interlacing in every direction, analogous to the sclerotic coat of the eye. It completely
invests the testicle, but not the epididymis. At the posterior part
of the gland it penetrates into its substance for a short distance,
and forms an incomplete vertical septum, termed, after the anatomist who first described it, ' *corpus Highmori*,' and subsequently,
by Sir A. Cooper, the ' *mediastinum testis* ' (fig. 138). This septum transmits the blood vessels of the gland, and contains, also,
the network of seminal ducts, called the rete testis, shown in
diagram 137.

From the mediastinum testis are given off in all directions a
number of slender fibrous cords, which traverse the interior of

the gland, and are attached to the inside of the tunica albuginea.
They serve to maintain the general shape of the testicle, to support
the numerous lobules of which its glandular substance is composed,
and to convey the blood vessels into it. These tie-beams (*trabeculæ
testis*), as well as the mediastinum from which they proceed, are
readily seen on making a transverse
section through the gland (fig. 138).

Respecting the so-called

Tunica
vasculosa.

tunica vasculosa, nothing
more need be said than that
it consists of a multitude of fine blood
vessels, formed by the ramifications of
the spermatic artery, and held together
by delicate cellular tissue. It lines the
inner surface of the tunica albuginea,
and gives off vessels which run with the
fibrous cords into the interior of the
gland.

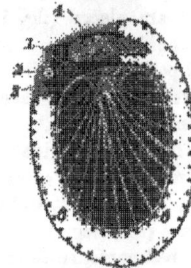

TRANSVERSE SECTION THROUGH
THE TESTICLE.

(Diagrammatic.)

1. Spermatic artery.
2. Vas deferens.
3. Deferential artery.
4. Epididymis.
5. Mediastinum testis.
6, 6. Cavity of tunica vaginalis.

(The dots show the reflections of the
tunica vaginalis.)

Glandular
structure.

When the testicle is cut
into, its interior looks soft
and pulpy, and of a reddish-
grey colour. It consists of an innume-
rable multitude of minute convoluted
tubes (*tubuli seminiferi*). For economy of space they are arranged in
lobules, between four and five hundred *
in number, of various sizes, and contained in the compartments
formed by the fibrous cords proceeding from the mediastinum
testis. Only a few of these lobules are shown in diagram 138.
Though disposed in lobules, still they communicate with each
other, and thus form one vast network of tubes. The secretion
from them is carried off by some forty or fifty straight vessels
(*vasa recta*), which penetrate the mediastinum testis, and there
form a plexus of seminal tubes, termed the ' *rete testis.*' This lies

* This estimate is according to Krause, Müller's Archiv. für Anat. 1837.

along the back of the gland. From the upper part of the rete the secretion is carried away to the large end of the epididymis by fifteen or twenty tubes, termed, ' *vasa efferentia*.' These, after forming a vast number of coils, termed ' *coni vasculosi*,' which collectively constitute the globus major of the epididymis, ultimately terminate, one after the other, in a single duct, the commencement of the vas deferens.

Commencing, then, in the globus major of the epididymis, the vas deferens descends, making a series of extremely tortuous coils, which alone form the globus minor.* From the lower part of the globus minor the vas deferens ascends, joins the other component parts of the spermatic cord, passes through the inguinal canal, winds round the back part of the bladder, and empties itself into the prostatic part of the urethra. The length of the vas deferens was estimated by Monro at upwards of thirty feet. The same anatomist calculated that the semen, before it arrived at the vas deferens, had to traverse a tube forty-two feet in length.

Spermatic cord.   The spermatic cord is composed of the spermatic vessels, nerves, and absorbents, of the vas deferens, with the little deferential artery (a branch of the superior vesical), of the cremaster muscle and the cremasteric artery. Its coverings have been described with the anatomy of the parts of hernia, p. 323.

The course of the spermatic arteries and veins have been described in the dissection of the Abdomen, p. 352. The artery is remarkably tortuous as it descends along the cord; it enters the back part of the testicle, and breaks up into a multitude of fine ramifications, which spread out on the inner surface of the tunica albuginea. The spermatic *veins* leave the testicle at its back part, and, as they ascend along the cord, become extremely tortuous, and form a plexus termed ' *pampiniform*.' It is usually stated that these veins are destitute of valves; and this fact is adduced as one of the reasons for the occurrence of ' varicocele.' But it is certain that the larger veins do contain valves.

* A little blind duct, called *vasculum aberrans*, is sometimes connected either to the epididymis or the vas deferens.

The *absorbents* of the testicle terminate in the lumbar glands; hence these glands become affected in malignant disease of the testicles.

The *nerves* of the testicle are derived from the sympathetic. They run down from the abdomen with the spermatic arteries (p. 356). This accounts for the stomach and intestines sympathising so readily with the testicle, and for the constitutional effects of an injury to it.

The testicle is originally developed in the lumbar region, immediately below the kidneys; and it is loosely attached to the back of the abdomen by a fold of peritoneum, termed the '*mesorchium*,' along which its vessels and nerves run up to it, as to any other abdominal viscus. From the lower end of the gland there proceeds to the bottom of the scrotum, a contractile cord termed the '*gubernaculum testis*.'* By the gradual contraction of this, the organ is brought into the scrotum. It begins to slide down from the loins about the fifth month, reaches the ring about the seventh, and about the ninth has entered the scrotum. Its original peritoneal coat is retained throughout; but, as it enters the inguinal canal, the peritoneal lining of the abdomen is pouched out before it, and eventually becomes the tunica vaginalis reflexa. Immediately after the descent of the testis, its serous bag communicates with the abdomen, and in the lower animals continues to do so through life.† But in the human subject the canal of communication soon begins to close. It begins to close at the top first, and the closure is generally complete in a child born at its full time.‡ The final

Descent of the testicle.

---

* Mr. Curling considers the gubernaculum testis to be a muscular cord. See his Observations on the Structure of the Gubernaculum, and on the Descent of the Testis in the Fœtus: Medical Gazette, April 10, 1841.

† According to Professor Owen, the African orang outan (*Simia troglodytes*) is the only exception to this rule. In this animal it is interesting to observe that the lower extremities are more fully developed as organs of support, and there is a ligamentum teres in the hip-joint.

‡ According to Camper, the canal on the right side is nearly always open at birth, whereas that on the left is nearly always closed. This fact explains the greater frequency of hernia on the right side in children under one year old. Thus out of

purpose of this is to provide against the occurrence of ruptures, to which man, from his erect attitude, is so much more exposed than animals. At the end of the first month after birth, the canal is entirely obliterated from the abdominal ring to the testis. Sometimes, however, this obliteration fails to take place, or is only partial; hence may arise congenital hernia, or hydrocele. The possible existence of a communication between the tunica vaginalis and the peritoneal cavity of the abdomen, is one of the reasons why hydroceles in infants are not treated by stimulating injections.

3,014 cases of right and left inguinal hernia, seen at the City of London Truss Society, 2,269 occurred on the right side, and 745 on the left; or in the proportion of 3 to 1.

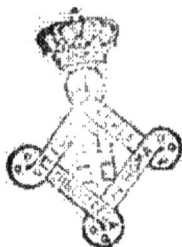

INDEX.

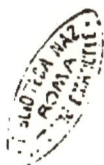

LONDON: PRINTED BY
SPOTTISWOODE AND CO., NEW-STREET SQUARE
AND PARLIAMENT STREET